Preclinical Animal Modeling in Medicine

Edited by Enkhsaikhan Purevjav, Joseph F. Pierre and Lu Lu

Published in London, United Kingdom

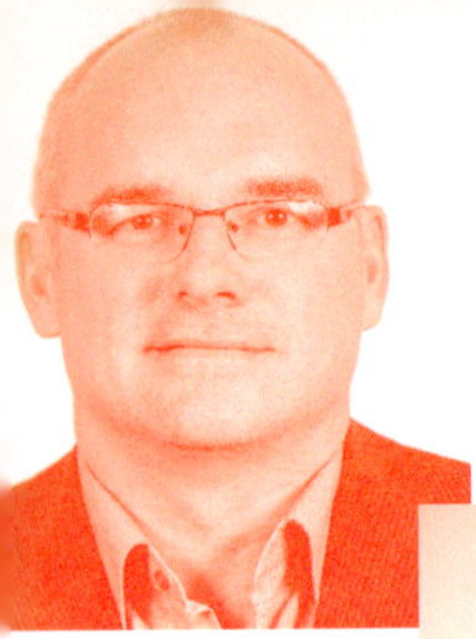
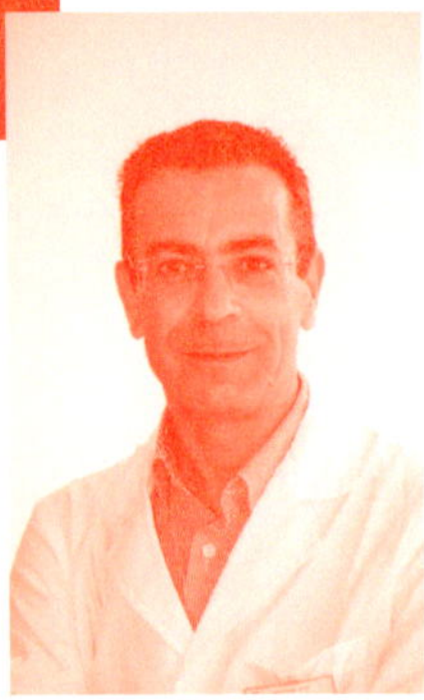
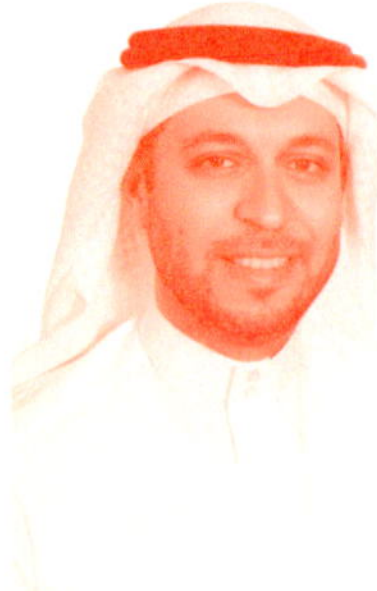
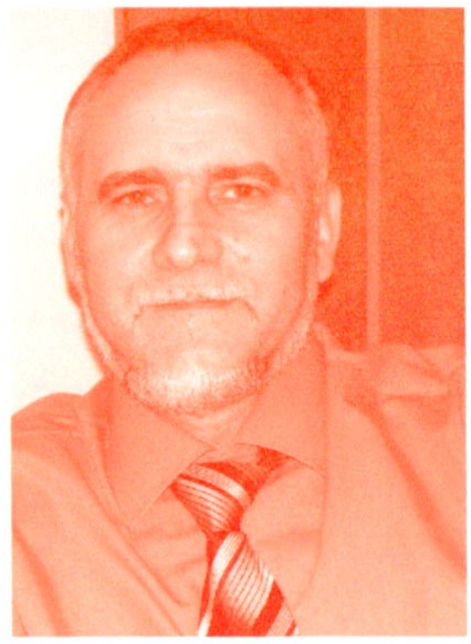
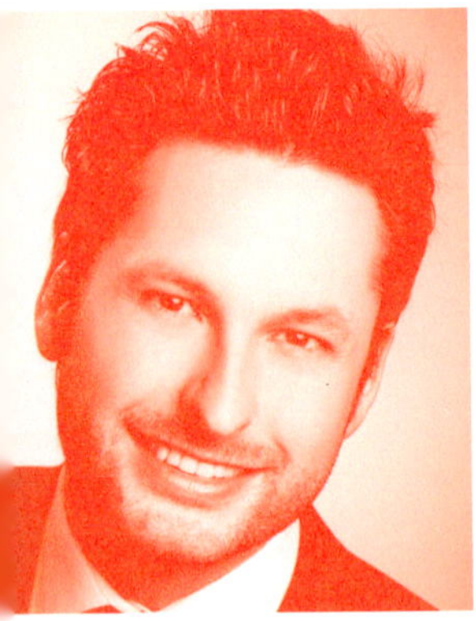
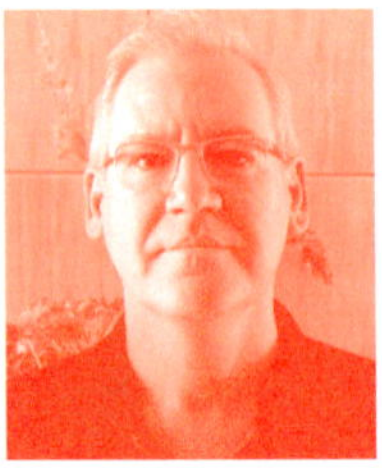
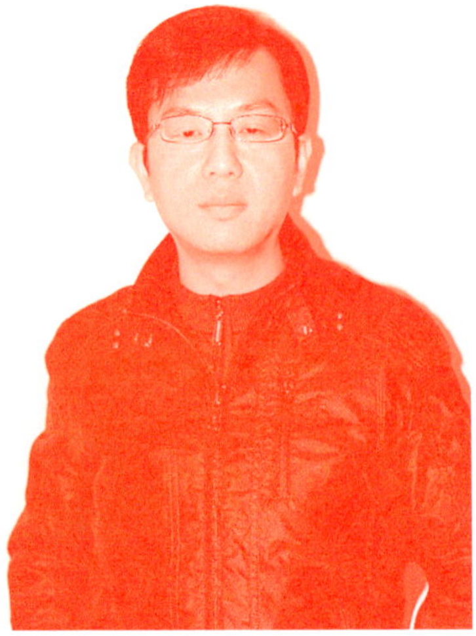

IntechOpen

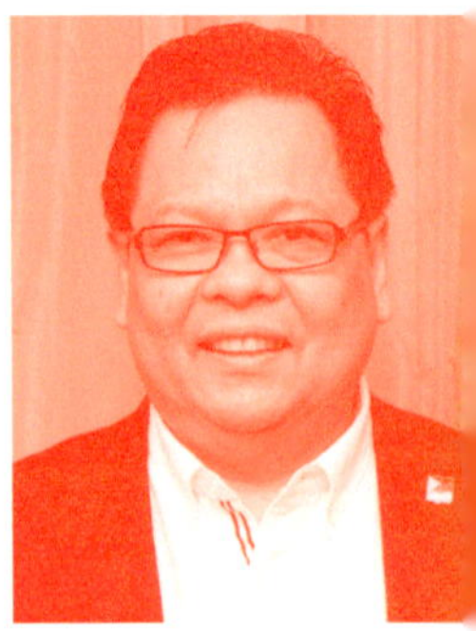
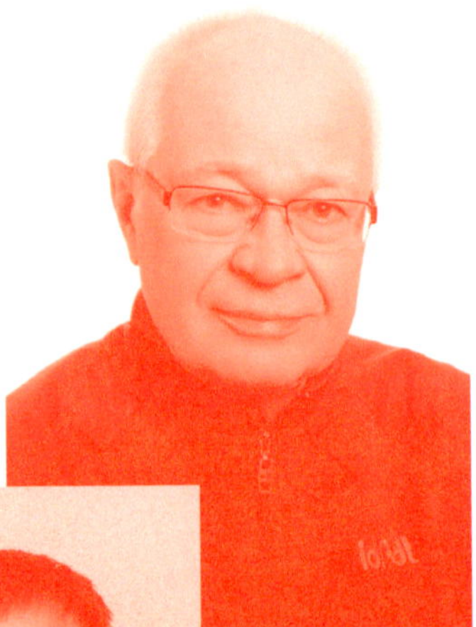
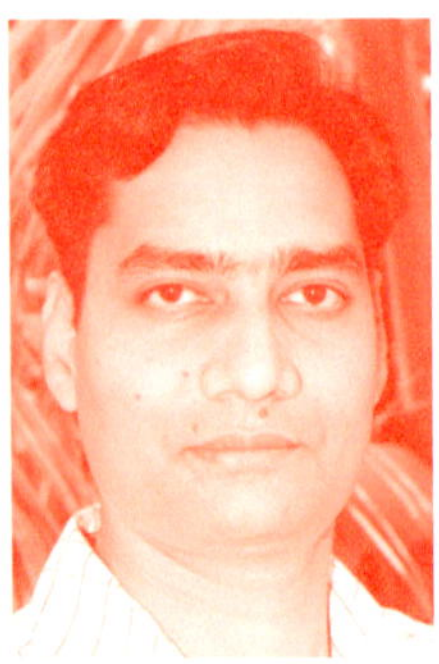
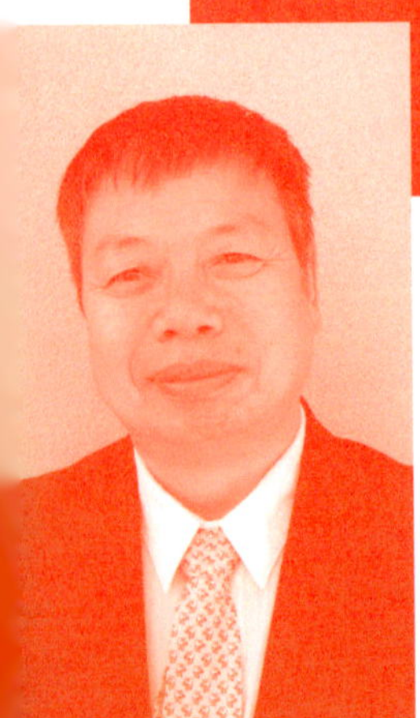
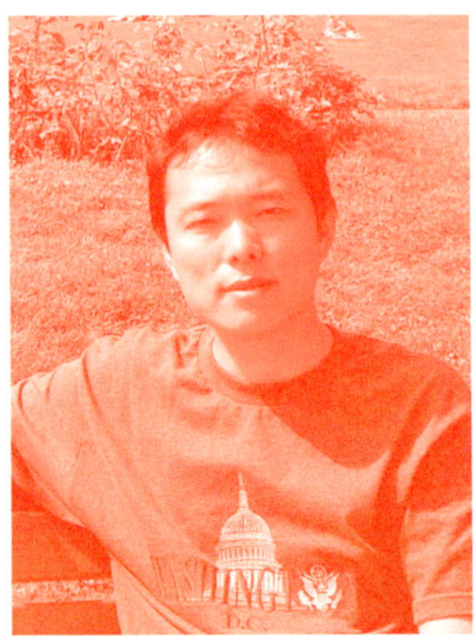
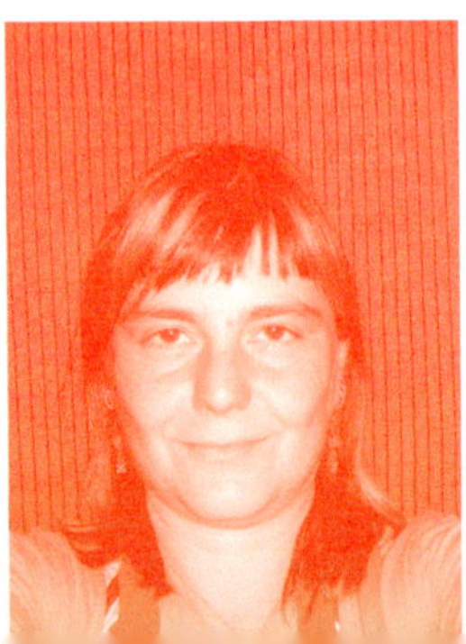

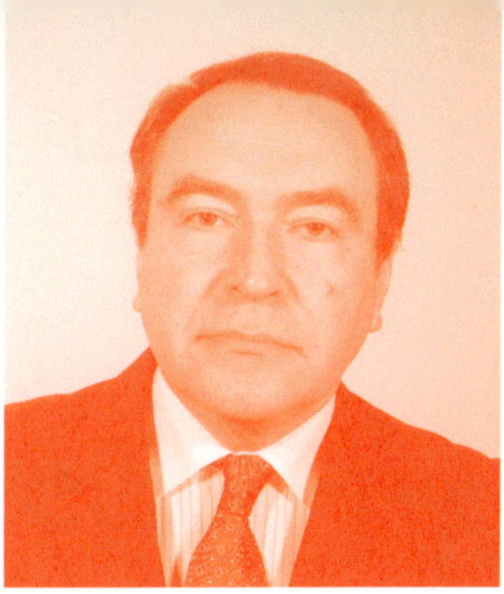
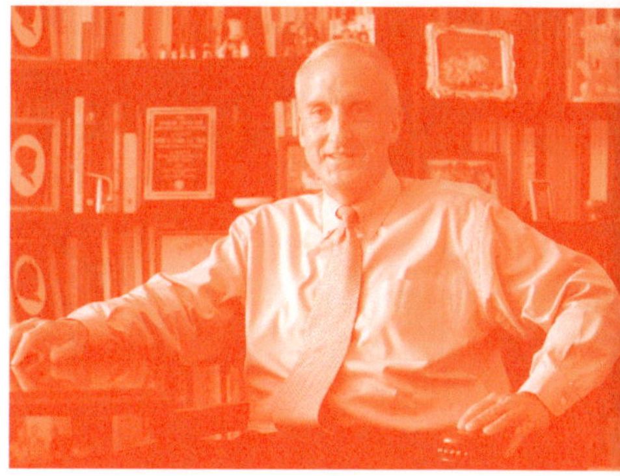
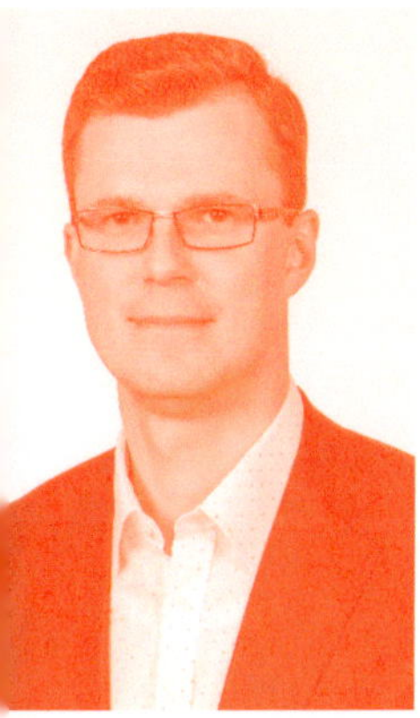
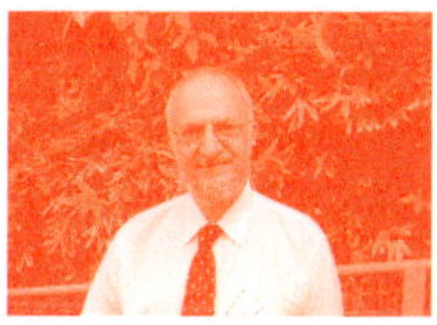
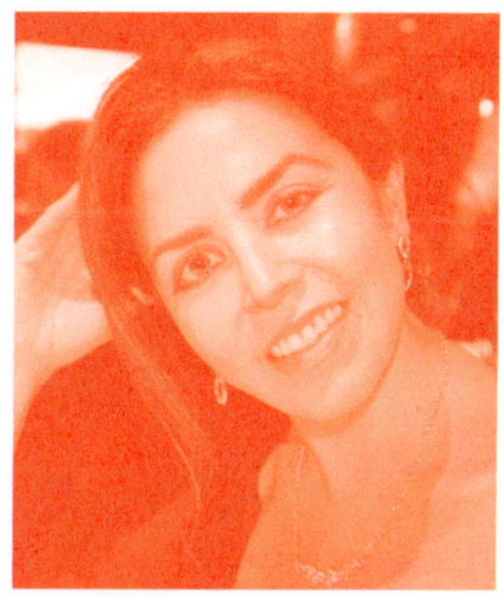

Supporting open minds since 2005

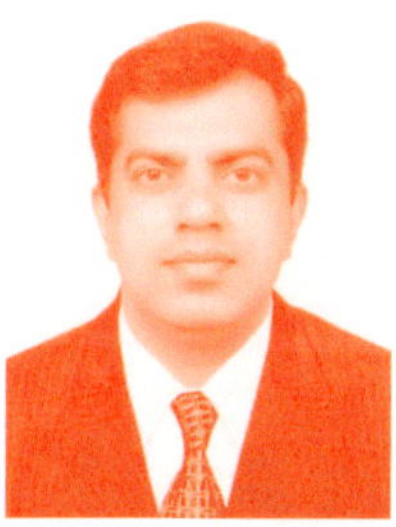
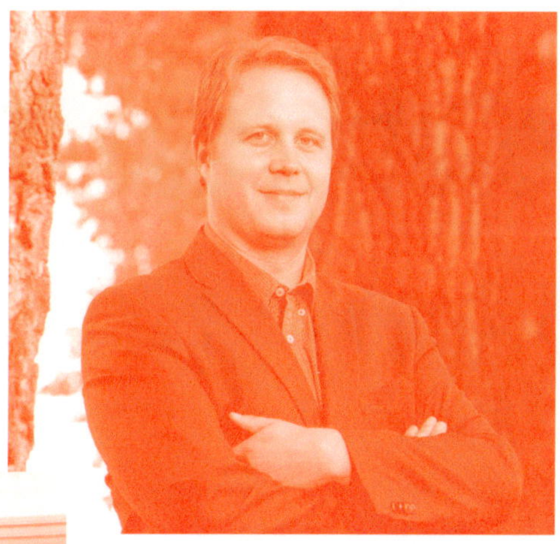
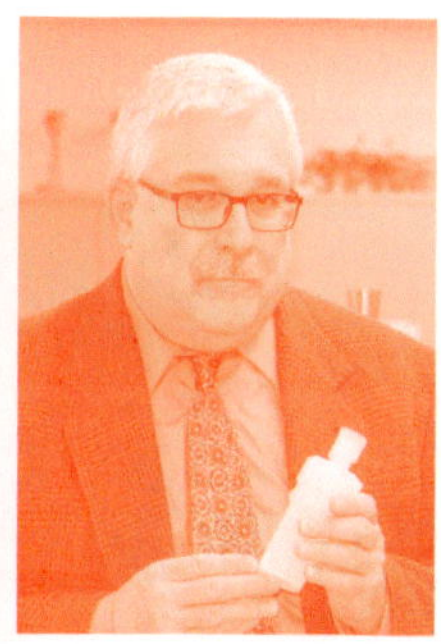
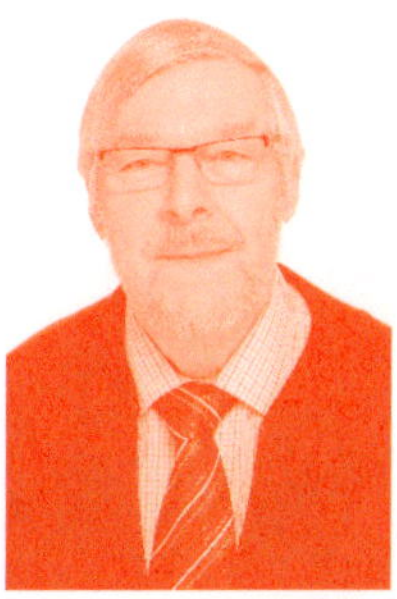
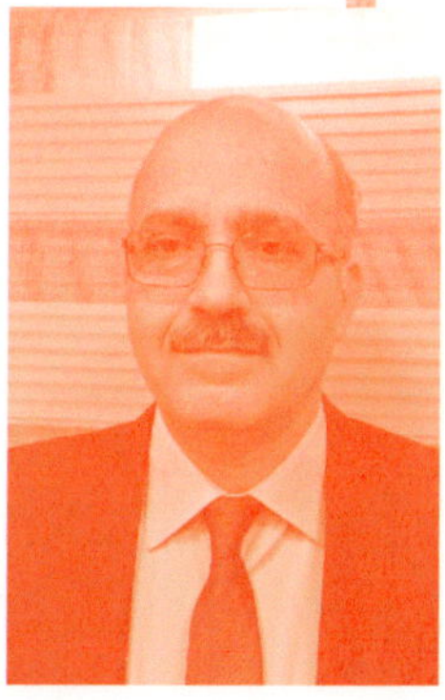
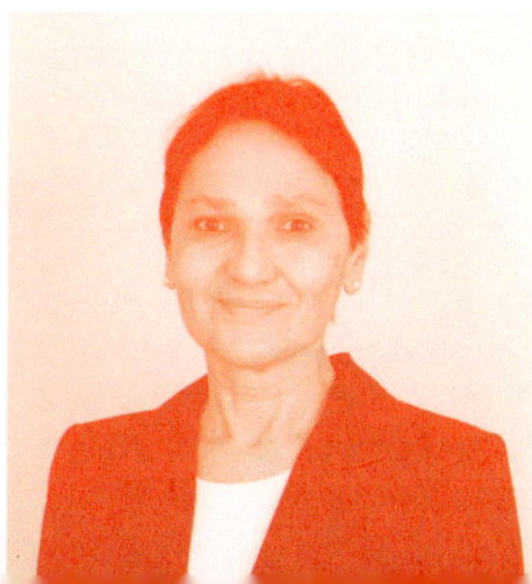
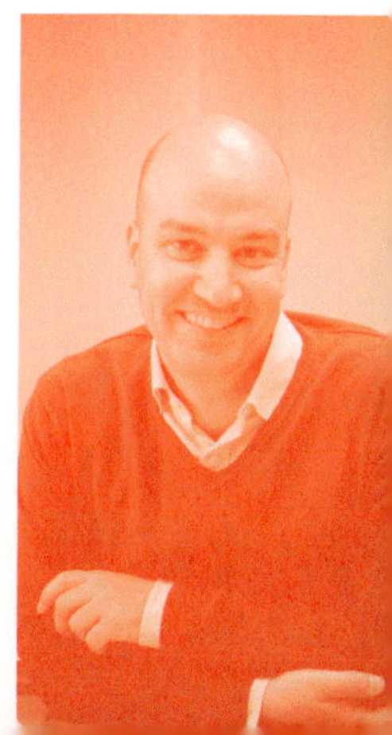

Preclinical Animal Modeling in Medicine
http://dx.doi.org/10.5772/intechopen.92923
Edited by Enkhsaikhan Purevjav, Joseph F. Pierre and Lu Lu

Contributors
Pinky Kain, Zoha Sadaqat, Shivam Kaushik, Joseph F. Pierre, Lydia M. Henry, Roshan Kumari, David L. Cedeño, Joseph M. Williams, Courtney A. Kelley, David C. Platt, Ricardo Vallejo, David G. Ashbrook, Lu Lu, Liang Gao, Xiaoyu Cai, Tao Xu, Maierdan Maimaiti, Tatiana V. Egorova, Anna V. Polikarpova, Ivan I. Galkin, Yulia V. Ivanova, Prabhakar Orsu, Y. Srihari, Monica M. Jablonski, Sophie Pilkinton, T.J. Hollingsworth, Brian Jerkins, Jonathan Rho, Paul Percelay, Ilyse Kornblau, Aman Bajwa, Navjot Pabla, Yogesh Scindia, Joseph Gigliotti, Enkhsaikhan Purevjav, Michelle Chintanaphol, Buyan-Ochir Orgil, Nelly R. Alberson, Jeffrey A. Towbin

First published in London, United Kingdom, 2022 by IntechOpen
IntechOpen is the global imprint of INTECHOPEN LIMITED, registered in England and Wales, registration number: 11086078, 5 Princes Gate Court, London, SW7 2QJ, United Kingdom
Printed in Croatia

British Library Cataloguing-in-Publication Data
A catalogue record for this book is available from the British Library

Additional hard and PDF copies can be obtained from orders@intechopen.com

Preclinical Animal Modeling in Medicine
Edited by Enkhsaikhan Purevjav, Joseph F. Pierre and Lu Lu
p. cm.
Print ISBN 978-1-83968-804-1
Online ISBN 978-1-83968-805-8
eBook (PDF) ISBN 978-1-83968-806-5

For EU product safety concerns:
IN TECH d.o.o., Prolaz Marije Krucifikse Kozulić 3, 51000 Rijeka, Croatia, info@intechopen.com or visit our website at intechopen.com.

Meet the editors

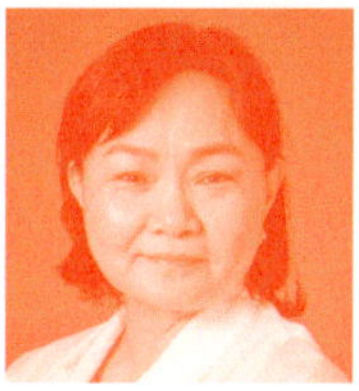

Dr. Enkhsaikhan Purevjav earned her MD from the Leningrad Pediatric Medical Institute (LMPI), Russia in 1989, followed by an internship and residency in pediatrics at the Mongolian National Medical University, a fellowship in pediatric cardiology at LPMI, and a Ph.D. in Medical Genetics and Molecular Biology from Shimane Medical University, Japan. Dr. Purevjav joined Baylor College of Medicine and Texas Children's Hospital as a postdoctoral trainee and instructor and then Cincinnati Children's Hospital Medical Center as an assistant professor. She currently works as an associate professor at the University of Tennessee Health Science Center where she continues to study the genetics of heart diseases, specifically focusing on pediatric cardiomyopathies and arrhythmias.

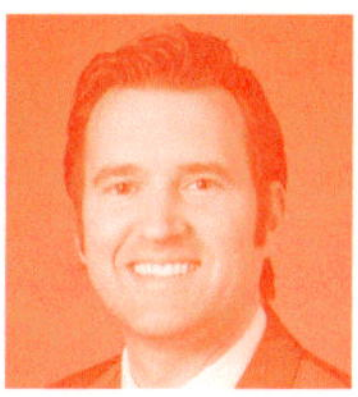

Dr. Joseph F. Pierre is currently an Assistant Professor of Nutritional Sciences and Surgery, University of Wisconsin-Madison. The Pierre lab addresses a range of basic, translational, and clinical research questions focused on the gastrointestinal microbiome, nutrition, and gut physiology and disease. Dr. Pierre utilizes experimental models that include bariatric surgery, parenteral and enteral nutrition, gnotobiotics, and organoid approaches. Where relevant, his research examines microbiome community composition and function to investigate host-microbial interactions. Dr. Pierre received his BS in Natural Science and Ph.D. in Nutritional Sciences from the University of Wisconsin-Madison before completing a postdoc fellowship in Gastroenterology, Hepatology, and Nutrition at the University of Chicago. He holds an adjunct faculty position at the University of Tennessee Health Science Center within the College of Medicine.

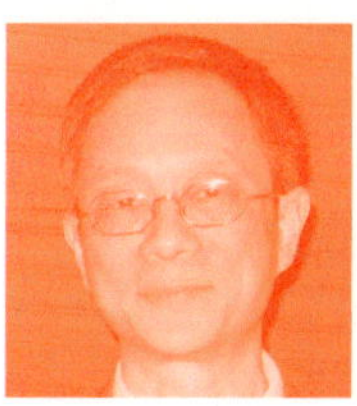

Dr. Lu Lu is a professor in the Department of Genetics, Genomics and Informatics, University of Tennessee Health Science Center (UTHSC). His research focuses on the examination of genetic effects on complex traits. He and his colleagues have developed large resources for the study of systems genetics that include the largest mouse genetic reference population, which includes BXD recombinant inbred lines, high-density genotypes, thousands of phenotypes, hundreds of transcriptomic data sets, and whole-genome sequence for all 152 inbred BXD strains. All these resources provide great power for genetic analysis of complex traits and are being used by many researchers for their studies of polygenetic diseases. As Principal Investigator, he has been funded by seven NIH R01 grants and has published ~200 science papers within the last seventeen years.

Contents

Preface

This book provides an overview of current preclinical research in various animals ranging from non-human primates and mammals to zebrafish and flies. It includes numerous animal models of complex and devastating human diseases such as Duchenne muscular dystrophy, left ventricular noncompaction cardiomyopathy, glaucoma, macular degeneration, acute kidney and cerebral injuries as well as Brucellar spondylodiscitis, which is difficult to diagnose in animals and humans. It reviews new diagnostic tools, pharmacological agents, and treatment devices in preclinical stages. The authors emphasize the importance of bidirectional research between human and preclinical models in improving the diagnosis of diseases and fine-tuning therapeutic interventions. Information on stem cell and viral therapies for tissue regeneration and repair will help researchers and medical personnel save millions of people and animals every year.

The modern design of translational animal modeling includes systems biological and omics approaches involving a large cohort of animal reference populations. Reviews on recombinant inbred populations of BXD strains and Drosophila melanogaster used for animal-to-human and human-to-animal translation provide intriguing information on how these animals are important for predictive and personalized medicine and biology and for clarifying gene-gene (epistasis), gene-age, gene-sex, gene-treatment, gene-environment, and organ–organ interactions that are relevant in the context of human pathologies including diabetes, obesity, neurodegenerative and cardiac diseases, gastrointestinal cancers, and aging. These animal resources are widely used for medical and biological research including open-web resources on omics (phenome, genome, transcriptome, epigenome, proteome, metabolome), hormones, and neuropeptides.

The book also highlights that the protection and welfare of animals utilized for experimental and scientific purposes are critical. Scientists have considered for decades the fundamental principles of the three "Rs": Replacement, Reduction, and Refinement. These principles include (1) avoiding or replacing the use of animals when other non-animal experimental approaches are available, (2) using the minimum number of animals for collecting essential scientific information, and (3) alleviating or minimizing any harm, pain, suffering, or distress, and improving the welfare and health of animals used in research. A chapter on the research of chronic pain describes rat and sheep models used for elucidating the mechanisms of pain and for advancing clinical outcomes in humans.

We are grateful to the authors for their expert contributions and hope this book will be a valuable and useful resource for scientists, researchers, and medical personnel, including medical educators and students.

Enkhsaikhan Purevjav, MD, Ph.D., FAHA
The Heart Institute,
Department of Pediatrics,
University of Tennessee Health Science Center,
Memphis, TN, USA

Joseph F. Pierre and Lu Lu
University of Tennessee Health Science Center,
Memphis, TN, USA

Section 1

Animal Models for Experimental Precision Medicine and Biology

Chapter 1

Recombinant Inbred Mice as Models for Experimental Precision Medicine and Biology

David G. Ashbrook and Lu Lu

Abstract

Recombinant inbred rodents form immortal genome-types that can be resampled deeply at many stages, in both sexes, and under multiple experimental conditions to model genome-environment interactions and to test genome-phenome predictions. This allows for experimental precision medicine, for which sophisticated causal models of complex interactions among DNA variants, phenotype variants at many levels, and innumerable environmental factors are required. Large families and populations of isogenic lines of mice and rats are now available and have been used across fields of biology. We will use the BXD recombinant inbred family and their derived diallel cross population as an example for predictive, experimental precision medicine and biology.

Keywords: BXD, experimental precision medicine, genome-by-environment, systems genetics, personalized medicine, recombinant inbred strains, diallel cross, prediction

1. Introduction

One of the major objectives of modern biology and medicine is prediction: being able to take information about an individual's genome and environment and accurately predict their phenotype. This effort has taken on many forms and many names in different fields over time including population genetics [1], statistical genetics, quantitative genetics [2], genetical genomics [3], complex trait analysis [4], systems genetics [5, 6], systems medicine [7, 8], personalized medicine [9], predictive medicine and precision medicine [10, 11]. In humans, this has been greatly constrained by the *N*-of-1 problem, by which we mean that each person is a unique individual [12] – even monozygotic twins will differ in their environment. This has made it impractical, if not impossible, to accurately predict at the individual level disease risk or best treatment options for most common diseases, especially across populations [13–18], although we can, of course, make generalizations within a population. As sample sizes for genome-wide association studies have grown, it has become increasingly clear that any single commonly segregating variant is likely to have a very small impact on disease risk [19–21]. Indeed, an omnigenic model has been proposed, whereby variants in every gene are likely to affect every phenotype [22]. Even for Mendelian disorders such as Huntington's disease, there are other alleles in the genetic background which modulate age of onset [23].

IntechOpen

How then, if there is so much complication in this one-to-one relationship (one gene variant to one phenotype), can we uncover the true many-to-many-to-many relationships that occur in biology? Phenotypes at many levels, including behavior, organ systems, cells, proteins, metabolites, and mRNAs, all interact together with sets of many gene variants, and with an individual's current and previous environmental exposures. We need to understand gene–gene (epistasis), gene-age, gene-sex, gene-treatment, and gene–environment interactions and all their combinations. One answer to this is through the use of recombinant inbred (RI) populations and their derivatives.

2. Recombinant inbred families

Recombinant inbred (RI) populations are a seemingly simple idea: two inbred strains are crossed, and their F1 progeny are then crossed again to produce an F2. Pairs of these F2 animals are mated, and new lines are established through repeated rounds of sib-mating (**Figure 1A**). By generation F20, we have a population of 99% inbred strains, each of which is a unique mosaic of homozygous genetic regions from both the parents, and for which an effectively infinite set of genetically identical individuals can be produced [24, 25]. This combination of genetic variability between strains but identical genome within strains allows the mapping of linkage between genotype and phenotype. The design has been expanded on in a variety of ways [26], such as increasing the number of parental strains (e.g. the 8 founders used for the Collaborative Cross mice [27, 28]) to increase the number

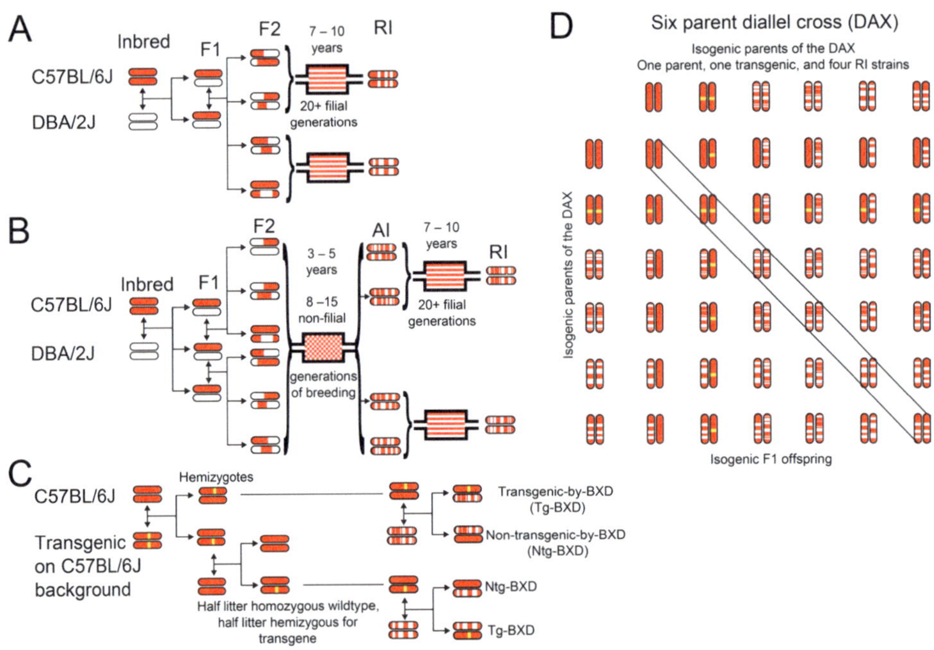

Figure 1.
Production of the BXD family, transgenic crosses, and diallel crosses. Approximately half of the BXD strains are from an F2 (A; epochs 1, 2, 4 and 6), and approximately half of the BXD strains are from advanced intercrosses (AI; B; epochs 3 and 5). Red represents regions of the genome coming from C57BL/6 J (B6), and white represents regions from the DBA/2 J (D2). Solid arrows have been used to represent a single generation of breeding. Trangenic and non-transgenic crosses for QTL mapping can be produced by crossing hemizygous transgenic mice to RI individuals, to produce litters containing both genotypes (C). The transgene is represented in yellow. A diallel cross (DAX) includes all combinations of genotypes, including the inbred 'diagonal', and all reciprical crosses (D). All offspring of the DAX are isogenic, meaning that genotypes are replicable.

of variants that segregates in the population, or using multiple rounds of crossing before inbreeding, producing so-called Advanced Intercross RI strains (AI-RI) to increase the number of recombinations, and therefore the precision of mapping (**Figure 1B**; [29]). Although RI strains were first developed in mice, and it is mice that we will concentrate on in this chapter, the design has now been used for a wide variety of organisms, including *Arabidopsis* [30, 31], *Zea mays* (maize) [32], barley [33], *Drosophila melanogaster* [34], *Drosophila simulans* [35], *Caenorhabditis elegans* [36] and rat [37].

These RI families are an essential complement to data collected in humans, allowing us to build experimental platforms for what is now called precision medicine. Each isogenic RI strain within a family is effectively an immortal genome-type. This is important because it allows the same genome to be resampled using any tissue, at any age, with any method, with any environmental exposure or treatment that the researcher cares to use. This allows us to model higher-order genome-environment interactions: the many-to-many-to-many problem stated above.

Whereas in human cohorts we have to imagine a counterfactual (e.g. what would have happened had I exercised more?), in isogenic strains we can effectively run this counterfactual – almost perfectly genomically and environmentally matched individuals can be phenotyped with only a single environmental perturbation between them. Even better, we can have multiple duplicates of these identical genome-types within each arm of the study, allowing us to reduce the effect of unwanted environmental perturbations, increasing our power to detect true associations [38]. However, in some sense, this is still an *N*-of-1 study, as only a single genome-type is being used. A problem many pre-clinical studies have had is that all experiments were carried out on a single genome-type and therefore effectively a single individual. The C57BL/6 J strain is often used to represent the entire mouse species [39, 40], when in fact its phenotype can often differ from even the closely related C57BL/6 N strain [41]. This may explain some of the failures to translate effects seen in mice to effects seen in humans, as in these studies only a single (genetic) individual is being examined, and then results extrapolated to the highly genetically diverse human population. RI families overcome this problem – many genome-types can be tested and many replicates within each genome-type. Therefore, we have a high-powered system to detect and test genome-phenome associations.

The goal is accurate genome-phenome prediction. With this goal in mind, we will use the BXD family of isogenic mouse strains as our example of how this can be achieved. The BXDs are by a wide margin the largest and most deeply phenotyped mammalian family and can be used as a testbed for experimental precision medicine.

3. The BXD family

The BXD family were among the first RI strains to be produced [24, 42, 43]. This work was started by Benjamin A. Taylor who crossed female C57BL/6 J (B6 or B) and male DBA/2 J (D2 or D) strains—hence BXD (**Figure 1A**). The first sets of BXDs were intended for mapping Mendelian loci [42, 44], but the family was also used to map complex traits such as cancer and cardiovascular disease [45–48], variation in CNS structure [49–52], and behavioral and pharmacological differences [53–62]. Twenty-seven of the original 32 BXD strains are still available from The Jackson Laboratory (JAX). In the mid-1990s, Taylor began the production of a second set of BXDs [44] and added nine new strains (BXD33–BXD42). BXD1-BXD42 carry the strain suffix "/TyJ".

We started production of another wave of BXDs at UTHSC in the late 1990s [29]. These new lines were derived from advanced intercross (AI) progeny that had accumulated chromosomal recombination events across 8 to 14 generations [63] (**Figure 1B**). These AI-derived BXDs incorporate roughly twice as many recombinations between parental genomes than do conventional F2-derived BXDs [63–67]. This improves mapping precision nearly two-fold. BXD strains BXD43 and above from UTHSC were donated to JAX once fully inbred, and carry the strain suffix "/RwwJ".

The BXD family has been used to define specific genes and even sequence variants corresponding to 20 or more QTLs. These include two tightly linked genes, *Iigp2* and *Irgb10,* for *Chlamydia* infectivity [68, 69], *Fmn2* as a master controller of tRNA synthetases in neurons [70], *Ubp1* for blood pressure [48], *Hc* for H5N1 influenza resistance [71], *Comt* as a master controller of neuropharmacological traits [72], *Alpl* for hypophosphatasia [73], *Mrps5* for longevity [74], *Bckdhb* for maple syrup urine disease, *Dhtkd1* for diabetes [75], *Hp1bp3* for cognitive aging [76], *Ahr* for locomotor activity [77], *Cacna2d1* for glaucoma [78] and *Gabra2* for behavioral traits [79]. Alleles discovered in the BXD have been successfully translated into medical applications in humans, such as stratified preclinical testing based on glaucoma risk alleles revealed in the BXDs [80, 81].

Two things now set the BXD family apart from all other recombinant inbred populations: the number of strains within the family, and the deep, coherent phenome that has been collected for them.

3.1 The largest mammalian recombinant inbred family

The BXD family is the largest mammalian recombinant inbred population, having expanded during its lifetime, from ~20 [42], to ~35 [44], to ~80 [29], to a total of 198 strains with data on GeneNetwork.org. There are 123 BXD strains currently distributed by The Jackson Laboratory (JAX) and an additional seventeen strains available at UTHSC, soon to be donated to JAX [82]. All 140 of these strains are available under a standard material transfer agreement. This expanded number of easily accessible strains increases the power and precision of linkage studies [82].

As the number of strains increases, there is an increase in the number of recombination junctions within the population, and consequently, quantitative trait loci (QTLs) can be narrowed down to smaller intervals. This is improved still further by the fact that approximately half of the BXD family are derived from advanced intercrosses, each of which will have a larger number of recombinations than their F2 derived cousins. We have demonstrated that when using approximately half of the family (60–80 strains), precision is close to 1 Mb for many traits [82]. This is also partially due to two other features of the family. The first, common to all RIs, is that the effective heritability of the trait can be boosted by resampling the same genome-type [38], and the second, that because there are two parents in the population, there is a well-balanced distribution of the two haplotypes across the genome (the mean minor allele frequency is ~0.44).

When carrying out QTL mapping the largest gain of power is given by increasing the number of genome-types tested [38, 73], and therefore, as the largest RI family, the BXD have the most power to detect genotype–phenotype linkage. A simple app has been produced to estimate power to detect QTL in the BXD, available at http://power.genenetwork.org [82]. When we examine power in the BXD family, we see a fact that might seem counter-intuitive to some: power is always increased more by increasing the number of strains compared to increasing the number of within strain biological replicates, even when heritability is low. Even at low-to-moderate heritabilities, increasing replicates above 6 within-strain gives very little improvement in power.

We should also note that the effect sizes seen in the BXD family (and other two-parent RIs), appear to be high, but this is correct, as effect size is highly dependent upon the population being studied. Effect sizes measured in families of inbred lines are typically much higher than those measured in an otherwise matched analysis of intercrosses, heterogeneous stock, or diversity outbred stock. Two factors contribute to the higher level of explained variance of loci when using inbred panels. The first reason is due to replicability. When effect size is treated as the proportion of total genomic variance explained by the QTL, effect size will increase as environmental effects decrease due to replication. That is, resampling decreases the standard error of the mean, suppressing environmental "noise" [38]. This is in addition to the increase in heritability above (i.e. an increase in total variance explained by the total genomic variance).

The second reason is that nearly all loci in inbred panels are homozygous and the same number of sampled animals will account for twice as much genetic variance as in an F2 cross, and four times as much variance as in a backcross [38]. When phenotyping with fully homozygous strains we are only examining the extreme ends of the distribution, providing a boost in power to detect additive effects. The downside is obvious: we cannot detect non-additive effects. However, if we add in members of the diallel cross population (DAX), we can now estimate both dominance and parent-of-origin effects. This is a topic we will come to later.

3.2 The deepest phenome for any family

As well as being the largest recombinant inbred family, the BXD are also the most deeply phenotyped. Over 40 years of data is now openly and publicly available at genenetwork.org, providing an unrivaled resource. This dense and well-integrated phenome consists of over 10,000 classical phenotypes [83]. The phenome begins with Taylor's 1973 analysis of cadmium toxicity, through to recent quantitative studies of addiction [84–86], behavior [87–90], vision [91], infectious disease [92–94], epigenetics [95, 96], and even indirect genetic effects [97–99]. The BXDs have been used to test specific developmental and evolutionary hypotheses [49, 100, 101]. They have allowed the study of gene-by-environmental interactions, with environmental exposures including alcohol and drugs of abuse [86, 102–105], infectious agents [71, 106–109], dietary modifications [110–115], and stress [116, 117]. The consequences of interventions and treatments as a function of genome, diet, age, and sex have been quantified [90, 96, 115, 118–120], and gene pleiotropy has been identified [121].

Beyond this, there is now extensive omics data for the BXD. Both parents have been fully sequenced [75, 122, 123], and deep linked-read and long-read sequencing of 152 members the BXD family is underway. Over 100 transcriptome datasets are available (e.g, [124, 125]), as well as more recent miRNA [84, 126], proteome [118, 120, 127], metabolome [75, 118, 125], epigenome [95, 128], and metagenome [93, 129] profiles. Nevertheless, much more is still to be done, as many of these measures have only been taken in the liver or in specific brain regions [118, 120]. However, as each of these new datasets is added, they will be fully coherent with previous datasets, multiplicatively increasing the usefulness of the whole phenome.

Access to this plethora of data is freely available from open-source web services, allowing users to download the data, or to make use of powerful statistical tools designed for global analyses that are integrated into websites (e.g. GeneNetwork.org, bxd.vital-it.ch, and Systems-Genetics.org) [125, 130, 131].

It cannot be overstated how important it is that those using the BXDs gain access to coherent genomes and quantitative phenomes generated under diverse laboratory and environmental conditions [83, 132]. New data can be compared to thousands of publicly available quantitative traits, and with each addition, the number of network connections grows quadratically—enabling powerful multi-systems analysis for all users [73, 111, 112, 118, 125, 133]. Causal pathways can be produced from genome variants, to gene expression, to metabolite levels, to phenotype [73]. Within minutes of finding a gene of interest, a researcher can look for correlations between its expression and thousands of other genes, across dozens of tissues. Enrichment analysis can then be carried out on these 'gene-friends' suggesting pathways and networks that your gene of interest may be associated with. Correlations can be found between the expression of your gene and over 10,000 phenotypes, giving suggestions of the role of the gene at the whole-organism level. Shared QTLs, where both the gene-expression and a phenotype of interest are associated with the same locus, provide strong evidence of a genetic link. Using GeneNetwork.org we can build biological networks, moving from genetic variant, to expression difference, to protein expression, to whole-system outcomes, with just a few keystrokes, and without touching a lab bench [134–136]. Entire manuscripts can be written without leaving a web browser [137]. This is a massive step forward that is under-appreciated by many.

The above demonstrates how the BXD can help us achieve our goal of predictive modeling of disease risk and the efficacy of interventions [138]. Indeed, the family has already been used to test specific functional predictions of behavior based on neuroanatomical variation [139]. The BXD family is well placed to address these questions that encompass both high levels of genetic variation and gene-environmental interactions: our many-to-many-to-many problem. This is bolstered by the family's easy extendibility into a massive diallel cross population (DAX).

4. Diallel crosses

The diallel cross is another simple idea that has been with us for over 60 years [140–142]. We now have the major opportunity to take full advantage of this approach using large panels of fully sequenced isogenic strains. A DAX is the set of all possible matings between several genome-types (**Figure 1D**). For the C57BL/6 J and DBA/2 J there are the two reciprocal F1s, and these have been used to study parent-of-origin effects and to estimate heritability (e.g. [53]). As the number of parental strains increases, the number of potential diallel crosses increases exponentially, and tools have been developed to deal with large DAXs [143]. Although we have learnt much about the genetic architecture of traits [53, 143–147], QTL mapping has been more difficult, given the relatively small number of strains used [148]. We can now imagine the full DAX for the BXD family of 140 strains – 19,460 replicable isogenic F1s, all of which have a reproducible, entirely defined genome, and any subset of which can be generated efficiently for *in vitro* and *in vivo* predictive biology and experimental precision medicine. Just as the C57BL/6 J and DBA/2 J are the parents of the BXDs, the BXD strains are the parents of a potentially huge isogenic DAX.

At the first level, this has important consequences for power and precision. The number of strains phenotyped can be increased massively, giving power to detect loci with even the weakest of effect sizes [148]. Precision can also be enhanced, as F1s can be produced which segregate for a narrow region of the genome, producing a small QTL interval containing fewer genes. All the data collected in these F1s can be coherently integrated into the phenome already aggregated for the BXD, meaning that every new phenotype measured adds quadratically to the phenome and that any user of this F1 has access to over 40 years of data.

At the next level up, it also allows us to detect, for example, dominance and parent-of-origin effects mentioned above. Small DAXs of mouse strains have been able to identify parent-of-origin effects, epistasis, and dominance, but have been unable to map the loci causing these effects [53, 143–146, 149, 150]. By using reciprocal crosses of inbred strains (e.g. BXD001xBXD002F1 vs. BXD002xBXD001F1), we can produce isogenic litters, the members of which are all genetically identical, and whose only differences are due to parent-of-origin effects [151] (**Figure 1C**). By building a large DAX of reciprocal crosses, the genomic loci causing these dominance, epistatic, and/or parent-of-origin effects can be identified. Mapping of these non-additive effects is a complete dark zone in fully homozygous inbred populations.

Finally, and most importantly, the DAX provides a population for the testing of predictions. Using the BXD family we have enough strains to make associations, whether gene-phenotype, environment-phenotype, or gene–environment-phenotype, with high power. However, using only the inbred BXD lines, we do not have a second population in which to test predicted associations. The BXD DAX provides a matrix of 19,600 isogenic genome-types. If only the 'diagonal' of inbred BXD strains are used to detect associations and make predictions, any of the 19,460 isogenic F1s are available to test these associations and predictions (**Figure 1D**).

We can expand the DAX even further using easily available isogenic strains. There are approximately 200 RI strains from other two-parent mouse populations, including AXB/BXA (29 strains), AKXD (20), BXH (11), BRX58N (7), CXB (19), ILSXISS (60), LGXSM (~18), NXSM (16) and SWXJ (12), plus approximately 55–75 strains from the Collaborative Cross 8-parent RI population [28]. From these inbred parents, there are over 152,100 isogenic F1s that can be produced and replicated. An additional expansion of this design is to cross RI families to genetically engineered disease models.

5. Diallele crosses to genetically modified strains

Genetically modified animals, including humanized, transgenic and knockout mouse models, have been a vital piece in uncovering genotype–phenotype associations, but they have often suffered from the same *N*-of-1 problem as above – for example, a knockout has been produced on a single genetic background, and then phenotyped. There is ample evidence that a genetic modification produced on one genetic background can have a different phenotypic effect compared to an identical modification on a different genetic background [152–165]. Expanding above this *N*-of-1 had been difficult, as each new isogenic strain had to be produced independently with a consequent near linear increase in effort. However, each of these genetically modified isogenic lines can be added into a DAX. Now, each of any of hundreds of F1 crosses is genetically defined, replicable and isogenic, but also contains one copy of the genetic modification (**Figure 1C** and **D**). Given that there are now thousands of knockout strains available (e.g. from the International Mouse Phenotyping Consortium [166, 167]), creating a DAX is a relatively cheap and quick method by which to test the effects of genetic background [158, 168–171]. By using an RI population, we can map the location of modifier loci, genes, and variants [172–174].

An excellent example of this already exists: the Alzheimer's disease BXD (AD-BXD) panel developed by Kaczorowski and colleagues [175, 176]. By crossing

C57BL/6J-congenic females hemizygous for the humanized 5xFAD transgene (JAX Stock No. 008730) to males from BXD strains, they produced litters, half of which had the 5xFAD transgene (the AD-BXD), and half of which did not have the 5xFAD transgene (non-transgenic-BXD). The whole litter is genetically and environmentally identical except for the presence of the transgene, giving an immediate and directly comparable control (**Figure 1C**). By crossing the humanized 5xFAD line on a single genetic background to a diverse but defined set of BXDs, they produced a population that incorporates high levels of sequence variation mirroring that of humans. They have mapped genetic and molecular causes of cognitive loss in AD-BXD mice [154, 175–179], including a broad spectrum of cognitive loss similar to that of humans with familial and late-onset AD [177]. The human transgenes in the 5XFAD line [180] sensitizes BXD hybrids to a greater or lesser degree—some begin to lose conditioned fear memory as early as 6 months; others well after a year [175], demonstrating a gene-by-gene-by-age interaction. Variation is highly heritable and mappable and gives a powerful means by which to define genetic causality and mechanisms of memory and non-cognitive loss and resilience to loss.

Neuner et al., were also able to demonstrate 'reverse translation' from human genomic data to mouse phenotype [175]. They generated a polygenic genetic risk score using 21 human genes which increase Alzheimer's disease risk, and showed that the allele dosage was significantly associated with cognitive outcomes in the AD-BXD. This confirms firstly, that naturally occurring variation in these networks has overlapping effects in mice and humans, and secondly that gene-phenotype associations translate across species. This approach can be applied to many other phenotypes.

Given that phenotypes from genetically engineered mice on a single genetic background cannot be reliably generalized to other mouse genetic backgrounds [158], it is unsurprising that there are difficulties in generalizing to other species. By crossing genetically modified lines to RI strains to produce a DAX, we overcome this problem and allow the integration and translation of data to other populations and other species.

6. Integration and translation with other populations

Compared to conventional F2s and advanced intercrosses (AIs), outcrossed heterogenous stock, or diversity outbred stock, the BXD are particularly advantageous when the heritability of a trait is moderate or low because the genetic signal can be boosted greatly by resampling isogenic members of the same line many times [38]. The drawbacks of the BXDs are lower precision, and a decreased amount of variation in the population compared to e.g. multiparent families (such as the Collaborative Cross and the Diversity Outbred), and a consequent decrease in the total phenotypic variance [181]. We consider this an acceptable drawback, as we have shown that medically relevant phenotypes have variation in the family and it is possible to achieve subcentimorgan mapping precision using only half of the full set of strains [82]. Beyond this level of precision, an efficient method to transition from QTLs to causal genes, variants, and mechanisms is to take advantage of complementary resources. These include sets of other murine mapping resources, efficient *in vitro* and *in vivo* screens [74, 132, 182], and human genome-wide association study (GWAS) data.

As a specific example of combining murine populations, Taylor's cadmium testicular toxicity mutation (BXD Phenotype 13035) that was unmappable in 1973 now maps to 3 Mb on GeneNetwork.org. When combined with SNP data for common strains, the variant can be restricted to a 400 Kb region that includes the causal *Slc39a8* gene, a heavy metal transporter expressed almost exclusively in the testes [183].

Mouse-to-human genetic translation has at least a 20-year history [184], but has taken off now that GWAS are routine [48, 78, 111, 112, 123, 125, 185, 186]. Human GWAS data can be used to refine QTL found in mice, e.g. taking advantage of the power to detect associations in the BXD to identify a homologous region in humans, and then using the precision of human GWAS to identify a candidate gene [185–187].

More importantly, mouse data can be used to determine the function and causal pathway for associations made in humans. Finding variant-phenotype associations for any phenotype with GWASs is now only limited by one's ability to collect phenotypes, but interpreting and determining the function of these variants is far more difficult, given the environmental and genetic variation in any human population. RI mice, such as the BXD, provide a method of 'reverse-translation', from human-to-mouse. Again, the work of Kaczorowski and colleagues above provides an excellent example [175] that can be applied to any other phenotypes.

7. Conclusions

Despite occasional arguments to the contrary [188, 189], mice, when used correctly, are a good model of human biology and medicine [12, 190–192]. Indeed, at least 40 Nobel Prizes have been awarded for research involving mice (http://www.animalresearch.info/en/medical-advances/nobel-prizes) [193], and their use has been vital in understanding the pathogenesis of many diseases. For true predictive medicine, we need to understand all gene-by-gene-by-environment-by-age-by-sex-by-treatment interactions [160], and animal models are the only way to do this at scale. The importance of using genetically diverse mice has often been overlooked, leading to difficulties with translation. RI families, such as the BXDs, and their expansions [130], including diallel crosses and reduced complexity crosses [194, 195], overcome this problem and are a vital step towards accurate, individualized, predictive medicine.

Acknowledgements

The UTHSC Center for Integrative and Translational Genomics (CITG) has supported production of the BXD colony at UTHSC and will continue to support this colony for the duration of the grant. The CITG also provides generous support for computer hardware and programming associated with GeneNetwork, and our Galaxy and UCSC Genome Browser instances. We thank the support of CITG, and funds from the UT-ORNL Governor's Chair, NIDA grant P30 DA044223, NIAAA U01 AA013499 and U01 AA016662, NHLBI R01 HL151438, and NIDDK R01 DK120567 for the work at UTHSC.

Conflict of interest

The authors have no conflicts of interest.

Author details

David G. Ashbrook* and Lu Lu*
Department of Genetics, Genomics and Informatics, University of Tennessee Health Science Center, Memphis, TN, USA

*Address all correspondence to: dashbrook@uthsc.edu and lulu@uthsc.edu

References

[1] Fisher R. Population genetics. Proc R Soc London Ser B, Biol Sci. 1953;141: 510-523. DOI: 10.1098/rspb.1953.0058

[2] Green EL. Quantitative genetics of skeletal variations in the mouse. I. Crosses between three short-ear strains (P, NB, SEC/2). J Natl Cancer Inst. 1954;15:609-627. Available from: http://www.ncbi.nlm.nih.gov/pubmed/13233912

[3] Jansen RC, Nap JP. Genetical genomics: the added value from segregation. Trends Genet. 2001;17: 388-391. DOI: 10.1016/S0168-9525(01)02310-1

[4] Threadgill DW. Meeting report for the 4th annual Complex Trait Consortium meeting: from QTLs to systems genetics. Mamm Genome. 2006;17:2-4. DOI: 10.1007/s00335-005-0153-5

[5] Morahan G, Williams RW. Systems genetics: the next generation in genetics research? Novartis Found Symp. 2007;281:181-8; discussion 188-91, 208-9. DOI: 10.1002/9780470062128.ch15

[6] Schughart K, Williams RW. Systems Genetics. Schughart K, Williams RW, editors. New York, NY: Springer New York; 2017. DOI: 10.1007/978-1-4939-6427-7

[7] Tao Y, Liu Y, Friedman C, Lussier YA. Information visualization techniques in bioinformatics during the postgenomic era. Drug Discov Today Biosilico. 2004;2:237-245. DOI: 10.1016/S1741-8364(04)02423-0

[8] Berlin R, Gruen R, Best J. Systems medicine-complexity within, simplicity without. J Healthc informatics Res. 2017;1:119-137. DOI: 10.1007/s41666-017-0002-9

[9] Langreth, Waldholz. New era of personalized medicine: targeting drugs for each unique genetic profile. Oncologist. 1999;4:426-427. DOI: 10.1634/theoncologist.4-5-426

[10] Wagner JB. Genomics and precision medicine to direct statin use in the young. Prog Pediatr Cardiol. 2009;54:101145. DOI: 10.1016/j.ppedcard.2019.101145

[11] Lloyd KCK, Meehan T, Beaudet A, Murray S, Svenson K, McKerlie C, et al. Precision medicine: Look to the mice. Science. 2015;349:390. DOI: 10.1126/science.349.6246.390-a

[12] Li H, Auwerx J. Mouse systems genetics as a prelude to precision medicine. Trends Genet. 2020;36:259-272. DOI: 10.1016/j.tig.2020.01.004

[13] Fisher AJ, Medaglia JD, Jeronimus BF. Lack of group-to-individual generalizability is a threat to human subjects research. Proc Natl Acad Sci U S A. 2018;115:E6106–E6115. DOI: 10.1073/pnas.1711978115

[14] Medaglia JD, Jeronimus BF, Fisher AJ. Reply to Adolf and Fried: Conditional equivalence and imperatives for person-level science. Proc Natl Acad Sci U S A. 2019;116:6542-6543. DOI: 10.1073/pnas.1820221116

[15] Adolf JK, Fried EI. Ergodicity is sufficient but not necessary for group-to-individual generalizability. Proc Natl Acad Sci U S A. 2019;116:6540-6541. DOI: 10.1073/pnas.1818675116

[16] Martin AR, Gignoux CR, Walters RK, Wojcik GL, Neale BM, Gravel S, et al. Human demographic history impacts genetic risk prediction across diverse populations. Am J Hum Genet. 2017;100:635-649. DOI: 10.1016/j.ajhg.2017.03.004

[17] Kim MS, Patel KP, Teng AK, Berens AJ, Lachance J. Genetic disease risks can be misestimated across global populations. Genome Biol. 2018;19:179. DOI: 10.1186/s13059-018-1561-7

[18] Mostafavi H, Harpak A, Agarwal I, Conley D, Pritchard JK, Przeworski M. Variable prediction accuracy of polygenic scores within an ancestry group. Elife. 2020;9. DOI: 10.7554/eLife.48376

[19] Wood AR, Esko T, Yang J, Vedantam S, Pers TH, Gustafsson S, et al. Defining the role of common variation in the genomic and biological architecture of adult human height. Nat Genet. 2014;46:1173-1186. DOI: 10.1038/ng.3097

[20] Schizophrenia Working Group of the Psychiatric Genomics Consortium. Biological insights from 108 schizophrenia-associated genetic loci. Nature. 2014;511:421-427. DOI: 10.1038/nature13595

[21] Huan T, Meng Q, Saleh MA, Norlander AE, Joehanes R, Zhu J, et al. Integrative network analysis reveals molecular mechanisms of blood pressure regulation. Mol Syst Biol. 2015;11:799. DOI: 10.15252/msb.20145399

[22] Boyle EA, Li YI, Pritchard JK. An expanded view of complex traits: From polygenic to omnigenic. Cell. 2017;169:1177-1186. DOI: 10.1016/j.cell.2017.05.038

[23] Long JD, Lee J-M, Aylward EH, Gillis T, Mysore JS, Abu Elneel K, et al. Genetic modification of Huntington disease acts early in the prediagnosis phase. Am J Hum Genet. 2018;103:349-357. DOI: 10.1016/j.ajhg.2018.07.017

[24] Crow JF. Haldane, Bailey, Taylor and recombinant-inbred lines. Genetics. 2007;176:729-732. Available from: http://www.ncbi.nlm.nih.gov/pubmed/17579238

[25] Bailey DW. Recombinant-inbred strains. An aid to finding identity, linkage, and function of histo compatibility and other genes. Transplantation. 1971;11:325-327. DOI: 10.1097/00007890-197103000-00013

[26] Teuscher F, Broman KW. Haplotype probabilities for multiple-strain recombinant inbred lines. Genetics. 2007;175:1267-1274. DOI: 10.1534/genetics.106.064063

[27] Churchill G a, Airey DC, Allayee H, Angel JM, Attie AD, Beatty J, et al. The Collaborative Cross, a community resource for the genetic analysis of complex traits. Nat Genet. 2004;36:1133-7. DOI: 10.1038/ng1104-1133

[28] Shorter JR, Najarian ML, Bell TA, Blanchard M, Ferris MT, Hock P, et al. Whole genome wequencing and progress toward full inbreeding of the mouse Collaborative Cross population. G3 (Bethesda). 2019;9:1303-1311. DOI: 10.1534/g3.119.400039

[29] Peirce JL, Lu L, Gu J, Silver LM, Williams RW. A new set of BXD recombinant inbred lines from advanced intercross populations in mice. BMC Genet. BioMed Central; 2004;5:7. DOI: 10.1186/1471-2156-5-7

[30] El-Din El-Assal S, Alonso-Blanco C, Peeters AJM, Raz V, Koornneef M. A QTL for flowering time in Arabidopsis reveals a novel allele of CRY2. Nat Genet. 2001;29:435-440. DOI: 10.1038/ng767

[31] Lister C, Dean C. Recombinant inbred lines for mapping RFLP and phenotypic markers in Arabidopsis thaliana. Plant J. 1993;4:745-750. DOI: 10.1046/j.1365-313X.1993.04040745.x

[32] Pan Q, Xu Y, Li K, Peng Y, Zhan W, Li W, et al. The genetic basis of plant architecture in 10 maize recombinant inbred line populations. Plant Physiol. 2017;175:858-873. DOI: 10.1104/pp.17.00709

[33] Yin X, Struik PC, Tang J, Qi C, Liu T. Model analysis of flowering phenology in recombinant inbred lines of barley. J Exp Bot. 2005;56:959-965. DOI: 10.1093/jxb/eri089

[34] Ruden DM, Chen L, Possidente D, Possidente B, Rasouli P, Wang L, et al. Genetical toxicogenomics in Drosophila identifies master-modulatory loci that are regulated by developmental exposure to lead. Neurotoxicology. 2009;30:898-914. DOI: 10.1016/j.neuro.2009.08.011

[35] Cochrane BJ, Windelspecht M, Brandon S, Morrow M, Dryden L. Use of recombinant inbred lines for the investigation of insecticide resistance and cross resistance in Drosophila simulans. Pestic Biochem Physiol. 1998;61:95-114. DOI: 10.1006/pest.1998.2355

[36] Snoek BL, Volkers RJM, Nijveen H, Petersen C, Dirksen P, Sterken MG, et al. A multi-parent recombinant inbred line population of C. elegans allows identification of novel QTLs for complex life history traits. BMC Biol. 2019;17:24. DOI: 10.1186/s12915-019-0642-8

[37] Printz MP, Jirout M, Jaworski R, Alemayehu A, Kren V. Genetic models in applied physiology. HXB/BXH rat recombinant inbred strain platform: a newly enhanced tool for cardiovascular, behavioral, and developmental genetics and genomics. J Appl Physiol. 2003;94:2510-2522. DOI: 10.1152/japplphysiol.00064.2003

[38] Belknap JK. Effect of within-strain sample size on QTL detection and mapping using recombinant inbred mouse strains. Behav Genet. 1998;28:29-38. DOI: 10.1023/A:1021404714631

[39] Johnson M. Laboratory Mice and Rats. Mater Methods. 2012;2. DOI: 10.13070/mm.en.2.113

[40] Miller RA. Not your father's, or mother's, rodent: Moving beyond B6. Neuron. 2016;91:1185-1186. DOI: 10.1016/j.neuron.2016.09.009

[41] Simon MM, Greenaway S, White JK, Fuchs H, Gailus-Durner V, Sorg T, et al. A comparative phenotypic and genomic analysis of C57BL/6J and C57BL/6N mouse strains. Genome Biol. 2013;14:R82. DOI: 10.1186/gb-2013-14-7-r82

[42] Taylor BA, Heiniger HJ, Meier H. Genetic analysis of resistance to cadmium-induced testicular damage in mice. Proc Soc Exp Biol Med. 1973;143:629-633. DOI: 10.3181/00379727-143-37380

[43] Morse HC, Chused TM, Hartley JW, Mathieson BJ, Sharrow SO, Taylor BA. Expression of xenotropic murine leukemia viruses as cell-surface gp70 in genetic crosses between strains DBA/2 and C57BL/6. J Exp Med. 1979;149:1183-1196. DOI: 10.1084/jem.149.5.1183

[44] Taylor BA, Wnek C, Kotlus BS, Roemer N, MacTaggart T, Phillips SJ. Genotyping new BXD recombinant inbred mouse strains and comparison of BXD and consensus maps. Mamm Genome. 1999;10:335-348. DOI: 10.1007/s003359900998

[45] Grizzle WE, Mountz JD, Yang P-A, Xu X, Sun S, Van Zant GE, et al. BXD recombinant inbred mice represent a novel T cell-mediated immune response tumor model. Int J cancer. 2002;101:270-279. DOI: 10.1002/ijc.10606

[46] Lee GH, Bennett LM, Carabeo RA, Drinkwater NR. Identification of hepatocarcinogen-resistance genes in DBA/2 mice. Genetics. 1995;139:387-395. Available from: http://www.ncbi.nlm.nih.gov/pubmed/7705639

[47] McGinnis JF, Lerious V, Pazik J, Elliott RW. Chromosomal assignment of the recoverin gene and cancer-associated retinopathy. Mamm Genome. 1993;4:43-45. DOI: 10.1007/BF00364662

[48] Koutnikova H, Laakso M, Lu L, Combe R, Paananen J, Kuulasmaa T, et al. Identification of the UBP1 locus as a critical blood pressure determinant using a combination of mouse and human genetics. PLoS Genet. 2009;5:e1000591. DOI: 10.1371/journal.pgen.1000591

[49] Seecharan DJ, Kulkarni AL, Lu L, Rosen GD, Williams RW. Genetic control of interconnected neuronal populations in the mouse primary visual system. J Neurosci. 2003;23:11178-11188. DOI: 10.1523/JNEUROSCI.23-35-11178.2003

[50] Rosen GD, Pung CJ, Owens CB, Caplow J, Kim H, Mozhui K, et al. Genetic modulation of striatal volume by loci on Chrs 6 and 17 in BXD recombinant inbred mice. Genes Brain Behav. 2009;8:296-308. DOI: 10.1111/j.1601-183X.2009.00473.x

[51] Belknap JK, Phillips TJ, O'Toole LA. Quantitative trait loci associated with brain weight in the BXD/Ty recombinant inbred mouse strains. Brain Res Bull. 1992;29:337-344. DOI: 10.1016/0361-9230(92)90065-6

[52] Zhou G, Williams RW. Eye1 and Eye2: gene loci that modulate eye size, lens weight, and retinal area in the mouse. Invest Ophthalmol Vis Sci. 1999;40:817-825. Available from: http://www.ncbi.nlm.nih.gov/pubmed/10102277

[53] Ashbrook DG, Roy S, Clifford BG, Riede T, Scattoni ML, Heck DH, et al. Born to cry: A genetic dissection of infant vocalization. Front Behav Neurosci. 2018;12:250. DOI: 10.3389/fnbeh.2018.00250

[54] Knoll AT, Jiang K, Levitt P. Quantitative trait locus mapping and analysis of heritable variation in affiliative social behavior and co-occurring traits. Genes Brain Behav. 2018;17:e12431. DOI: 10.1111/gbb.12431

[55] Belknap JK, Crabbe JC, Plomin R, McClearn GE, Sampson KE, O'Toole LA, et al. Single-locus control of saccharin intake in BXD/Ty recombinant inbred (RI) mice: Some methodological implications for RI strain analysis. Behav Genet. 1992;22:81-100. DOI: 10.1007/BF01066794

[56] Belknap JK, Metten P, Helms ML, O'Toole LA, Angeli-Gade S, Crabbe JC, et al. Quantitative trait loci (QTL) applications to substances of abuse: physical dependence studies with nitrous oxide and ethanol in BXD mice. Behav Genet. 1993;23:213-222. DOI: 10.1007/BF01067426

[57] Grisel JE, Belknap JK, O'Toole LA, Helms ML, Wenger CD, Crabbe JC. Quantitative trait loci affecting methamphetamine responses in BXD recombinant inbred mouse strains. J Neurosci. 1997;17:745-754. DOI: 10.1523/JNEUROSCI.17-02-00745.1997

[58] Weimar WR, Lane PW, Sidman RL. Vibrator (vb): a spinocerebellar system degeneration with autosomal recessive inheritance in mice. Brain Res. 1982;251:357-364. DOI: 10.1016/0006-8993(82)90754-5

[59] Phillips TJ, Belknap JK, Buck KJ, Cunningham CL. Genes on mouse chromosomes 2 and 9 determine variation in ethanol consumption.

Mamm Genome. 1998;9:936-941. DOI: 10.1007/s003359900903

[60] Palmer AA, Lessov-Schlaggar CN, Ponder CA, McKinnon CS, Phillips TJ. Sensitivity to the locomotor-stimulant effects of ethanol and allopregnanolone: a quantitative trait locus study of common genetic influence. Genes Brain Behav. 2006;5:506-517. DOI: 10.1111/j.1601-183X.2005.00198.x

[61] Jones LC, McCarthy KA, Beard JL, Keen CL, Jones BC. Quantitative genetic analysis of brain copper and zinc in BXD recombinant inbred mice. Nutr Neurosci. 2006;9:81-92. DOI: 10.1080/00268970600691365

[62] Rodriguez LA, Plomin R, Blizard DA, Jones BC, McClearn GE. Alcohol acceptance, preference, and sensitivity in mice. I. Quantitative genetic analysis using BXD recombinant inbred strains. Alcohol Clin Exp Res. 1994;18:1416-1422. DOI: 10.1111/j.1530-0277.1994.tb01444.x

[63] Darvasi A. Experimental strategies for the genetic dissection of complex traits in animal models. Nat Genet. 1998;18:19-24. DOI: 10.1038/ng0198-19

[64] Williams RW, Gu J, Qi S, Lu L. The genetic structure of recombinant inbred mice: high-resolution consensus maps for complex trait analysis. Genome Biol. 2001;2:RESEARCH0046. DOI: 10.1186/gb-2001-2-11-research0046

[65] Parker CC, Sokoloff G, Cheng R, Palmer AA. Genome-wide association for fear conditioning in an advanced intercross mouse line. Behav Genet. 2012;42:437-448. DOI: 10.1007/s10519-011-9524-8

[66] Parker CC, Cheng R, Sokoloff G, Palmer AA. Genome-wide association for methamphetamine sensitivity in an advanced intercross mouse line. Genes Brain Behav. 2012;11:52-61. DOI: 10.1111/j.1601-183X.2011.00747.x

[67] Pandey AK, Williams RW. Genetics of gene expression in CNS. Int Rev Neurobiol. 2014;116:195-231. DOI: 10.1016/B978-0-12-801105-8.00008-4

[68] Miyairi I, Tatireddigari VRRA, Mahdi OS, Rose LA, Belland RJ, Lu L, et al. The p47 GTPases Iigp2 and Irgb10 regulate innate immunity and inflammation to murine Chlamydia psittaci infection. J Immunol. 2007;179:1814-24. DOI: 179/3/1814 [pii]

[69] Miyairi I, Ziebarth J, Laxton JD, Wang X, van Rooijen N, Williams RW, et al. Host genetics and Chlamydia disease: prediction and validation of disease severity mechanisms. PLoS One. 2012;7:e33781. DOI: 10.1371/journal.pone.0033781

[70] Mozhui K, Ciobanu DC, Schikorski T, Wang X, Lu L, Williams RW. Dissection of a QTL hotspot on mouse distal chromosome 1 that modulates neurobehavioral phenotypes and gene expression. PLoS Genet. 2008;4:e1000260. DOI: 10.1371/journal.pgen.1000260

[71] Boon ACM, Williams RW, Sinasac DS, Webby RJ. A novel genetic locus linked to pro-inflammatory cytokines after virulent H5N1 virus infection in mice. BMC Genomics. 2014;15:1017. DOI: 10.1186/1471-2164-15-1017

[72] Li Z, Mulligan MK, Wang X, Miles MF, Lu L, Williams RW. A transposon in Comt generates mRNA variants and causes widespread expression and behavioral differences among mice. Hoheisel J, editor. PLoS One. 2010;5:e12181. DOI: 10.1371/journal.pone.0012181

[73] Andreux PA, Williams EG, Koutnikova H, Houtkooper RH, Champy M-F, Henry H, et al. Systems genetics of metabolism: the use of the BXD murine reference panel for multiscalar integration of traits. Cell.

2012;150:1287-1299. DOI: 10.1016/j.cell.2012.08.012

[74] Houtkooper RH, Mouchiroud L, Ryu D, Moullan N, Katsyuba E, Knott G, et al. Mitonuclear protein imbalance as a conserved longevity mechanism. Nature. 2013;497:451-457. DOI: 10.1038/nature12188

[75] Wu Y, Williams EG, Dubuis S, Mottis A, Jovaisaite V, Houten SM, et al. Multilayered genetic and omics dissection of mitochondrial activity in a mouse reference population. Cell. 2014;158:1415-1430. DOI: 10.1016/j.cell.2014.07.039

[76] Neuner SM, Garfinkel BP, Wilmott LA, Ignatowska-Jankowska BM, Citri A, Orly J, et al. Systems genetics identifies Hp1bp3 as a novel modulator of cognitive aging. Neurobiol Aging. 2016;46:58-67. DOI: 10.1016/j.neurobiolaging.2016.06.008

[77] Williams EG, Mouchiroud L, Frochaux M, Pandey A, Andreux P a, Deplancke B, et al. An evolutionarily conserved role for the aryl hydrocarbon receptor in the regulation of movement. PLoS Genet. 2014;10:e1004673. DOI: 10.1371/journal.pgen.1004673

[78] Chintalapudi SR, Maria D, Di Wang X, Bailey JNC, NEIGHBORHOOD consortium, International Glaucoma Genetics consortium, et al. Systems genetics identifies a role for Cacna2d1 regulation in elevated intraocular pressure and glaucoma susceptibility. Nat Commun. 2017;8:1755. DOI: 10.1038/s41467-017-00837-5

[79] Mulligan MK, Abreo T, Neuner SM, Parks C, Watkins CE, Houseal MT, et al. Identification of a functional non-coding variant in the GABAA Receptor α2 subunit of the C57BL/6J mouse reference genome: Major implications for neuroscience research. Front Genet. 2019;10:188. DOI: 10.3389/fgene.2019.00188

[80] Chen D-S, Dai J-Q, Han S-C. Identification of the pheromone biosynthesis genes from the sex pheromone gland transcriptome of the diamondback moth, Plutella xylostella. Sci Rep. 2017;7:16255. DOI: 10.1038/s41598-017-16518-8

[81] Ibrahim MM, Maria DN, Mishra SR, Guragain D, Wang X, Jablonski MM. Once daily pregabalin eye drops for management of glaucoma. ACS Nano. 2019;13:13728-13744. DOI: 10.1021/acsnano.9b07214

[82] Ashbrook DG, Arends D, Prins P, Mulligan MK, Roy S, Williams EG, et al. The expanded BXD family of mice: A cohort for experimental systems genetics and precision medicine. bioRxiv. 2019;672097. DOI: 10.1101/672097

[83] Ashbrook DG, Mulligan MK, Williams RW. Post-genomic behavioral genetics: From revolution to routine. Genes Brain Behav. 2018;17:e12441. DOI: 10.1111/gbb.12441

[84] Mulligan MK, Dubose C, Yue J, Miles MF, Lu L, Hamre KM. Expression, covariation, and genetic regulation of miRNA Biogenesis genes in brain supports their role in addiction, psychiatric disorders, and disease. Front Genet. 2013;4:126. DOI: 10.3389/fgene.2013.00126

[85] Dickson PE, Miller MM, Calton MA, Bubier JA, Cook MN, Goldowitz D, et al. Systems genetics of intravenous cocaine self-administration in the BXD recombinant inbred mouse panel. Psychopharmacology (Berl). 2016;233:701-714. DOI: 10.1007/s00213-015-4147-z

[86] Dickson PE, Roy TA, McNaughton KA, Wilcox TD, Kumar P, Chesler EJ. Systems genetics of

sensation seeking. Genes Brain Behav. 2019;18:e12519. DOI: 10.1111/gbb.12519

[87] Graybeal C, Bachu M, Mozhui K, Saksida LM, Bussey TJ, Sagalyn E, et al. Strains and stressors: an analysis of touchscreen learning in genetically diverse mouse strains. Zhuang X, editor. PLoS One. 2014;9:e87745. DOI: 10.1371/journal.pone.0087745

[88] Mulligan MK, Williams RW. Systems genetics of behavior: a prelude. Curr Opin Behav Sci. 2015;2:108-115. DOI: 10.1016/j.cobeha.2015.01.014

[89] Carhuatanta KAK, Shea CJA, Herman JP, Jankord R. Unique genetic loci identified for emotional behavior in control and chronic stress conditions. Front Behav Neurosci. 2014;8:341. DOI: 10.3389/fnbeh.2014.00341

[90] Philip VM, Duvvuru S, Gomero B, Ansah TA, Blaha CD, Cook MN, et al. High-throughput behavioral phenotyping in the expanded panel of BXD recombinant inbred strains. Genes Brain Behav. 2010;9:129-159. DOI: 10.1111/j.1601-183X.2009.00540.x

[91] Geisert EE, Williams RW. Using BXD mouse strains in vision research: A systems genetics approach. Mol Vis. 2020;26:173-187. Available from: http://www.ncbi.nlm.nih.gov/pubmed/32180682

[92] Hayes KS, Hager R, Grencis RK. Sex-dependent genetic effects on immune responses to a parasitic nematode. BMC Genomics. 2014;15:193. DOI: 10.1186/1471-2164-15-193

[93] McKnite AM, Perez-Munoz ME, Lu L, Williams EG, Brewer S, Andreux PA, et al. Murine gut microbiota is defined by host genetics and modulates variation of metabolic traits. White BA, editor. PLoS One. 2012;7:e39191. DOI: 10.1371/journal.pone.0039191

[94] Wang J, Yoon TW, Read R, Yi A-K, Williams RW, Fitzpatrick EA. Genetic variability of T cell responses in hypersensitivity pneumonitis identified using the BXD genetic reference panel. Am J Physiol Lung Cell Mol Physiol. 2020;318:L631–L643. DOI: 10.1152/ajplung.00120.2019

[95] Baker CL, Walker M, Arat S, Ananda G, Petkova P, Powers NR, et al. Tissue-specific trans regulation of the mouse epigenome. Genetics. 2019;211:831-845. DOI: 10.1534/genetics.118.301697

[96] Sandoval-Sierra JV, Helbing AHB, Williams EG, Ashbrook DG, Roy S, Williams RW, et al. Body weight and high-fat diet are associated with epigenetic aging in female members of the BXD murine family. Aging Cell. 2020;e13207. DOI: 10.1111/acel.13207

[97] Ashbrook DG, Sharmin N, Hager R. Offspring genes indirectly influence sibling and maternal behavioural strategies over resource share. Proceedings Biol Sci. 2017;284:20171059. DOI: 10.1098/rspb.2017.1059

[98] Ashbrook DG, Gini B, Hager R. Genetic variation in offspring indirectly influences the quality of maternal behaviour in mice. Elife. 2015;4:e11814. DOI: 10.7554/eLife.11814

[99] Baud A, Mulligan MK, Casale FP, Ingels JF, Bohl CJ, Callebert J, et al. Genetic variation in the social environment contributes to health and disease. Feldman MW, editor. PLoS Genet. 2017;13:e1006498. DOI: 10.1371/journal.pgen.1006498

[100] Hager R, Lu L, Rosen GD, Williams RW. Genetic architecture supports mosaic brain evolution and independent brain-body size regulation. Nat Commun. 2012;3:1079. DOI: 10.1038/ncomms2086

[101] Oren Y, Nachshon A, Frishberg A, Wilentzik R, Gat-Viks I. Linking traits based on their shared molecular mechanisms. Elife. 2015;4. DOI: 10.7554/eLife.04346

[102] Théberge ET, Baker JA, Dubose C, Boyle JK, Balce K, Goldowitz D, et al. Genetic influences on the amount of cell death in the neural tube of BXD mice exposed to acute ethanol at midgestation. Alcohol Clin Exp Res. 2019;43:439-452. DOI: 10.1111/acer.13947

[103] Zhou D, Zhao Y, Hook M, Zhao W, Starlard-Davenport A, Cook MN, et al. Ethanol's effect on Coq7 expression in the hippocampus of mice. Front Genet. 2018;9:602. DOI: 10.3389/fgene.2018.00602

[104] Mulligan MK, Zhao W, Dickerson M, Arends D, Prins P, Cavigelli SA, et al. Genetic contribution to initial and progressive alcohol intake among recombinant inbred strains of mice. Front Genet. 2018;9:370. DOI: 10.3389/fgene.2018.00370

[105] Wang LS, Jiao Y, Huang Y, Liu XY, Gibson G, Bennett B, et al. Critical evaluation of transcription factor Atf2 as a candidate modulator of alcohol preference in mouse and human populations. Genet Mol Res. 2013;12:5992-6005. DOI: 10.4238/2013.November.26.9

[106] Chella Krishnan K, Mukundan S, Alagarsamy J, Hur J, Nookala S, Siemens N, et al. Genetic architecture of group a streptococcal necrotizing soft tissue infections in the mouse. Bessen DE, editor. PLoS Pathog. 2016;12:e1005732. DOI: 10.1371/journal.ppat.1005732

[107] Russo LM, Abdeltawab NF, O'Brien AD, Kotb M, Melton-Celsa AR. Mapping of genetic loci that modulate differential colonization by Escherichia coli O157:H7 TUV86-2 in advanced recombinant inbred BXD mice. BMC Genomics. 2015;16:947. DOI: 10.1186/s12864-015-2127-7

[108] Nedelko T, Kollmus H, Klawonn F, Spijker S, Lu L, Heßman M, et al. Distinct gene loci control the host response to influenza H1N1 virus infection in a time-dependent manner. BMC Genomics. 2012;13:411. DOI: 10.1186/1471-2164-13-411

[109] Boon ACM, DeBeauchamp J, Hollmann A, Luke J, Kotb M, Rowe S, et al. Host genetic variation affects resistance to infection with a highly pathogenic H5N1 influenza A virus in mice. J Virol. 2009;83:10417-10426. DOI: 10.1128/JVI.00514-09

[110] Rodrigues B de A, Muñoz VR, Kuga GK, Gaspar RC, Nakandakari SCBR, Crisol BM, et al. Obesity increases mitogen-activated protein kinase phosphatase-3 levels in the hypothalamus of mice. Front Cell Neurosci. 2017;11:313. DOI: 10.3389/fncel.2017.00313

[111] Jha P, McDevitt MT, Gupta R, Quiros PM, Williams EG, Gariani K, et al. Systems analyses reveal physiological roles and genetic regulators of liver lipid species. Cell Syst. 2018;6:722-733.e6. DOI: 10.1016/j.cels.2018.05.016

[112] Jha P, McDevitt MT, Halilbasic E, Williams EG, Quiros PM, Gariani K, et al. Genetic regulation of plasma lipid species and their association with metabolic phenotypes. Cell Syst. 2018;6:709-721.e6. DOI: 10.1016/j.cels.2018.05.009

[113] Jones BC, Jellen LC. Systems genetics analysis of iron and its regulation in brain and periphery. Methods Mol Biol. 2017;1488:467-480. DOI: 10.1007/978-1-4939-6427-7_22

[114] Reyes Fernandez PC, Replogle RA, Wang L, Zhang M, Fleet JC. Novel genetic loci control calcium absorption

and femur bone mass as well as their response to low calcium intake in male BXD recombinant inbred mice. J Bone Miner Res. 2016;31:994-1002. DOI: 10.1002/jbmr.2760

[115] Fleet JC, Replogle RA, Reyes-Fernandez P, Wang L, Zhang M, Clinkenbeard EL, et al. Gene-by-Diet interactions affect serum 1,25-Dihydroxyvitamin D levels in male BXD recombinant inbred mice. Endocrinology. 2016;157:470-481. DOI: 10.1210/en.2015-1786

[116] Diessler S, Jan M, Emmenegger Y, Guex N, Middleton B, Skene DJ, et al. A systems genetics resource and analysis of sleep regulation in the mouse. Kramer A, editor. PLoS Biol. 2018;16: e2005750. DOI: 10.1371/journal.pbio.2005750

[117] Jung SH, Brownlow ML, Pellegrini M, Jankord R. Divergence in Morris Water Maze-based cognitive performance under chronic stress Is associated with the hippocampal whole transcriptomic modification in mice. Front Mol Neurosci. 2017;10:275. DOI: 10.3389/fnmol.2017.00275

[118] Williams EG, Wu Y, Jha P, Dubuis S, Blattmann P, Argmann CA, et al. Systems proteomics of liver mitochondria function. Science. 2016;352:aad0189. DOI: 10.1126/science.aad0189

[119] Roy S, Sleiman MB, Jha P, Williams EG, Ingels JF, Chapman CJ, et al. Gene-by-environmental modulation of longevity and weight gain in the murine BXD family. bioRxiv. 2020;776559. DOI: 10.1101/776559

[120] Williams EG, Roy S, Statzer C, Ingels J, Bohl C, Hasan M, et al. The molecular landscape of the aging mouse liver. bioRxiv Syst Biol. 2020;2020.08.20.222968. DOI: 10.1101/2020.08.20.222968

[121] Wang L, Jiao Y, Wang Y, Zhang M, Gu W. Self-confirmation and ascertainment of the candidate genomic regions of complex trait loci - A none-experimental solution. Kulwal PL, editor. PLoS One. 2016;11:e0153676. DOI: 10.1371/journal.pone.0153676

[122] Keane TM, Goodstadt L, Danecek P, White MA, Wong K, Yalcin B, et al. Mouse genomic variation and its effect on phenotypes and gene regulation. Nature. 2011;477:289-294. DOI: 10.1038/nature10413

[123] Wang X, Pandey AK, Mulligan MK, Williams EG, Mozhui K, Li Z, et al. Joint mouse-human phenome-wide association to test gene function and disease risk. Nat Commun. 2016;7:10464. DOI: 10.1038/ncomms10464

[124] King R, Lu L, Williams RW, Geisert EE. Transcriptome networks in the mouse retina: An exon level BXD RI database. Mol Vis. 2015;21:1235-1251. Available from: http://www.ncbi.nlm.nih.gov/pubmed/26604663

[125] Li H, Wang X, Rukina D, Huang Q, Lin T, Sorrentino V, et al. An integrated systems genetics and omics toolkit to probe gene function. Cell Syst. 2018;6:90-102.e4. DOI: 10.1016/j.cels.2017.10.016

[126] Parsons MJ, Grimm C, Paya-Cano JL, Fernandes C, Liu L, Philip VM, et al. Genetic variation in hippocampal microRNA expression differences in C57BL/6 J X DBA/2 J (BXD) recombinant inbred mouse strains. BMC Genomics. 2012;13:476. DOI: 10.1186/1471-2164-13-476

[127] Williams EG, Wu Y, Wolski W, Kim JY, Lan J, Hasan M, et al. Quantifying and localizing the mitochondrial proteome across five tissues in a mouse population. Mol Cell Proteomics. 2018;17:1766-1777. DOI: 10.1074/mcp.RA118.000554

[128] Sandoval-Sierra JV, Helbing AHB, Williams EG, Ashbrook DG, Roy S, Williams RW, et al. Influence of body weight at young adulthood on the epigenetic clock and lifespan in the BXD murine family. bioRxiv. 2019;791582. DOI: 10.1101/791582

[129] Perez-Munoz ME, McKnite AM, Williams EG, Auwerx J, Williams RW, Peterson DA, et al. Diet modulates cecum bacterial diversity and physiological phenotypes across the BXD mouse genetic reference population. Wilson BA, editor. PLoS One. 2019;14:e0224100. DOI: 10.1371/journal.pone.0224100

[130] Williams RW, Williams EG. Resources for systems genetics. In: Schughart K, Williams RW, editors. Syst Genet Methods Protoc. New York, NY: Springer New York; 2017. p. 3-29. DOI: 10.1007/978-1-4939-6427-7_1

[131] Sloan Z, Arends D, W. Broman K, Centeno A, Furlotte N, Nijveen H, et al. GeneNetwork: framework for web-based genetics. J Open Source Softw. 2016;1:25. DOI: 10.21105/joss.00025

[132] Williams EG, Auwerx J. The convergence of systems and reductionist approaches in complex trait analysis. Cell. 2015;162:23-32. DOI: 10.1016/j.cell.2015.06.024

[133] Chesler EJ, Wang J, Lu L, Qu Y, Manly KF, Williams RW. Genetic correlates of gene expression in recombinant inbred strains: a relational model system to explore neuro behavioral phenotypes. Neuro informatics. 2003;1:343-357. DOI: 10.1385/NI:1:4:343

[134] Parker CC, Dickson PE, Philip VM, Thomas M, Chesler EJ. Systems genetic analysis in GeneNetwork.org. Curr Protoc Neurosci. Hoboken, NJ, USA: John Wiley & Sons, Inc.; 2017;79:8.39.1-8.39.20. DOI: 10.1002/cpns.23

[135] Mulligan MK, Mozhui K, Prins P, Williams RW. GeneNetwork: A Toolbox for Systems Genetics. K. S, R. W, editors. Methods Mol Biol. New York, NY: Humana Press; 2017;1488:75-120. DOI: 10.1007/978-1-4939-6427-7_4

[136] Watson PM, Ashbrook DG. GeneNetwork: a continuously updated tool for systems genetics analyses. bioRxiv. 2020;2020.12.23.424047. DOI: 10.1101/2020.12.23.424047

[137] Ashbrook DG, Delprato A, Grellmann C, Klein M, Wetzel R, Overall RW, et al. Transcript co-variance with Nestin in two mouse genetic reference populations identifies Lef1 as a novel candidate regulator of neural precursor cell proliferation in the adult hippocampus. Front Neurosci. Frontiers Research Foundation; 2014;8:418. DOI: 10.3389/fnins.2014.00418

[138] Hood L, Flores M. A personal view on systems medicine and the emergence of proactive P4 medicine: predictive, preventive, personalized and participatory. N Biotechnol. 2012;29:613-624. DOI: 10.1016/j.nbt.2012.03.004

[139] Yang RJ, Mozhui K, Karlsson R-M, Cameron HA, Williams RW, Holmes A. Variation in mouse basolateral amygdala volume is associated with differences in stress reactivity and fear learning. Neuropsychopharmacology. 2008;33:2595-2604. DOI: 10.1038/sj.npp.1301665

[140] Griffing B. Concept of general and specific combining ability in relation to diallel crossing systems. Aust J Biol Sci. 1956;9:463. DOI: 10.1071/BI9560463

[141] Kempthorne O. The theory of the diallel cross. Genetics. 1956;41:451-459. Available from: http://www.ncbi.nlm.nih.gov/pubmed/17247640

[142] Hayman BI. The theory and analysis of diallel crosses. Genetics. 1954;39:789-809. Available from: http://www.ncbi.nlm.nih.gov/pubmed/17247520

[143] Lenarcic AB, Svenson KL, Churchill GA, Valdar W. A general Bayesian approach to analyzing diallel crosses of inbred strains. Genetics. 2012;190:413-435. DOI: 10.1534/genetics.111.132563

[144] Percival CJ, Liberton DK, Pardo-Manuel de Villena F, Spritz R, Marcucio R, Hallgrímsson B. Genetics of murine craniofacial morphology: diallel analysis of the eight founders of the Collaborative Cross. J Anat. 2015; DOI: 10.1111/joa.12382

[145] Crowley JJ, Kim Y, Lenarcic AB, Quackenbush CR, Barrick CJ, Adkins DE, et al. Genetics of adverse reactions to haloperidol in a mouse diallel: a drug-placebo experiment and Bayesian causal analysis. Genetics. 2014;196:321-347. DOI: 10.1534/genetics.113.156901

[146] Airey DC, Lu L, Shou S, Williams RW. Genetic sources of individual differences in the cerebellum. Cerebellum. 2002;1:233-240. DOI: 10.1080/147342202320883542

[147] Maurizio PL, Ferris MT, Keele GR, Miller DR, Shaw GD, Whitmore AC, et al. Bayesian diallel analysis reveals Mx1-dependent and Mx1-independent effects on response to influenza A cirus in mice. G3 (Bethesda). 2018;8:427-445. DOI: 10.1534/g3.117.300438

[148] Williams RW, Threadgill DW, Airey DC, Gu J, Lu L. RIX Mapping: a demonstration using CXB RIX hybrids to map QTLs modulating brain weight in mice. Soc Neurosci Abst. 2001;27.

[149] Green EL. Quantitative gnetics of skeletal variations in the mouse. II. Crosses between four inbred strains (C3H, DBA, C57BL, BALB/c). Genetics. 1962;47:1085-1096. Available from: http://www.ncbi.nlm.nih.gov/pubmed/13950066

[150] Shorter JR, Maurizio PL, Bell TA, Shaw GD, Miller DR, Gooch TJ, et al. A diallel of the mouse Collaborative Cross founders reveals strong strain-specific maternal effects on litter size. G3 (Bethesda). 2019;9:1613-1622. DOI: 10.1534/g3.118.200847

[151] Ashbrook DG, Hager R. Empirical testing of hypotheses about the evolution of genomic imprinting in mammals. Front Neuroanat. 2013;7:6. DOI: 10.3389/fnana.2013.00006

[152] Acevedo-Arozena A, Kalmar B, Essa S, Ricketts T, Joyce P, Kent R, et al. A comprehensive assessment of the SOD1G93A low-copy transgenic mouse, which models human amyotrophic lateral sclerosis. Dis Model Mech. 2011;4:686-700. DOI: 10.1242/dmm.007237

[153] Heiman-Patterson TD, Sher RB, Blankenhorn EA, Alexander G, Deitch JS, Kunst CB, et al. Effect of genetic background on phenotype variability in transgenic mouse models of amyotrophic lateral sclerosis: a window of opportunity in the search for genetic modifiers. Amyotroph Lateral Scler. 2011;12:79-86. DOI: 10.3109/17482968.2010.550626

[154] O'Connell KMS, Ouellette AR, Neuner SM, Dunn AR, Kaczorowski CC. Genetic background modifies CNS-mediated sensorimotor decline in the AD-BXD mouse model of genetic diversity in Alzheimer's disease. Genes Brain Behav. 2019;18:e12603. DOI: 10.1111/gbb.12603

[155] Cowin R-M, Bui N, Graham D, Green JR, Yuva-Paylor LA, Weiss A, et al. Genetic background modulates behavioral impairments in R6/2 mice and suggests a role for dominant genetic

modifiers in Huntington's disease pathogenesis. Mamm Genome. 2012;23:367-377. DOI: 10.1007/s00335-012-9391-5

[156] Fetterman JL, Zelickson BR, Johnson LW, Moellering DR, Westbrook DG, Pompilius M, et al. Mitochondrial genetic background modulates bioenergetics and susceptibility to acute cardiac volume overload. Biochem J. 2013;455:157-167. DOI: 10.1042/BJ20130029

[157] Sisay S, Pryce G, Jackson SJ, Tanner C, Ross RA, Michael GJ, et al. Genetic background can result in a marked or minimal effect of gene knockout (GPR55 and CB2 receptor) in experimental autoimmune encephalomyelitis models of multiple sclerosis. Furlan R, editor. PLoS One. 2013;8:e76907. DOI: 10.1371/journal.pone.0076907

[158] Sittig LJ, Carbonetto P, Engel KA, Krauss KS, Barrios-Camacho CM, Palmer AA. Genetic background limits generalizability of genotype-phenotype relationships. Neuron. 2016;91:1253-1259. DOI: 10.1016/j.neuron.2016.08.013

[159] Buchner DA, Trudeau M, Meisler MH. SCNM1, a putative RNA splicing factor that modifies disease severity in mice. Science. 2003;301:967-969. DOI: 10.1126/science.1086187

[160] Nair RR, Corrochano S, Gasco S, Tibbit C, Thompson D, Maduro C, et al. Uses for humanised mouse models in precision medicine for neurodegenerative disease. Mamm Genome. 2019;30:173-191. DOI: 10.1007/s00335-019-09807-2

[161] Hahn H, Nitzki F, Schorban T, Hemmerlein B, Threadgill D, Rosemann M. Genetic mapping of a Ptch1-associated rhabdomyosarcoma susceptibility locus on mouse chromosome 2. Genomics. 2004;84:853-858. DOI: 10.1016/j.ygeno.2004.07.002

[162] Doetschman T. Influence of genetic background on genetically engineered mouse phenotypes. Methods Mol Biol. 2009;530:423-433. DOI: 10.1007/978-1-59745-471-1_23

[163] Phillips TJ, Hen R, Crabbe JC. Complications associated with genetic background effects in research using knockout mice. Psychopharmacology (Berl). 1999;147:5-7. DOI: 10.1007/s002130051128

[164] Threadgill DW, Dlugosz AA, Hansen LA, Tennenbaum T, Lichti U, Yee D, et al. Targeted disruption of mouse EGF receptor: effect of genetic background on mutant phenotype. Science. 1995;269:230-234. DOI: 10.1126/science.7618084

[165] Sanford LP, Kallapur S, Ormsby I, Doetschman T. Influence of genetic background on knockout mouse phenotypes. Methods Mol Biol. New Jersey: Humana Press; 2001;158:217-225. DOI: 10.1385/1-59259-220-1:217

[166] Cacheiro P, Haendel MA, Smedley D, International Mouse Phenotyping Consortium and the Monarch Initiative. New models for human disease from the International Mouse Phenotyping Consortium. Mamm Genome. 2019;30:143-150. DOI: 10.1007/s00335-019-09804-5

[167] Lloyd KCK, Adams DJ, Baynam G, Beaudet AL, Bosch F, Boycott KM, et al. The Deep Genome Project. Genome Biol. 2020;21:18. DOI: 10.1186/s13059-020-1931-9

[168] Lifsted T, Le Voyer T, Williams M, Muller W, Klein-Szanto A, Buetow KH, et al. Identification of inbred mouse strains harboring genetic modifiers of mammary tumor age of onset and metastatic progression. Int J cancer. 1998;77:640-644. DOI: 10.1002/(sici)1097-0215(19980812)77:4<640::aid-ijc26>3.0.co;2-8

[169] Dorman A, Baer D, Tomlinson I, Mott R, Iraqi FA. Genetic analysis of intestinal polyp development in Collaborative Cross mice carrying the Apc (Min/+) mutation. BMC Genet. 2016;17:46. DOI: 10.1186/s12863-016-0349-6

[170] Nnadi SC, Watson R, Innocent J, Gonye GE, Buchberg AM, Siracusa LD. Identification of five novel modifier loci of Apc(Min) harbored in the BXH14 recombinant inbred strain. Carcinogenesis. 2012;33:1589-1597. DOI: 10.1093/carcin/bgs185

[171] Bennett BJ, Davis RC, Civelek M, Orozco L, Wu J, Qi H, et al. Genetic architecture of atherosclerosis in mice: A systems genetics analysis of common inbred strains. Barsh GS, editor. PLoS Genet. 2015;11:e1005711. DOI: 10.1371/journal.pgen.1005711

[172] Crawford NPS, Hunter KW. Germline variation and other host determinants of metastatic potential. In: Lyden D, Welch DR, Psaila B, editors. Cancer Metastasis. Cambridge: Cambridge University Press; 2011. p. 96-104. DOI: 10.1017/CBO9780511976117.011

[173] Yang H, Crawford N, Lukes L, Finney R, Lancaster M, Hunter KW. Metastasis predictive signature profiles pre-exist in normal tissues. Clin Exp Metastasis. 2005;22:593-603. DOI: 10.1007/s10585-005-6244-6

[174] Hunter KW, Broman KW, Voyer TL, Lukes L, Cozma D, Debies MT, et al. Predisposition to efficient mammary tumor metastatic progression is linked to the breast cancer metastasis suppressor gene Brms1. Cancer Res. 2001;61:8866-8872. Available from: http://www.ncbi.nlm.nih.gov/pubmed/11751410

[175] Neuner SM, Heuer SE, Huentelman MJ, O'Connell KMS, Kaczorowski CC. Harnessing genetic complexity to enhance translatability of Alzheimer's disease mouse models: A path toward precision medicine. Neuron. 2019;101:399-411.e5. DOI: 10.1016/j.neuron.2018.11.040

[176] Neuner SM, Heuer SE, Zhang J-G, Philip VM, Kaczorowski CC. Identification of pre-symptomatic gene signatures that predict resilience to cognitive decline in the genetically diverse AD-BXD model. Front Genet. 2019;10:35. DOI: 10.3389/fgene.2019.00035

[177] Neuner SM, Wilmott LA, Hope KA, Hoffmann B, Chong JA, Abramowitz J, et al. TRPC3 channels critically regulate hippocampal excitability and contextual fear memory. Behav Brain Res. 2015;281:69-77. DOI: 10.1016/j.bbr.2014.12.018

[178] Neuner SM, Wilmott LA, Hoffmann BR, Mozhui K, Kaczorowski CC. Hippocampal proteomics defines pathways associated with memory decline and resilience in normal aging and Alzheimer's disease mouse models. Behav Brain Res. 2017;322:288-298. DOI: 10.1016/j.bbr.2016.06.002

[179] Hyman B, Tanzi RE. Effects of species-specific genetics on Alzheimer's mouse models. Neuron. 2019;101:351-352. DOI: 10.1016/j.neuron.2019.01.021

[180] Oakley H, Cole SL, Logan S, Maus E, Shao P, Craft J, et al. Intraneuronal beta-amyloid aggregates, neurodegeneration, and neuron loss in transgenic mice with five familial Alzheimer's disease mutations: potential factors in amyloid plaque formation. J Neurosci. 2006;26:10129-10140. DOI: 10.1523/JNEUROSCI.1202-06.2006

[181] Abu-Toamih Atamni HJ, Iraqi FA. Efficient protocols and methods for high-throughput utilization of the Collaborative Cross mouse model for dissecting the genetic basis of complex

traits. Anim Model Exp Med. 2019;2:137-149. DOI: 10.1002/ame2.12074

[182] Smemo S, Tena JJ, Kim K-H, Gamazon ER, Sakabe NJ, Gómez-Marín C, et al. Obesity-associated variants within FTO form long-range functional connections with IRX3. Nature. 2014;507:371-375. DOI: 10.1038/nature13138

[183] Dalton TP, He L, Wang B, Miller ML, Jin L, Stringer KF, et al. Identification of mouse SLC39A8 as the transporter responsible for cadmium-induced toxicity in the testis. Proc Natl Acad Sci U S A. 2005;102:3401-3406. DOI: 10.1073/pnas.0406085102

[184] Stoll M, Kwitek-Black AE, Cowley AW, Harris EL, Harrap SB, Krieger JE, et al. New target regions for human hypertension via comparative genomics. Genome Res. 2000;10:473-482. DOI: 10.1101/gr.10.4.473

[185] Ashbrook DG, Williams RW, Lu L, Stein JL, Hibar DP, Nichols TE, et al. Joint genetic analysis of hippocampal size in mouse and human identifies a novel gene linked to neurodegenerative disease. BMC Genomics. 2014;15:850. DOI: 10.1186/1471-2164-15-850

[186] Ashbrook DG, Williams RW, Lu L, Hager R. A cross-species genetic analysis identifies candidate genes for mouse anxiety and human bipolar disorder. Front Behav Neurosci. 2015;9:171. DOI: 10.3389/fnbeh.2015.00171

[187] Ashbrook DG, Cahill S, Hager R. A cross-species systems genetics analysis links APBB1IP as a candidate for schizophrenia and prepulse inhibition. Front Behav Neurosci. 2019;13:266. DOI: 10.3389/fnbeh.2019.00266

[188] Seok J, Warren HS, Cuenca AG, Mindrinos MN, Baker H V, Xu W, et al. Genomic responses in mouse models poorly mimic human inflammatory diseases. Proc Natl Acad Sci U S A. 2013;110:3507-3512. DOI: 10.1073/pnas.1222878110

[189] Pound P, Bracken MB. Is animal research sufficiently evidence based to be a cornerstone of biomedical research? BMJ. 2014;348:g3387. DOI: 10.1136/bmj.g3387

[190] Conejero L, Potempa K, Graham CM, Spink N, Blankley S, Salguero FJ, et al. The blood transcriptome of experimental melioidosis reflects disease severity and shows considerable similarity with the human disease. J Immunol. 2015;195:3248-3261. DOI: 10.4049/jimmunol.1500641

[191] Takao K, Miyakawa T. Genomic responses in mouse models greatly mimic human inflammatory diseases. Proc Natl Acad Sci U S A. 2015;112:1167-1172. DOI: 10.1073/pnas.1401965111

[192] Nadeau JH, Auwerx J. The virtuous cycle of human genetics and mouse models in drug discovery. Nat Rev Drug Discov. 2019;18:255-272. DOI: 10.1038/s41573-018-0009-9

[193] Festing MFW, Fisher EMC. Mighty mice. Nature. 2000;404:815. DOI: 10.1038/35009167

[194] Bryant CD, Smith DJ, Kantak KM, Nowak TS, Williams RW, Damaj MI, et al. Facilitating complex trait analysis via reduced complexity crosses. Trends Genet. 2020;36:549-562. DOI: 10.1016/j.tig.2020.05.003

[195] Bryant CD, Ferris MT, De Villena FPM, Damaj MI, Kumar V, Mulligan MK. Reduced complexity cross design for behavioral genetics. In: Gerlai RT, editor. Mol Stat Tech Behav Neural Res. Elsevier; 2018. p. 165-190. DOI: 10.1016/B978-0-12-804078-2.00008-8

Chapter 2

Parenteral Nutrition Modeling and Research Advances

Roshan Kumari, Lydia M. Henry and Joseph F. Pierre

Abstract

Parenteral nutrition (PN) provides nutritional support intravenously to individuals who have gastrointestinal (GI) failure or contraindication to enteral feeding. Since the initial development of PN, researchers have developed specialized formulas with complete macronutrients, micronutrients, vitamins, minerals, and electrolytes to support patients' metabolic needs. These formulas prevent malnutrition and optimize patient health, especially under long-term feeding circumstances. Although PN is commonly used and essential in preterm and malnourished patients, complications associated with PN feeding include gastrointestinal defects, infection, and other metabolic abnormalities such as liver injury and brain related disorders. In this chapter, we highlight an overview of PN and its association with abnormalities of microbiome composition as well as with gastrointestinal (GI), immune, hepatic, and neuronal disfunction. Within the gut, PN influences the number and composition of gut-associated lymphoid tissue (GALT) cells, altering adaptive immune responses. PN also modulates intestinal epithelium cell turnover, secretions, and gut barrier function, as well as the composition of the intestinal microbiome leading to changes in gut permeability. Collectively, these changes result in increased susceptibility to infection and injury. Here, we highlight animal models used to examine parenteral nutrition, changes that occur to the major organ systems, and recent advancement in using enteric nervous system (ENS) neuropeptides or microbially derived products during PN, which may improve GI, immune cell, hepatic, and neuronal function.

Keywords: parenteral nutrition, animal models, gastrointestinal immunity, Paneth cells, microbiome, mucosal immunity, parenteral nutrition associated liver disease (PNALD), neurodevelopmental disorder

1. Introduction

Parenteral nutrition (PN) is a clinical nutrition strategy that provides patients with essential calories, macronutrients, and micronutrients needed for metabolic function through vascular access. PN is necessary in preterm babies and malnourished adult patients who are unable to feed, such as following gut trauma or general surgery, or in instances where the bowel requires rest under chronic inflammatory conditions. 'Parenteral' derives from the English *para* (beside) and ancient Greek *enteron* (intestine) and is usually administered via the central vein (jugular or subclavian vein). The formulation typically contains vital nutrients such as dextrose (D-glucose), amino acid cocktails, electrolytes, vitamins, tracer elements, and usually emulsified lipids in a hypertonic solution that is added just before administration. When lipids are added, the term total parenteral nutrition (TPN) is applied. PN helps preserve lean body mass, supports immune functions, and reduces metabolic complications and oxidative stress in patients who are otherwise unable to consume and digest food by GI [1]. In the United States today, approximately 40,000 patients remain permanently dependent upon TPN and another 350,000 require transient PN for the treatment of or to prevent malnutrition [2]. Prior to the clinical use of PN, thousands of individuals developed severe malnutrition and while others starved when faced with GI failure.

2. History of parenteral nutrition development

The complexity of PN technique proved challenging and successful long-term administration was not performed until 1968, even though PN is now considered an essential clinical strategy in modern medicine [3]. Interestingly, NASA accelerated the field by attempting to formulate standardized elemental nutrition solutions during the Mercury space program. For almost 400 years prior, clinicians attempted to administer numerous solutions intravenously, including salt water, milk, and wine, with limited success [4]. The first successful use of PN in humans was performed by *Dudrick and Wilmore* when they intravenously supported an infant with PN for 6 weeks [3]. This development led to the rapid use of PN in clinical settings. Early on, PN was administered prophylactically to many patients in pre- and post-surgical settings regardless of their nutrition status. In today's practice, patients are first assessed for whether the risks outweigh the benefits of either short-term or long-term PN feeding. The decision to use PN has become more selective because long-term PN confers certain clinical risks related to vascular access, inflammatory bowel disease, catheter site infections, improper brain development (in neonatal settings), and other metabolic complications such as hepatic steatosis and cholestasis related to the continuous hypertonic glucose solution entering circulation compared with intermittent enteral feeding. When PN is used in otherwise healthy and well-nourished patients, these individuals are exposed to these risks without room for significant nutritional benefit [5–8].

Several clinical trials supported the shift to reserving PN for those with GI failure or malnutrition. In one trial, 400 general surgery patients were preoperatively randomized to receive either PN alongside *ad lib* oral feeding or *ad lib* oral intake alone [9]. The results demonstrated that PN elevated the risk of major infections and did not reduce non-infectious complications between treatment groups. However, further analysis demonstrated that subjects with existing malnutrition in the cohort did benefit from PN by exhibiting improved wound healing compared with the control group [9]. These results showed that PN provides the greatest benefit in malnourished patients, and that nutritionally replete patients could be exposed to harm from PN complications with minimal benefit. Clinicians are still faced with challenges, since definitions of nutrient status and malnutrition vary across the life span, clinical settings, and between disease states, making exact categorization of patient nutritional status and risk-benefit balance difficult [10]. With these challenges in mind, PN is generally targeted to surgery patients with existing malnutrition or individuals who are not expected to feed enterally for 7–10 days, since loss of lean muscle begins within 2 weeks following lack of enteral intake.

In addition to general surgery settings, another common setting of nutritional deficiency occurs in patients with hypermetabolic states following acute infection or those with traumatic injuries where rapid proliferation of immune and organ cells is required [1]. The average human typically maintains 1200 kcals in hepatic glycogen storage, before lean muscle mass and peripheral fat are utilized to support

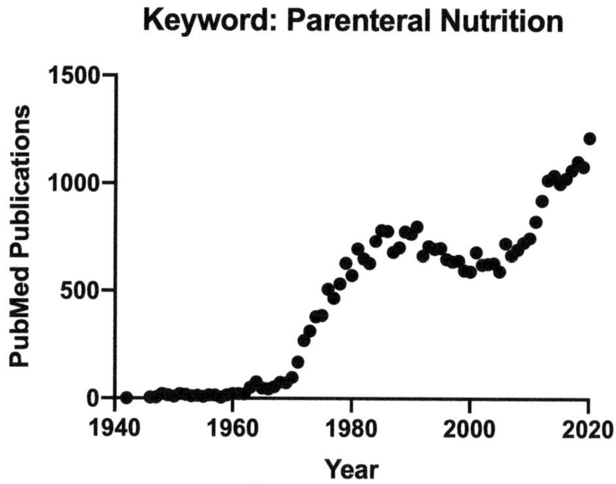

Figure 1.
The rise in parenteral nutrition biomedical research publications determined by pubmed keywords used between 1940 and 2020.

energy requirements [11]. Under acute infectious or injurious challenge, enhanced immune activation, increased oxygen consumption, and elevated muscle catabolism rapidly results in negative nitrogen balances. Even patients with no existing nutritional deficiencies may require PN when their energy needs are increased beyond their stored nutrient capacity. These settings also present challenges to the clinician, as it is established that a greater degree of injury leads to a higher risk of malnutrition [12, 13].

It is now accepted that enteral nutrition with a functional GI tract is the preferred route of nutrition in stable patients who can feed or tolerate feeding of either normal diet or standardized formula. Enteral nutrition is not without challenges, especially in patients where obtaining enteral access is difficult and the intestine requires time to adapt to calories. Specific to the latter case, enteral feeding also increases the risk of diarrhea, gut distention and upset. When tolerated, enteral nutrition leads to better clinical outcomes, including decreased risk of intra-abdominal abscess and respiratory infection, total length of stay, medical costs, and mortality [5, 9, 13–19]. PN remains essential for patients who cannot feed enterally, but these risks must always be considered. This chapter will discuss how PN impacts the gut immune system and microbiome, gut-liver axis, gut-brain axis, and future opportunities in PN research (**Figure 1**).

3. Models used to study parenteral nutrition

Animal have become a valuable preclinical model for nutritional studies. This includes mice, rats, rabbits, guinea pigs, dogs, and pigs [20–22]. As with all models, some species are considered to be more physiologically relevant to humans, and hence better models for understanding mechanistic pathways influenced by PN in pediatric and adult patients.

Rodents (mice and rats) have many similarities to humans including stages of development, anatomical features, immune responses, and associated physiology. Mice share many common genes, many of which can be knocked out or modified, as well as similar metabolic pathways compared with humans. Rodents are also cost effective and easily manipulated in a controlled environment, with a relatively short gestational period (19–22 days). These animals also offer a valuable tool for easy genetic/transgenic manipulation. These practical considerations make rodents suitable for many studies. One important difference to note is that the poorly developed guts and brains of pups at birth mature gradually during the early lactational period before weaning, whereas human infants show mature guts at full gestational birth. This feature of mice pups offers a great model to compare rodent guts with the guts of premature human infants. This allows the modeling of PN under the premature setting following a short time protocol [23]. Neonatal dogs are also used to determine the effect of enteral and parenteral feeding on GI growth and maturation because of immature intestines at birth relative to mature newborn human intestines [24–26].

Rabbit models have been used to characterize the nutritional value of different combinations to determine the effect of different TPN components on hepatic cholestasis and bacterial translocation. This includes characterization of nutrition supplements using different solutions such as carbohydrate-based solution, lipid-based solution, enriched amino acid-based solution, and protein deficient solution on newly born rabbits. Rabbits with protein deficient calories developed cholestasis after 7 days of administration [27]. Additionally, newborn rabbits provided with protein deficient solution had increased bacterial translocation [28]. Guinea pigs have been used to study multivitamin mixed lipid emulsion vs. amino-acid and dextrose based mixed solution [29]. Additionally, guinea pigs have been used to study the effect of light exposure on multivitamin mixed lipid emulsion which generates peroxide free radicals and induces oxidative stress in the lung [30].

Extensive research has demonstrated that premature neonatal piglets are a preferred model over rodents to study long term PN related chronic and acute effects on organ size and developmental outcome. This includes effects on tissue components such as immune cells, hepatocytes, neurons, and other metabolic tissues. In particular, the neonatal pig, unlike rodents, rabbits, guinea pigs, and dogs, has been shown to be highly homologous with the human neonate regarding the function of numerous organ systems, especially the liver and the gastrointestinal tract, several aspects of metabolism, and stages of development [22, 31]. Although the piglet has a slightly immature digestive system and shorter gestational length (~115 days) compared with humans, it offers a very good animal model to study the effect of enteral/parenteral nutrition in early life on postnatal growth and development [20]. In early postnatal days, the rapid intestinal growth, adaptation to food, bacterial colonization and improved nutrient absorption provides an elegant model to study PN related issues in premature children. Newborn piglets have been used to study gut maturation and functional changes in preterm piglets (107 day of gestation) and full-term piglets (115 day of gestation) because they are physiologically similar to human preterm infants [20, 22, 31]. Further, preterm neonatal piglets are a well-established model to study PN associated PNALD including hepatic cholestasis and brain related disorders [32, 33]. In late postnatal days, the growth of the intestine is gradual, reflecting the transition from milk-feeding to solid-food feeding. This may provide a model for TPN in immature children/neonates and adults. The piglet model is also favored over other model organisms because of body size, which allows for extensive surgical manipulation.

4. Importance of enteral feeding

In the 1970s and 1980s, early researchers focused on sepsis found that enterally-fed, well-nourished animals had a 70% survival rate, whereas animals given PN had only a 10% survival rate, regardless of whether they were malnourished [34]. Initially this observation was hypothesized to occur from a lack of essential nutrients in the PN formulation. However, further experiments showed that animal survival improved when the same volume and composition of PN components were provided orally [35, 36]. This outcome demonstrated the importance of gut stimulation and homeostasis.

5. Overview of gastrointestinal innervation and immunity

The gastrointestinal (GI) tract has several vital functions, acting as not only a digestive organ but also as an important endocrine and immune organ. The GI tract handles the breakdown and acquisition of nutrients as well as influences peripheral nutrient handling. The GI tract is home to vital neurological networks, including both the autonomic nervous system (with sympathetic and parasympathetic fibers that communicate with the spinal cord and central nervous system (CNS) through the dorsal root ganglia) and the unique enteric nervous system (ENS) [37]. The ENS, unlike the autonomic nervous system, is autonomous from the CNS and is comprised of over 10^8 sensory, motor, and interneurons that release acetylcholine and neuropeptides [38]. In response to ingested nutrients and bulk, GRP triggers enteroendocrine cell hormone release that regulate intestinal motility, digestive enzyme release from the pancreas, bile acid and bicarbonate release, stimulation of splanchnic blood flow, and electrolyte balances, each of which shape the stability and composition of the gut microbial ecology [39].

Approximately, 70 and 80% of all active immune cells in the body are innervated by ENS fibers connected to the epithelial and immune cells that make up the gut's huge surface area of over 400 m^2 [40]. This immune function is the vital barrier between the host and its environment. The gut and other mucosal surfaces are tasked with defending against dietary, microbial, and environmental products through innate barriers, adaptive immunity, and stable microbial colonizers. Barriers include ranging from simple cellular layers, complex secreted products such as antimicrobial peptides and glycoproteins, specific and non-specific immunoglobulins (IgA), and maintenance of the gut microbiome [38]. During periods of both feeding and fasting, the defenses provided by ENS-innervated immune cells facilitate digestion, maintenance of immune response, and the prevention of pathogens from entering systemic circulation.

6. Changes in gastrointestinal immunity following PN

6.1 The gut-associated lymphoid tissues (GALT) following PN

The Gut-Associated Lymphoid Tissues (GALT), a compartment which contains an astonishing 70–80% of all active immune cells, consists of both innate and adaptive cells residing beneath the epithelium and sampling the intestinal lumen [41]. The GALT facilitates release of sIgA on mucosal surfaces throughout the body. sIgA serves as an opsonin that can bind pathogens either specifically or non-specifically [42]. sIgA can mediate tolerance leading to attenuated inflammatory responses and induction of Treg lymphocytes [43]. One of the major detrimental effects of PN is GALT atrophy which occurs quickly after cessation of enteral feeding, and is driven by changes in blood flow, decreased expression of leukocyte binding, and decreased cellularity throughout the splanchnic bed. Grossly, PN-induced gut atrophy is observed with decreased organ wet and smaller bowel circumference approaching declines of 10% [44].

In rodent models of PN, Peyer's patch lymphocyte numbers begin to decline within 1–2 days of PN, where 75% of total cells are lost by 3 days compared with controls [45]. While total cellularity decreases, the ratios of T to B-lymphocytes, CD4+ to CD8+ cells, and relative percentages of memory, activated, and naïve cells remain stable [46]. In normal Peyer's patch function, specialized microfold cells cover Peyer's patches and sample luminal antigen to present to dendritic cells and naïve αβ+ T and B-lymphocytes within underlying germinal centers [47]. The naïve cells are localized to the Peyer's patches via expression of the integrins L-selectin and to a lesser extent α4β7. The integrins interact with mucosal addressing cellular adhesion molecule-1 (MadCAM-1) [41]. Diapedesis of the naïve cells into the Peyer's patch is facilitated by the chemokines CXCL13, CCL19, and CCL21 [48].

PN alters MAdCAM-1 expression within the Peyer's patch tissues by altering two MAdCAM-1 regulatory networks, through the lymphotoxin β receptor (LTβR) and noncanonical NFkB signaling pathways [49]. In the LTβR pathway, lymphotoxin α and β on the surface of systemic lymphocytes bind LTβR within the GALT tissues, elevating MAdCAM-1 and Th2 cytokines including IL-4 [50]. Following PN, Peyer's patch and GALT expression of LTβR rapidly declines, leading to decreased MAdCAM-1 within 4 h [51]. Mechanistically, inhibition of LTβR alone with blocking antibodies significantly decreases MAdCAM-1 expression. Conversely, providing stimulation of the LTβR under PN feeding through anti-LTβR monoclonal antibodies increase Peyer's patch lymphocyte numbers and mucosal release of sIgA in the gut and respiratory tract [44].

The second MAdCAM-1 regulatory signaling pathway is noncanonical NFkB, which is regulated in-part through lymphoid receptors and LTβR signaling described above. The canonical (or classical) NFkB pathway is stimulated in infectious and injurious insults, driving inflammatory tissue responses. In contrast, noncanonical NFkB triggers nuclear P52/RelB dimer formation and subsequently elevation of MAdCAM-1. Animal studies providing PN have demonstrated that both the canonical and noncanonical NFkB pathways are reduced during PN feeding [52]. Experimental inhibition of LTβR signaling significantly decreases nuclear P52/RelB dimerization and leads to lower MAdCAM-1, CCL19, CCL20, and CCL25 expression, but blockade of LTβR does not affect canonical NFkB protein levels [51]. Experimental stimulation of LTβR with agonists during PN drives expression of MAdCAM-1, P52/RelB, and IL-10. On the other hand, blocking ligands administered to control animals result in less MadCAM-1, L-selectin, and α4β7 [51]. These studies highlight the changes that occur in gut signaling following PN with lack of enteral stimulation. Fortunately, providing enteral stimulation drives normalization of these parameters in experimental animals within 2 days [53].

Peyer's patches serve as important induction sites for gut immune responses, where cells subsequently enter the lymphatics and circulation before returning to mucosal effector sites throughout the body. During transit through these compartments, plasma cells are activated and return producing IgA [54]. Through the same anatomical transit, T helper lymphocytes subpopulations are stimulated, including Th1, Th2, Th17, Th22, and Treg [55]. Th2 lymphocytes generate IL-4, IL-5, IL-6, IL-9, IL-10, IL-13, and IL-25, which plasma cell IgA production by plasma cells. These cytokines also have important roles in driving epithelial machinery that is required to translocate IgA to the luminal surface, such as polymeric immunoglobulin receptor (pIgR) [56]. Enterocyte pIgR bonds with a dimeric for of IgA where endocytosis moves the complex to the luminal surface before releasing secretory IgA (sIgA). The ratios of cytokines expressed in the lamina propria balance the release of sIgA production and release. For instance, IL-10, IL-17, and TGF-β drives plasma cell IgA production and pIgR expression, while IL-2, IFN-γ, and TNFα decrease pIgR expression [57, 58]. Of these cytokines, TGF-β appears to be critical, as mutant animals lacking TGF-β fail to present sIgA at mucosal surfaces, perhaps in part due to the need for this cytokine in plasma cell maturation [59].

By reducing the expression of α4β7, the integrin that binds MadCAM-1to help localize lymphocytes to the lamina propria, PN functionally results in reduced systemic lymphocytes dedicated for mucosal defense (CD4+CD25+) as well as resident lymphocytes in GALT tissues [46]. Furthermore, the activated lymphocyte population has a reduced capacity for tolerance or memory of self-antigens, as evidenced by reduced expression of Treg (CD4+CD25+Foxp3+) and memory (CD44+). The reduction in Treg cells also results in less TGFβ and IL-10 are produced, which usually support plasma cell function by counteracting the pro-inflammatory Th1 cytokine IFN-γ. PN decreases GALT IL-4 and IL-10 levels [45].

PN alters Th1:Th2 ratios by reducing the production of Th2 but not Th1 cytokines. Implications are increased neutrophil recruitment through ICAM-1 expression due to loss of IL-4 and IL-10 with stable IFN levels [60, 61]. Following PN, elevates neutrophils are observed in multiple organs, which may result in greater injury following hemorrhagic shock, ischemia, and sepsis. Experimental injury demonstrates that the percentage of activated neutrophils is significantly higher following PN, functionally resulting in greater mortality (50%) than enterally fed controls (5%).

Mucosal IgA responses are specific and vital, as has been shown in IgA mucosal vaccination studies for poliovirus and enterotoxigenic *Escherichia coli*, where specific sIgA appears at all body surfaces following mucosal exposure [62, 63].

Viral and bacterial challenges in rodent models have shown that functionally, PN leads to lower IgA-mediated immunity for antigen recognition and elimination of pathogens. Immunizing mice against *Pseudomonas (Ps) aeruginosa* leads to 90% survival when exposed to an intra-tracheal challenge compared with only 10% survival in control animals [64]. Given the dramatic effect of PN on adaptive immune responses, immunized animals provided PN survive intra-tracheal Ps at the rate of unimmunized animals. Similar results were obtained with influenza shedding studies, illustrating the loss of adaptive immunity to specific pathogens in the absence of gut feeding [65]. These findings draw a larger working schematic that PN feeding, without enteral intake, functionally alters the GALT compartment into a state that is far less protective. Unfortunately, these adaptive immune changes occur in parallel with increased pro-inflammatory neutrophil infiltrates that make any subsequent injury or infection more severe.

7. Changes in gut barrier defense following PN

The epithelial barrier of the intestine, which turns over rapidly due to highly proliferative pluripotent Lgr5+ stem cells in the intestinal crypts, serve as the first line of defense against the external environment of the gut. The epithelium turns over every 3–5 days [66]. One cell type that does not turn over rapidly are small intestinal Paneth cells, that turn over every 20–30 days. The selective barrier allows absorption of water, electrolytes, and some macromolecules via tight-junction proteins, including zonulins, occludins, and claudins between enterocytes. Epithelial permeability increases significantly during PN feeding [67, 68], in parallel with a loss of tight-junction proteins [69]. In addition to the physical barrier along the gut lining, subepithelial dendritic cells extend dendrites between epithelial cells, which are hypothesized to sample luminal antigens and augment barrier responses [70]. A smaller proportion (10%) of intestinal cells secretory cells, including enteroendocrine cells and mucous secreting goblet cells [47].

The epithelium's contribution to defense includes not only physical barrier formation, but release of antimicrobial molecules that influence microbial community composition and membership. Enterocytes comprise 90% of total epithelial cells in the gut and release β-defensins and RegIIIγ enzymes that limit microbial growth at the mucous barrier [71]. The far less abundant Paneth cells, found at the crypt bases, produce a large array of antimicrobial peptides and enzymes, including lysozyme, RegIIIγ, secretory PLA_2, Angiogenin4, and α-defensins (murine cryptdins) [72]. These cationic antimicrobials localize to the negatively-charged mucous surface and work by targeting conserved aspects of microbial cell walls and membranes [67]. Studies demonstrate Paneth cell antimicrobial molecules reach 15–100 mg/mL within intestinal crypts, exceeding antimicrobial concentrations [73]. The colon exhibits two layers of mucous, an inner sterile layer and an outer more loosely colonized layer.

Paneth cell antimicrobial release is regulated by Th2 cytokines, including IL-4, IL-9, and IL-13, GLP-2, and insulin [37, 74, 75]. Stimulatory triggers include the ligands TLRs and NOD2 and parasympathetic cholinergic stimulation [76]. PN decreases antimicrobial production through lower levels of intestinal IL-4 and IL-13 [77, 78]. Enterocyte release of RegIIIγ is also lost during PN [79]. Exogenous administration of IL-25 stimulates production of IL-4 and IL-13 cytokines and levels of Lysozyme, $sPLA_2$, and RegIIIγ compared with PN feeding alone [80]. Following PN, mucosal secretions contain less Paneth cell antimicrobial products, leading to decreased killing of bacteria in vitro [76]. Tissue explants from PN fed animals have been demonstrated to be more susceptible to enteroinvasive *E. coli* compared with controls [81].

The function of goblet cells is to produce the mucous barrier, composed of glycoprotein mucins. These proteins have numerous carbohydrate residues including *O*-glycosylation, *N*-actyl-galactosamine, galactose, and *N*-actyl-glucosamines [82]. Functionally, mucins mucous serves as a selective physical barrier that allows for movement of luminal digesta, absorption of nutrients, and limiting bacterial access to the gut wall. Mucins also help concentrate Paneth cell antimicrobial molecules and sIgA through charge interactions [83]. The importance of mucins is demonstrated by in mutant animals lacking the more abundant mucin, MUC2, which leads to inflammatory enteritis and increased risk of tumor formation [45].

PN decreases the release of MUC2, RELMβ, and trefoil factor 3 (TFF3) in neonatal piglets and adult mice [75, 84]. TFF3 promotes epithelial response to injury. Animals deficient in RELMβ display increased susceptibility to *Citrobacter rodentium* challenge. The release of goblet cell products are influenced by Th2 cytokines, including IL-4 and IL-13, which are decreased under PN feeding [85]. Exogenous administration of the Th2 stimulating cytokine, IL-25, elevates luminal MUC2 levels [77].

Although only 1% of the total intestinal epithelial cells are enteroendocrine cells (EECs), they collectively make up the largest endocrine organ, expressing almost 2 dozen peptide hormones that shape metabolism, immunity, and behavior [86, 87]. EECs respond to enteral nutrients as well as microbial ligands [88]. EECs are also intricately linked to innate immunity, indirectly activating and recruiting immune cells by producing the chemokines CXCL-1, CXCL-3, and the cytokine IL-32. EEC hormones can also influence epithelial cell function in the gut, including Paneth cell release of antimicrobial molecules. GLP-2 mutant animals are at increased susceptibility to gut infection than wild-type littermates [37].

8. Changes in the gut microbiome under PN

The microbial communities within the gut contain vast numbers of microorganisms from the domains of bacteria, archeae, yeasts and fungi, protists, and virus. The number of individual microbial cells rivals that of the human host and contains upwards of 150 fold the genetic content of the mammalian host [89]. The bacterial population, which accounts for >99% of all microbial DNA, contains trillions of organisms from numerous phyla, including *Firmicutes*, *Bacteroidetes*, and *Actinobacteria*. The basic role of the microbes in digestion is to breakdown nutrients and to synthesize novel compounds—including short chain fatty acids (SCFAs) and vitamins, including vitamin K and numerous B vitamins. Intestinal colonizers play complex roles in gut colonization and community establishment, creating barriers to intruding pathobionts and serve the host through modification of secreted molecules, including bile acids, and consumption of secreted glycoproteins. *O*-glycosylated mucin glycoproteins secreted by the host serve both as nutrients for the microorganisms and as a substrate for colonization by *Akkermansia muciniphila*, *Bacteroides thetaiotaomicron*, and *Bacteroides fragilis* [89].

PN challenges the host with a unique set of circumstances. On one hand, elemental nutrients are plentiful in the bloodstream, yet the physiology required for host adaptation are bypassed. From a gastrointestinal standpoint, lack of central intake only occurs during hibernation and prolonged fasting or starvation. These circumstances are associated with catabolism. However, the goal of PN is to prevent catabolism and drive stable metabolic homeostasis or anabolism. Given the close interdependence of the gut microbiome and diet, it is unsurprising that the primary driver of microbial community structure is host nutrition [90]. Resident got colonizers are adapted to metabolize the breakdown of indigestible fiber and play important roles in coordinating host responses to dietary intake, influencing incretins, bile acid pools, and gut enterohormones [91]. Some of these hormones have direct effects on the pancreatic islet and acinar cells (GLP-1, secretin), liver homeostasis (FGF15/19), and gall bladder (CCK).

Given that *Firmicutes* are efficient degraders of dietary carbohydrate, this phylum is decreased under PN while increased relative abundance of *Proteobacteria* are frequently observed [92]. *Proteobacteria* can digest alternate food sources, such as amino acids and various host secretions, making them more resilient in a fasted or starved state. Prior work showed that elemental nutrients from PN enter the gut lumen in low abundance through the use of tracers and that these nutrients are utilized by resident *Enterobacteriaceae* [93]. Since PN reaches the lumen, it is perhaps unsurprising that dirurnal variations in host metabolism may also influence gut community structure, even in the absence of dietary intake. Leone et al. demonstrated that the intestinal microbiome oscillates in composition over 24-h circadian rhythms, regardless of whether the host is enterally fed or PN [79]. This finding further illustrates the role of the diet, host, and combined metabolites in shaping and selecting for gut microbial community members.

In the absence of enteral feeding, pathogens may proliferate in the setting of PN due to decreased commensal nutrition that would usually lead to an ecology capable of outcompeting with them. Under PN feeding *Proteobacteria* blooms include many pathogens such as *E. coli*, *Salmonella*, *Yersinia*, *Helicobacter*, and *Vibrio* [92, 94]. In addition to providing competitive exclusion, other beneficial bacteria, including *Bacteroides fragilis*, are decreased. The presence of *B. fragilis* can support sIgA release [95]. The problematic changes in gut microbiome communities occur in concert with a loss of gut barrier, innate, and adaptive immune responses which can render the gut susceptible to a source of infection. Fecal microbiome transplantation (FMT) have demonstrated PN microbiome communities alone can decrease gut inflammation and decrease tight junction protein expression when placed into enterally fed previously germ-free animals [93].

In addition to bacteria, PN also reduces resistance to fungal pathogens, such as *Candida albicans* [96]. While *C. albicans* is found in healthy humans, it can become virulent in the gut and oral cavity, eventually entering systemic circulation, and causing disease. Experimental inoculation of *C. albicans* during PN results in increased gut translocation systemic infection of *C. albicans* compared with control animals [97]. As with bacteria, it is likely that changes in innate and adaptive immune arms underscore the increased susceptibility to otherwise harmless gut microbes [40, 98].

9. Changes in liver function during PN

PN is a valuable clinical method supporting complete nutrition in the case of intestinal failure. However, PN can lead to serious metabolic complications including gut atrophy and dysfunction and hepatic abnormalities. Liver dysfunction is common in infant and adult patients receiving PN for both short- and long-term. Prolonged PN feeding can lead to PN associated liver disease (PNALD), fibrosis, steatosis, and eventually liver failure [99, 100].

Depending on the patient's age and duration of the PN administration, PNALD can be classified into three types: hepatic steatosis, cholestasis and gallbladder sludge [101, 102]. PN associated steatosis is mostly seen in adult patients with higher caloric intake from carbohydrates such as dextrose or carbohydrate-nitrogen imbalance with elevated triglyceride synthesis in the liver. PN associated cholestasis is more common among premature newborns (40–60%) and infants receiving short-term and long-term PN than adults. PN associated cholestasis was first reported in premature infants receiving TPN. Cholestasis occurs when bile flow is impaired with an elevation in bilirubin level > 2 mg/dL. Other hepatic enzymes including alkaline phosphatase (ALP) and gamma glutamyl aminotransferase (GGT) involved in the synthesis and secretion of bile are also impaired. This occurs within 1–5 weeks of PN administration [103]. Gallbladder sludge is seen in both adults and children and develops due to bile storage in the bladder for an extended period. Biliary sludge develops in patients having PN between 3 and 6 weeks [104].

Several risk factors have been shown to contribute to the development of PNALD including poor nutrition with inappropriate ratio of dextrose, lipid, and amino acid, premature birth, duration of PN, bacterial/fungal infection and short bowel syndrome. Evidence from the literature suggests that PN associated liver dysfunction can be improved by avoiding excess calories and maintaining dextrose/lipid/amino acid balance. This will promote fatty acid oxidation, avoiding hyperinsulinemia in the liver and reducing the risk for the development of PN associated fatty liver disease [105].

Another key factor for the prevention or reversal of PNALD includes either fish oil-based lipid emulsion or lipid emulsion infusion of fish oil, soybean oil and olive oil mixture rather than a soybean oil-based formulation. Pro-inflammatory ω-6 fatty acids having a high amount of phytosterols in soybean oil promotes the proliferation of Kupffer cells and development of PNALD by impairing bile secretion and activating excessive secretion of pro-inflammatory cytokines such as TNF-α, IL-6, IL-1β, IFN-γ, and reactive oxygen species (ROS) [106]. Soybean oil derived lipid component phytosterols alter the intestinal microbial composition including the overgrowth of specific bacterial components associated with PNALD [7]. Farnesoid X receptor (FXR) is known to inhibit bacterial overgrowth and induce the expression of genes involved in the protection of gut [107]. Soybean-derived phytosterols are FXR agonists. TPN studies in piglet and mouse models have suggested that alteration in the bile acid mediated FXR-FGF19 axis may lead to the pathophysiology of PNALD [108, 109].

Alternatively, fish oil-based lipid emulsion or lipid emulsion of fish oil, olive oil and soybean oil mixture can reverse the development of PNALD. Anti-inflammatory ω-3 polyunsaturated fatty acids (PUFA) in fish oil, which have a high amount of omegaven and a low amount of phytosterols, can reduce the development of PNALD by suppressing the cytokine TNF-α [103, 110–114]. Additionally, a study from Harris, JK et al., shows that parenteral nutrition associated liver injury (PNALI) mice receiving fish oil derived lipid emulsion with a high amount of Omegaven harbor a specific composition of fecal microbiota. Specifically, there is a reduction in *Erysipelotrichaceae,* which appears to prevent the activation of Kupffer cells and subsequent PNALD as compared to soybean oil based lipid emulsions [32, 106]. Further, piglet studies have shown that replacing soybean oil based PN with fish oil based PN in neonatal piglets results in lower bilirubin, alanine transferase (ALT), aspartate transferase (AST) and improved PNALD [115, 116].

As mentioned, bacterial overgrowth and bacterial translocation is another potential cause of PNALD, which can be augmented with antibiotics such as metronidazole. Metronidazole administration in a rat model showed reduced fat accumulation with lower alkaline phosphatase (ALP), aspartate aminotransferase (AAT), and gamma glutamyl transpeptidase in the metronidazole treated group relative to the control group receiving PN [117, 118]. Further glutamine supplementation, an essential energy source for the gut, prevented liver steatosis in a PN rat model [119]. Considering the importance of a healthy gut microbiome in early life on immune development and metabolic growth, it remains unclear what the implications of antibiotic administration in neonates have on long-term growth and development.

10. Challenges in supporting healthy neonatal growth during PN

The ultimate goal of NICU physicians is to support optimal infant growth and maturation until the child is stable for discharge. This goal is complicated by increased metabolic needs in infants who commonly have infectious stresses and underdeveloped GI and immune organs function. Preterm infants do not require the same nutrition intake as weight-matched term infants; they often require greater caloric intake due to weight loss after birth and high metabolic rates [120]. Despite the years of research and clinical trial and error that have gone into creating the PN formulas used in NICUs today, several developmental delays are still noted in neonates during PN. Among these are neurodevelopmental delays, which have been widely observed, but the underlying mechanisms remain poorly characterized [121]. There are also delays in development of the immune system and the closely related enteric nervous system in the intestine. PN infants also show slowing of intestinal and hepatic development.

Developmental outcomes for preterm infants have mostly only been studied during the NICU stay. What is less clear is the longer-term effects of neonatal growth delay. Several studies have examined the effects of too little growth and/or the deficiency of certain nutrients during infancy on height, BMI z-scores, and other developmental factors measured later in life. In a cohort study of preterm infants receiving either standard or energy-enhanced PN (meaning an increased calorie:protein ratio), no significant difference in growth was found at 24 months of life. Both types of PN did, however, cause PN-related complications in 98% of patients [122]. Other studies have shown little or no significant difference in the effects of different protein or fat compositions of neonatal formula on height or BMI after 1 year of age [123]. It has, however, been found that breast feeding reproducibly leads to a higher IQ in childhood compared to formula feeding, and by extension PN. As discussed in Section 12, supplementation of PN with DHA may help alleviate some detriments of neurological development [123].

Though most of the focus is on supporting adequate growth in the neonate, some researchers have questioned the effect of overcompensation and accelerated growth on later life. It has been observed that overly accelerated growth in infants may lead to increased incidence of obesity and other related diseases later in life. This appears to be true whether the infants are term or premature [124]. These long-term effects are thought to occur through "nutritional programming"; that is, the nutrients received in certain key developmental periods can lastingly alter endocrine function, immune function, and other health indices via epigenetic responses to early life nutrients [123]. A cohort study in the UK identified several risk factors in children who were obese at 7 years of age. In that study, neonatal "catch up" growth was identified as an independent risk factor for obesity. However, large birth weight was also an independent risk factor, suggesting a trade-off between these two variables [125]. The clinical goal is to strike a balance between providing enough nutrition to prevent neurodevelopmental delays and prevent hyperalimentation associated with long term obesity risk. It is also important to note that most of these studies have focused on accelerated growth with enteral feeding (either breast milk or formula), so little is known about the compound effects of over-accelerated growth on PN.

11. Changes in brain development during PN

Preterm infants on PN long-term are at high risk of having compromised brain development and delayed cognitive skills. Neurodevelopmental delays and defects are commonly seen among 40–50% of preterm infants [121]. Preterm babies born during late second and third trimesters (30 weeks) with extremely low body weight < 1 kg with poorly developed GI tracts show delayed brain development and maturation. These preterm babies rely on PN for proper growth and development. Magnetic resonance imaging (MRI) technology has shown that the total brain development including white and gray matter happens around 25–37 weeks of gestation with cerebellum enlargement [126–129]. PMID: 17151398 showed that using a preterm pig model with EN vs. PN, preterm pigs on PN for 10 days had neurodevelopment delays, smaller brains, immature myelination patterns and compromised motor skills compared to those on EN [8]. In addition, PN pigs had smaller cerebellums with slower locomotion than EN pigs regardless of similar body weight. These results suggest that maintaining preterm infants on PN long-term may be detrimental for optimal brain development [8].

The effect of soybean derived fat components of PN and their association with fatty liver disease was discussed in an earlier section. Here, we discuss the effect of soybean derived oil on the brain in PN patients. Neurodevelopmental disorders among PN infants occurs due to the effects of soybean oil derived PN and its association with the gut microbiome, and the development of gut microbiome-brain axis [130].

This raises the prudence of replacing soybean oil derived lipid emulsions with fish oil derived lipid emulsions for protection against PNALD and to ensure support of optimal brain growth and development. It has also been shown that dietary ω-3 fatty acid docosahexaenoic acid (DHA) and arachidonic acid in fish oil modulate brain development in piglets [131–133]. To date, there are no specific clinical models established to study PN associated neurodevelopmental disorders in preterm infants and children. Therefore, further studies are needed to identify the cause of PN associated neurodevelopmental disorders.

12. Metabolite supplements for restoring homeostasis during PN

PN is required in patients with progressive malnutrition, which is exacerbated by infectious and injurious challenge, leading to hypermetabolism. A major goal of recent research has been to find combinations of PN additives that will reduce the detrimental impact on the gut's immune and metabolic functions, as well as on the mucous composition in the intestinal and respiratory tract. Immune enhancing nutrition formulations include the addition of glutamine, arginine, cysteine, tyrosine, leucine, choline, ω-3 fatty acids, nucleotides, and micronutrients (vitamin C, selenium, and tracer elements including iron and zinc). Glutamine has been studied most extensively as the most prominent free amino acid that supports normal metabolism but becomes limited during gut atrophy and critical illness [134]. Recent reviews have concentrated on the effects of these additives in basic and clinical work [135]. Outside of macronutrients classes, targets that stimulate aspects of immune and neuronal signaling have promise in mediating elevated immune and barrier response when PN is necessary.

12.1 Enteric nervous system molecules

Outside of the central nervous system, the enteric nervous system contains an enormous number of autonomous neurons and glial cells that coordinate the physiological functions of digestion, gut immune homeostasis, and diverse numbers of epithelial functions. Among the targets of ENS neuropeptides, including gastrin-releasing peptide (GRP), substance P, and VIP, are GALT immune cells. During normal feeding, ENS fibers release GRP, stimulating a cascade of digestion and immune cell responses [136]. Analogues for GRP, including bombesin (BBS), have been used to efficiently stimulate the GRP receptor and mimic gut feeding responses. Administration of BBS to mice on PN significantly elevates intestinal blood flow, Peyer's patch lymphocytes [46], activated and memory lymphocytes in the lamina propria, and elevated pIgR and luminal IgA [137–139]. BBS also drives increased expression of Paneth cell antimicrobial enzymes. Functionally these changes following BBS results in increased resistance to infectious organisms, including respiratory H1N1 and *Pseudomonas* [140], and intestinal enteroinvasive *E. coli* [141], compared with PN alone. Outside of the immune compartment, BBS stimulates GI motility and pancreatic secretions during PN that are otherwise attenuated [142].

In summary, providing rodents with exogenous neuropeptides, for example BBS, can compensate for the loss of normal enteral nutrient stimulation that drives gut physiological and immunological responses. Artificial stimulation of these gut functions may hold promise in patients where prolonged periods of PN are needed and patients may otherwise be at increased risk of mucosal immune atrophy and infectious microorganisms.

12.2 AHR molecules

Given the loss of microbial community structure and function in the absence of enteral feeding, disturbances in the gut microbiota occur rapidly following PN. One such change is the loss of microbial Aryl hydrocarbon receptor (Ahr) ligands production that normally stimulate IL-22 production. IL-22 generates epithelail barrier responses, including antimicrobial molecule production [143]. Ahr deficient animals are at increased susceptibility to infectious challenge, including *Citrobacter rodentium*. Prior work demonstrates that microbial Ahr production elevates bone marrow B cell maturation [144, 145].

12.3 SCFAs

Short chain fatty acids (SCFAs) Are generated by microbial fermentation of dietary carbohydrates. SCFAs phase can reach 130 mmol/kg in the distal gut where they stimulate the receptors, GRP41, GPR42, and GPR109a, shaping immune responses and modifying the release of enteroendocrine hormones. Exogenous administration of SCFAs stimulates the number of IgA+ producing plasma cells in the gut and elevates circulating immunoglobulins [146]. Functionally, the importance of these metabolites in immune stimulation have been demonstrated through experimental studies administering SCFA to mice during infection with *Citrobacter rodentium*, and enhanced IgA levels and pathogen clearance was observed. In addition to driving antibodies at mucosal surfaces, SCFAs mitigate pro-inflammatory responses and stimulate tolerance by inducing Treg cells [147]. Isolated plasma cells enhance production of IgG and IgA when exposed to SCFAs, demonstrating the direct effect of these metabolites on immune function [146]. At the mucosal barrier, through GRP receptors, SCFAs stimulate goblet cell mucin gene expression and improve tight junction protein expression [148, 149]. Dietary SCFAs administration improves diet induced metabolic complications including liver dysfunction via the G-protein coupled receptor FFAR3 and prevents *de-novo* lipogenesis in mice [150, 151]. SCFAs modulate gut microbiome-brain communication by crossing the blood-brain barrier and regulating signaling pathways involved in central nervous system (CNS) production of neurotransmitters such as dopamine and serotonin [152]. SCFAs alleviate blood-brain barrier permeability and microglia maturation and function [153]. Also, dietary administration of SCFAs increases serum plasma of GLP-1 and protects mice from diet-induced obesity [154].

12.4 Polyamines

Polyamines are a unique class of polycationic metabolites produced by many lifeforms. Diets lacking polyamines lead to slowing of intestinal development and atrophy of the mucosa [155]. By enhancing expression of occludin and E-cadherin, polyamines improve epithelial tight-junction function in addition to improving mucous glycoprotein release [156, 157]. Polyamines are also demonstrated to drive IgA levels and increase lamina propria CD4+ T cells [158, 159]. Considering the importance of these molecules in normal gut homeostasis, this class of molecules represents one area of innovation for researchers investigating PN additives for improved outcomes.

12.5 Bile acid agonists (INT-777, INT-747): supporting liver function and gut epithelial signaling

Bile acids play a crucial role in maintaining lipid and glucose metabolism via G-protein coupled receptor (TGR5) and farnesoid X receptor (FXR) signaling. FXR regulates key pathways involved in metabolism in the liver. Alteration in bile acid signaling reduces bile acid synthesis in the liver and leads to hepatic cholestasis and inflammation [160, 161]. Recent literature suggests that altered bile acid signaling increases insulin resistance and promotes hepatic gluconeogenesis [162, 163]. TGR5 activates the cAMP/PKA pathway to regulate lipid metabolism. INT-777 and INT-747, novel and selective agonists of TGR5 and FXR respectively, stimulate bile flow. INT-777/TGR5 activation inhibits nuclear translocation of NFkB and displays an anti-inflammatory effect by reducing the secretion of TNF-α, IL-6, IL-1β and IFN-γ. Bile acids activate FXR, which regulates the transcription of FGF19 and binds to FGFR4. FGFR4 blocks CYP7A1 and represses bile acid synthesis [164, 165].

Treatment using bile acid receptor agonists INT-777 (TGR5) and obeticholic acid/INT-747 (FXR) can attenuate hepatic steatosis and improve the overall metabolic profile induced by high fat diet (HFD). Animal models show that INT-747 and INT-777 supplementation promote fatty acid oxidation in the liver by regulating the expression of key genes (*acyl-CoA oxidase* and *carnitine palmitoyltransferase*) involved in fatty acid metabolism [166, 167].

12.6 Lipid formulations (soy vs fish oil lipid emulsions); enhancing brain growth, normalizing PNALD

For decades, intravenous soybean oil-based lipid formulations have been used extensively in PN patients in the United States. However, the use of soybean oil-based lipid emulsion may not be optimal for the safety and benefit of PN patients. While this is a great source of essential fatty acids, soybean oil based lipid contains a higher amount of proinflammatory ω-6 PUFA including oleic acid, linoleic acid (18:2), and phytosterols [168]. A high amount of linoleic acid in ω-6 fatty acid has inflammatory properties [169]. Plant based phytosterols inhibit bile flow, increase triglyceride storage, increase hepatic cholestasis, and increase neurological disorders [170, 171]. Phytosterols are thought to be toxic to hepatocytes, but if they are taken enterally, they are absorbed by GI tract.

Over the years, PN with a fish oil-based lipid emulsion or a mixture of fish, soybean, and olive oil derived lipid emulsions have been preferred. Recent literature supports the idea of considering the use of fish oil based lipids solely, or a mixture of fish, olive and soybean oil based lipid emulsions as an alternative as significant improvements have been observed using fish oil based composition. This especially applies to preterm babies with immature brains and pediatric patients with PNALD. Fish oil or mixed oil lipid emulsions have increased antioxidant properties because the triglycerides formed from each lipid emulsion differ based on the fatty acid content, such as long vs. short chain fatty acid chains (LCFAs vs. SCFAs) and unsaturated vs. saturated. Different length FAs have different biological properties and clinical outcomes. Fish oil based lipid emulsions contain a high concentration of anti-inflammatory ω-3 unsaturated fatty acids with small amounts of linoleic acid and higher amounts of Omegaven, docosahexaenoic acid (DHA) and eicosapentaenoic (EPA). These have been shown reduce oxidative stress and inflammation by blocking proinflammatory cytokines to prevent or reverse PNALD with cholestasis in neonates as well as in the setting of intestinal failure [172–174]. DHA and EPA are the major metabolites of ω-3 fatty acids highly enriched in fish oil. DHA plays an important role in reducing inflammation by suppressing inflammatory markers [110]. Additionally, DHA present in Omegaven modulates the liver X-receptor involved in bile regulation [175, 176]. Further, DHA and arachidonic acid present in fish-oil or mixed lipid modulate neuronal development and brain maturation in piglets and preterm infants [132, 133, 177]. Alternatively, olive oil-based lipid emulsions have been proven as another alternative because they have a low amount of ω-6 fatty acid which reduces oxidative stress with no major changes in liver enzymes [178].

13. Future directions in PN research

Although PN is highly effective in pediatric and adult patients, the pathophysiology of its association with PNALD and neurological disorders and the underlying mechanisms are not well understood and are of high priority in the clinical setting. Over the years, most of the research has emphasized understanding the maturation of the GI tract in PN patients. There are no specific safer therapies yet established for the prevention or treatment of multifactorial PNALD or brain abnormalities in PN patients. There are challenges to overcome in terms of the characterization and standardization of PN supplements for optimal nutrition to promote normal brain development trajectories and normal liver function. PN is essential but detrimental in preterm babies and infant patients on long term feeding, and they are at high risk for liver and brain abnormalities. Optimal nutrition with minimal side effects is highly important in early neonates for their developing brain and normal liver function. Several key questions need to be addressed including (1) the revision of PN components, (2) the characterization of current PN components, (3) the use of ω-3 fatty acid enriched fish-oil based lipid or mixed oil based lipid rather than soyabean oil based lipid, 4) the inclusion of essential short chain FA (SCFAs) and essential amino acids, and 5) the effects of specific dietary solutions in the rapidly developing brain in early life.

There is a need to consider cyclic PN (cPN) rather than continuous PN for long term in infants. Studies in neonates suggest that patients on cyclic (cPN) have delayed liver dysfunction compared to continuous PN [179]. Another study from Costadel Sol Hospital in Spain shows that patients ≥18 years had delayed hepatic abnormalities on cPN for 12–15 days compared to patients on continuous PN. The cPN patients showed significant reduction in hepatic enzymes such as Bilirubin, AST, ALT and GGT with no change in ALP [180]. However, the limitations of this study were the exclusion of patients having early liver abnormalities and sample size [180]. Future studies involving cPN instead of continuous PN administration will help in addressing early hepatic and brain related issues.

There is also the possibility for improvement of the route of PN, including partial enteral nutrition (EN) that may reduce the risk of developing PNALD. Given the limitations of current therapies, more research is needed for the optimization of current nutritional components and advancement in PN associated with neurological disorders and PNALD. The next key question in the field is to identify the driving factors and associated cellular and molecular mechanisms that modulate neurodevelopmental outcomes in the rapidly developing brain of preterm neonates and infants.

Another key factor to consider is how to maintain bacterial diversity (*Bacteriodities* vs. *Firmicuties*) and prevent unwanted bacterial overgrowth. Additionally, we need to focus on understanding the molecular mechanisms driving gut-brain maturation in pediatric patients on PN. In summary, there are several challenges remaining in clinical trials to optimize efficacy and safety of PN for patients.

14. Conclusions

The work that has been done in animal models to both characterize the molecular effects of PN on the body and to optimize PN additives has influenced the development of safer PN for patients. PN is essential and life-saving, so it is important that GI, immune, hepatic, and nervous system complications be minimized. Researchers have described the changes in intestinal cellularity, mucous composition, microbial population, innate immune function, enterohepatic circulation, and brain development induced by PN. Even though many patients requiring PN are critically ill and often malnourished making them predisposed to infection and underlying metabolic complications, a vast body of work demonstrates that route of feeding can dramatically alter the gut immune system, gut microbiome, metabolic handling, and organ function, which may contribute to the pathophysiology observed in PN settings. The elegant work demonstrating the mechanisms by through mucosal immune cell signaling is altered under PN show that these alterations are targetable. Several additives have been explored that show promise in restoring normal function in the absence of enteric stimulation. For example, immune-enhancing metabolites like glutamine are helpful in patients with hypermetabolism. A major area of investigation has been using exogenous ENS neuropeptides to stimulate normal GALT function. Elsewhere, bile acid agonists and the use of fish oil lipid emulsions have been shown to support normal gut-liver feedback and reduce the incidence of PNALD in PN patients. Explorations of administering microbial metabolites, such as bile acid analogues, SCFAs, and polyamines are promising areas of research that can be further deliniated using translational models of PN feeding in the laboratory setting.

Funding

NIH R01CA253329, NIH R21AI163503 (JFP).

Author details

Roshan Kumari[1], Lydia M. Henry[1] and Joseph F. Pierre[2*]

1 Department of Pediatrics-Neonatology, College of Medicine, University of Tennessee Health Science Center, Memphis, TN, United States

2 Department of Nutritional Sciences, University of Wisconsin-Madison, Madison, WI, USA

*Address all correspondence to: jpierre@wisc.edu

References

[1] Mizock BA. Immunonutrition and critical illness: An update. Nutrition. 2010;**26**(7-8):701-707. Available from: http://www.ncbi.nlm.nih.gov/pubmed/20381315

[2] Pfuntner A, Wier LM, Elixhauser A. Overview of Hospital Stays in the United States, 2011: Statistical Brief #166 [Internet]. Healthcare Cost and Utilization Project (HCUP) Statistical Briefs. US: Agency for Healthcare Research and Quality; 2006 [cited 2017 Jan 18]. Available from: http://www.ncbi.nlm.nih.gov/pubmed/24404630

[3] Dudrick SJ, Wilmore DW, Vars HM, Rhoads JE. Long-term total parenteral nutrition with growth, development, and positive nitrogen balance. Surgery. 1968;**64**(1):134-42. Available from: http://www.ncbi.nlm.nih.gov/pubmed/4968812

[4] Wretlind A, Szczygieł B. Total parenteral nutrition. History. Present time. Future. Polski Merkuriusz Lekarski. 1998;**4**(22):181-185. Available from: http://www.ncbi.nlm.nih.gov/pubmed/9770991

[5] Peter JV, Moran JL, Phillips-Hughes J. A metaanalysis of treatment outcomes of early enteral versus early parenteral nutrition in hospitalized patients. Critical Care Medicine. 2005;**33**(1):213-220; discussion 260-261. Available from: http://www.ncbi.nlm.nih.gov/pubmed/15644672

[6] Zhan L, Yang I, Kong B, Shen J, Gorczyca L, Memon N, et al. Dysregulation of bile acid homeostasis in parenteral nutrition mouse model. American Journal of Physiology. Gastrointestinal and Liver Physiology. 2016;**310**(2):G93-G102. Available from: http://www.ncbi.nlm.nih.gov/pubmed/26564717

[7] Cahova M, Bratova M, Wohl P. Parenteral nutrition-associated liver disease: The role of the gut microbiota. Nutrients. 2017;**9**(9):1-19. Available from: https://pubmed.ncbi.nlm.nih.gov/28880224/

[8] Choudhri AF, Sable HJ, Chizhikov VV, Buddington KK, Buddington RK. Parenteral nutrition compromises neurodevelopment of preterm pigs. The Journal of Nutrition. 2014;**144**(12):1920-1927. Available from: https://pubmed.ncbi.nlm.nih.gov/25342697/

[9] The Veterans Affairs Total Parenteral Nutrition Cooperative Study Group. Perioperative total parenteral nutrition in surgical patients. The New England Journal of Medicine. 1991;**325**(8):525-532. Available from: http://www.ncbi.nlm.nih.gov/pubmed/1906987

[10] Meijers JMM, van Bokhorst-de van der Schueren MAE, Schols JMGA, Soeters PB, Halfens RJG. Defining malnutrition: Mission or mission impossible? Nutrition. 2010;**26**(4):432-440. Available from: http://www.ncbi.nlm.nih.gov/pubmed/19954929

[11] Wernerman J, Hammarqvist F, Gamrin L, Essén P. Protein metabolism in critical illness. Baillière's Clinical Endocrinology and Metabolism. 1996;**10**(4):603-615. Available from: http://www.ncbi.nlm.nih.gov/pubmed/9022954

[12] Borlase BC, Moore EE, Moore FA. The abdominal trauma index--a critical reassessment and validation. The Journal of Trauma. 1990;**30**(11):1340-1344. Available from: http://www.ncbi.nlm.nih.gov/pubmed/2231802

[13] Moore FA, Moore EE, Jones TN, McCroskey BL, Peterson VM. TEN versus TPN following major abdominal trauma--reduced septic morbidity. The Journal of Trauma. 1989;**29**(7):916-922; discussion

922-923. Available from: http://www.ncbi.nlm.nih.gov/pubmed/2501509

[14] Moore EE, Jones TN. Benefits of immediate jejunostomy feeding after major abdominal trauma--a prospective, randomized study. The Journal of Trauma. 1986;**26**(10):874-881. Available from: http://www.ncbi.nlm.nih.gov/pubmed/3095557

[15] Moore FA, Feliciano D V, Andrassy RJ, McArdle AH, Booth F V, Morgenstein-Wagner TB, et al. Early enteral feeding, compared with parenteral, reduces postoperative septic complications. The results of a meta-analysis. Annals of Surgery. 1992;**216**(2):172-183. Available from: http://www.pubmedcentral.nih.gov/articlerender.fcgi?artid=1242589&tool=pmcentrez&rendertype=abstract

[16] Kondrup J, Rasmussen HH, Hamberg O, Stanga Z. Nutritional risk screening (NRS 2002): A new method based on an analysis of controlled clinical trials. Clinical Nutrition. 2003;**22**(3):321-336. Available from: http://www.ncbi.nlm.nih.gov/pubmed/12765673

[17] Sherrington A, Newham JJ, Bell R, Adamson A, McColl E, Araujo-Soares V. Systematic review and meta-analysis of internet-delivered interventions providing personalized feedback for weight loss in overweight and obese adults. Obesity Reviews. 2016;**17**(6):541-551. Available from: http://www.ncbi.nlm.nih.gov/pubmed/26948257

[18] Kudsk KA, Croce MA, Fabian TC, Minard G, Tolley EA, Poret HA, et al. Enteral versus parenteral feeding. Effects on septic morbidity after blunt and penetrating abdominal trauma. Annals of Surgery. 1992;**215**(5):503-511; discussion 511-513. Available from: http://www.pubmedcentral.nih.gov/articlerender.fcgi?artid=1242485&tool=pmcentrez&rendertype=abstract

[19] Marik PE, Zaloga GP. Meta-analysis of parenteral nutrition versus enteral nutrition in patients with acute pancreatitis. BMJ. 2004;**328**(7453):1407. Available from: http://www.bmj.com/content/328/7453/1407

[20] Puiman P, Stoll B. Animal models to study neonatal nutrition in humans. Current Opinion in Clinical Nutrition and Metabolic Care. 2008;**11**(5):601-606. Available from: https://pubmed.ncbi.nlm.nih.gov/18685456/

[21] Kudsk KA. Jonathan E Rhoads lecture: Of mice and men... and a few hundred rats. JPEN Journal of Parenteral and Enteral Nutrition. 2008;**32**(4):460-473. Available from: http://www.pubmedcentral.nih.gov/articlerender.fcgi?artid=2596714&tool=pmcentrez&rendertype=abstract

[22] Sangild PT, Thymann T, Schmidt M, Stoll B, Burrin DG, Buddington RK. Invited review: The preterm pig as a model in pediatric gastroenterology. Journal of Animal Science. 2013;**91**(10):4713-4729. Available from: https://pubmed.ncbi.nlm.nih.gov/23942716/

[23] Sangild PT. Gut responses to enteral nutrition in preterm infants and animals. Experimental Biology and Medicine (Maywood, N.J.). 2006;**231**(11):1695-1711. Available from: https://pubmed.ncbi.nlm.nih.gov/17138756/

[24] Owens L, Burrin DG, Berseth CL. Minimal enteral feeding induces maturation of intestinal motor function but not mucosal growth in neonatal dogs. The Journal of Nutrition. 2002;**132**(9):2717-2722. Available from: https://pubmed.ncbi.nlm.nih.gov/12221235/

[25] Lippert AC, Fulton Jr RB, Parr AM. A retrospective study of the use of total parenteral nutrition in dogs and cats. Journal of Veterinary Internal Medicine.

1993;**7**(2):52-64. Available from: https://pubmed.ncbi.nlm.nih.gov/8501697/

[26] Chandler ML, Guilford WG, Maxwell A, Barter L. A pilot study of protein sparing in healthy dogs using peripheral parenteral nutrition. Research in Veterinary Science. 2000;**69**(1):47-52. Available from: https://pubmed.ncbi.nlm.nih.gov/10924393/

[27] Hata S, Kamata S, Nezu R, Takagi Y, Okada A. A newborn rabbit model for total parenteral nutrition: Effects of nutritional components on cholestasis. JPEN Journal of Parenteral and Enteral Nutrition. 1989;**13**(3):265-271. Available from: https://pubmed.ncbi.nlm.nih.gov/2503636/

[28] Yamanouchi T, Suita S, Masumoto K. Non-protein energy overloading induces bacterial translocation during total parenteral nutrition in newborn rabbits. Nutrition. 1998;**14**(5):443-447. Available from: https://pubmed.ncbi.nlm.nih.gov/9614309/

[29] Chessex P, Friel J, Harison A, Rouleau T, Lavoie JC. The mode of delivery of parenteral multivitamins influences nutrient handling in an animal model of total parenteral nutrition. Clinical Nutrition. 2005;**24**(2):281-287. Available from: https://pubmed.ncbi.nlm.nih.gov/15784490/

[30] Lavoie J-C, Chessex P, Rouleau T, Tsopmo A, Friel J. Shielding parenteral multivitamins from light increases vitamin A and E concentration in lung of newborn guinea pigs. Clinical Nutrition. 2007;**26**(3):341-347. Available from: https://pubmed.ncbi.nlm.nih.gov/17306907/

[31] Sanglid PT, Petersen YM, Schmidt M, Elnif J, Petersen TK, Buddington RK, et al. Preterm birth affects the intestinal response to parenteral and enteral nutrition in newborn pigs. The Journal of Nutrition. 2002;**132**(9):3786-3794. Available from: https://pubmed.ncbi.nlm.nih.gov/12221228/

[32] Harris JK, El Kasmi KC, Anderson AL, Devereaux MW, Fillon SA, Robertson CE, et al. Specific microbiome changes in a mouse model of parenteral nutrition associated liver injury and intestinal inflammation. PLoS One. 2014;**9**(10):1. Available from: https://pubmed.ncbi.nlm.nih.gov/25329595/

[33] Bergström A, Kaalund SS, Skovgaard, Andersen AD, Pakkenberg B, Rosenørn A, et al. Limited effects of preterm birth and the first enteral nutrition on cerebellum morphology and gene expression in piglets. Physiological Reports. 2016;**4**(14):1. Available from: https://pubmed.ncbi.nlm.nih.gov/27462071/

[34] Petersen SR, Kudsk KA, Carpenter G, Sheldon GE. Malnutrition and immunocompetence: Increased mortality following an infectious challenge during hyperalimentation. The Journal of Trauma. 1981;**21**(7):528-533. Available from: http://www.ncbi.nlm.nih.gov/pubmed/6788958

[35] Kudsk KA, Carpenter G, Petersen S, Sheldon GF. Effect of enteral and parenteral feeding in malnourished rats with *E. coli*-hemoglobin adjuvant peritonitis. The Journal of Surgical Research. 1981;**31**(2):105-110. Available from: http://www.ncbi.nlm.nih.gov/pubmed/6790873

[36] Kudsk KA, Stone JM, Carpenter G, Sheldon GF. Enteral and parenteral feeding influences mortality after hemoglobin-*E. coli* peritonitis in normal rats. The Journal of Trauma. 1983;**23**(7):605-609. Available from: http://www.ncbi.nlm.nih.gov/pubmed/6410081

[37] Lee S-J, Lee J, Li KK, Holland D, Maughan H, Guttman DS, et al. Disruption of the murine Glp2r impairs Paneth cell function and increases susceptibility to small bowel enteritis. Endocrinology. 2012;**153**(3):1141-1151

[38] Ottaway CA. Neuroimmunomodulation in the intestinal mucosa. Gastroenterology Clinics of North America. 1991;**20**(3):511-529. Available from: http://www.ncbi.nlm.nih.gov/pubmed/1717380

[39] Debas HT, Mulvihill SJ. Neuroendocrine design of the gut. American Journal of Surgery. 1991;**161**(2):243-249. Available from: http://www.ncbi.nlm.nih.gov/pubmed/1671322

[40] Devkota S, Wang Y, Musch MW, Leone V, Fehlner-Peach H, Nadimpalli A, et al. Dietary-fat-induced taurocholic acid promotes pathobiont expansion and colitis in Il10-/- mice. Nature. 2012;**487**(7405):104-108

[41] Suzuki K, Kawamoto S, Maruya M, Fagarasan S. GALT: Organization and dynamics leading to IgA synthesis. Advances in Immunology. 2010;**107**:153-185. Available from: http://www.ncbi.nlm.nih.gov/pubmed/21034974

[42] Macpherson AJ, McCoy KD, Johansen F-E, Brandtzaeg P. The immune geography of IgA induction and function. Mucosal Immunology. 2008;**1**(1):11-22. Available from: http://www.ncbi.nlm.nih.gov/pubmed/19079156

[43] Fagarasan S. Evolution, development, mechanism and function of IgA in the gut. Current Opinion in Immunology. 2008;**20**(2):170-177. Available from: http://www.ncbi.nlm.nih.gov/pubmed/18456485

[44] Kang W, Gomez FE, Lan J, Sano Y, Ueno C, Kudsk KA. Parenteral nutrition impairs gut-associated lymphoid tissue and mucosal immunity by reducing lymphotoxin Beta receptor expression. Annals of Surgery. 2006;**244**(3):392-399. Available from: http://www.pubmedcentral.nih.gov/articlerender.fcgi?artid=1856545&tool=pmcentrez&rendertype=abstract

[45] Li J, Kudsk KA, Gocinski B, Dent D, Glezer J, Langkamp-Henken B. Effects of parenteral and enteral nutrition on gut-associated lymphoid tissue. The Journal of Trauma. 1995;**39**(1):44-51; discussion 51-52. Available from: http://www.ncbi.nlm.nih.gov/pubmed/7636909

[46] Jonker MA, Heneghan AF, Fechner JH, Pierre JF, Sano Y, Lan J, et al. Gut lymphocyte phenotype changes after parenteral nutrition and neuropeptide administration. Annals of Surgery. 2015;**262**(1):194-201. Available from: http://www.ncbi.nlm.nih.gov/pubmed/25563877

[47] Mabbott NA, Donaldson DS, Ohno H, Williams IR, Mahajan A. Microfold (M) cells: Important immunosurveillance posts in the intestinal epithelium. Mucosal Immunology. 2013;**6**(4):666-677

[48] Zhai S-K, Volgina V V, Sethupathi P, Knight KL, Lanning DK. Chemokine-mediated B cell trafficking during early rabbit GALT development. Journal of Immunology. 2014;**193**(12):5951-5959. Available from: http://www.ncbi.nlm.nih.gov/pubmed/25385821

[49] Connor EM, Eppihimer MJ, Morise Z, Granger DN, Grisham MB. Expression of mucosal addressin cell adhesion molecule-1 (MAdCAM-1) in acute and chronic inflammation. Journal of Leukocyte Biology. 1999;**65**(3):349-355. Available from: http://www.ncbi.nlm.nih.gov/pubmed/10080539

[50] Dejardin E, Droin NM, Delhase M, Haas E, Cao Y, Makris C, et al. The

lymphotoxin-beta receptor induces different patterns of gene expression via two NF-kappaB pathways. Immunity. 2002;**17**(4):525-535. Available from: http://www.ncbi.nlm.nih.gov/pubmed/12387745

[51] Ikeda S, Kudsk KA, Fukatsu K, Johnson CD, Le T, Reese S, et al. Enteral feeding preserves mucosal immunity despite in vivo MAdCAM-1 blockade of lymphocyte homing. Annals of Surgery. 2003;**237**(5):677-685; discussion 685. Available from: http://www.pubmedcentral.nih.gov/articlerender.fcgi?artid=1514523&tool=pmcentrez&rendertype=abstract

[52] Lan J, Heneghan AF, Sano Y, Jonker MA, Omata J, Xu W, et al. Parenteral nutrition impairs lymphotoxin β receptor signaling via NF-κB. Annals of Surgery. 2011;**253**(5):996-1003. Available from: http://www.pubmedcentral.nih.gov/articlerender.fcgi?artid=3079800&tool=pmcentrez&rendertype=abstract

[53] Janu P, Li J, Renegar KB, Kudsk KA. Recovery of gut-associated lymphoid tissue and upper respiratory tract immunity after parenteral nutrition. Annals of Surgery. 1997;**225**(6):707-715; discussion 715-717. Available from: http://www.pubmedcentral.nih.gov/articlerender.fcgi?artid=1190874&tool=pmcentrez&rendertype=abstract

[54] Parrott DM. The gut as a lymphoid organ. Clinics in Gastroenterology. 1976;**5**(2):211-228. Available from: http://www.ncbi.nlm.nih.gov/pubmed/798640

[55] Luckheeram RV, Zhou R, Verma AD, Xia B. $CD4^+$T cells: Differentiation and functions. Clinical & Developmental Immunology. 2012;**2012**:925135. Available from: http://www.pubmedcentral.nih.gov/articlerender.fcgi?artid=3312336&tool=pmcentrez&rendertype=abstract

[56] Kaetzel CS. The polymeric immunoglobulin receptor: Bridging innate and adaptive immune responses at mucosal surfaces. Immunological Reviews. 2005;**206**(1):83-99. Available from: http://www.ncbi.nlm.nih.gov/pubmed/16048543

[57] Cao AT, Yao S, Gong B, Elson CO, Cong Y. Th17 cells upregulate polymeric Ig receptor and intestinal IgA and contribute to intestinal homeostasis. Journal of Immunology. 2012;**189**(9):4666-4673. Available from: http://www.pubmedcentral.nih.gov/articlerender.fcgi?artid=3478497&tool=pmcentrez&rendertype=abstract

[58] Bowcutt R, Malter LB, Chen LA, Wolff MJ, Robertson I, Rifkin DB, et al. Isolation and cytokine analysis of lamina propria lymphocytes from mucosal biopsies of the human colon. Journal of Immunological Methods. 2015;**421**:27-35. Available from: http://www.ncbi.nlm.nih.gov/pubmed/25769417

[59] Feng T, Elson CO, Cong Y. Treg cell-IgA axis in maintenance of host immune homeostasis with microbiota. International Immunopharmacology. 2011;**11**(5):589-592. Available from: http://www.pubmedcentral.nih.gov/articlerender.fcgi?artid=3078992&tool=pmcentrez&rendertype=abstract

[60] Chang Y-J, Holtzman MJ, Chen C-C. Interferon-gamma-induced epithelial ICAM-1 expression and monocyte adhesion. Involvement of protein kinase C-dependent c-Src tyrosine kinase activation pathway. The Journal of Biological Chemistry. 2002;**277**(9):7118-7126. Available from: http://www.ncbi.nlm.nih.gov/pubmed/11751911

[61] Fukatsu K, Kudsk KA, Zarzaur BL, Sabek O, Wilcox HG, Johnson CD. Increased ICAM-1 and beta2 integrin expression in parenterally fed mice after a gut ischemic insult. Shock. 2002;**18**(2):119-124. Available from:

http://www.ncbi.nlm.nih.gov/pubmed/12166773

[62] Jertborn M, Svennerholm AM, Holmgren J. Saliva, breast milk, and serum antibody responses as indirect measures of intestinal immunity after oral cholera vaccination or natural disease. Journal of Clinical Microbiology. 1986;**24**(2):203-209. Available from: http://www.pubmedcentral.nih.gov/articlerender.fcgi?artid=268875&tool=pmcentrez&rendertype=abstract

[63] Nathavitharana KA, Catty D, Raykundalia C, McNeish AS. Presence of secretory IgA antibodies to an enteric bacterial pathogen in human milk and saliva. Archives of Disease in Childhood. Fetal and Neonatal Edition. 1995;**72**(2):F102-F106. Available from: http://www.pubmedcentral.nih.gov/articlerender.fcgi?artid=2528391&tool=pmcentrez&rendertype=abstract

[64] King BK, Kudsk KA, Li J, Wu Y, Renegar KB. Route and type of nutrition influence mucosal immunity to bacterial pneumonia. Annals of Surgery. 1999;**229**(2):272-278. Available from: http://www.pubmedcentral.nih.gov/articlerender.fcgi?artid=1191641&tool=pmcentrez&rendertype=abstract

[65] Kudsk KA, Li J, Renegar KB. Loss of upper respiratory tract immunity with parenteral feeding. Annals of Surgery. 1996;**223**(6):629-635; discussion 635-638. Available from: http://www.pubmedcentral.nih.gov/articlerender.fcgi?artid=1235201&tool=pmcentrez&rendertype=abstract

[66] Barker N. Adult intestinal stem cells: Critical drivers of epithelial homeostasis and regeneration. Nature Reviews. Molecular Cell Biology. 2014;**15**(1):19-33. Available from: http://www.ncbi.nlm.nih.gov/pubmed/24326621

[67] Yang H, Feng Y, Sun X, Teitelbaum DH. Enteral versus parenteral nutrition: Effect on intestinal barrier function. Annals of the New York Academy of Sciences. 2009;**1165**(1):338-346. Available from: http://doi.wiley.com/10.1111/j.1749-6632.2009.04026.x

[68] Kansagra K, Stoll B, Rognerud C, Niinikoski H, Ou C-N, Harvey R, et al. Total parenteral nutrition adversely affects gut barrier function in neonatal piglets. American Journal of Physiology. Gastrointestinal and Liver Physiology. 2003;**285**(6):G1162-G1170. Available from: http://www.ncbi.nlm.nih.gov/pubmed/12969831

[69] Krug SM, Schulzke JD, Fromm M. Tight junction, selective permeability, and related diseases. Seminars in Cell & Developmental Biology. 2014;**36**:166-176. Available from: http://www.ncbi.nlm.nih.gov/pubmed/25220018

[70] Lelouard H, Fallet M, de Bovis B, Méresse S, Gorvel J-P. Peyer's patch dendritic cells sample antigens by extending dendrites through M cell-specific transcellular pores. Gastroenterology. 2012;**142**(3):592-601.e3. Available from: http://www.ncbi.nlm.nih.gov/pubmed/22155637

[71] Vaishnava S, Yamamoto M, Severson KM, Ruhn KA, Yu X, Koren O, et al. The antibacterial lectin RegIIIgamma promotes the spatial segregation of microbiota and host in the intestine. Science. 2011;**334**(6053):255-258. Available from: http://www.pubmedcentral.nih.gov/articlerender.fcgi?artid=3321924&tool=pmcentrez&rendertype=abstract

[72] Salzman NH, Bevins CL. Dysbiosis--a consequence of Paneth cell dysfunction. Seminars in Immunology. 2013;**25**(5):334-341. Available from: http://www.ncbi.nlm.nih.gov/pubmed/24239045

[73] Ayabe T, Satchell DP, Wilson CL, Parks WC, Selsted ME, Ouellette AJ. Secretion of microbicidal

alpha-defensins by intestinal Paneth cells in response to bacteria. Nature Immunology. 2000;**1**(2):113-118. Available from: http://www.ncbi.nlm.nih.gov/pubmed/11248802

[74] Clevers HC, Bevins CL. Paneth cells: Maestros of the small intestinal crypts. Annual Review of Physiology. 2013;**75**:289-311. Available from: http://www.ncbi.nlm.nih.gov/pubmed/23398152

[75] Steenwinckel V, Louahed J, Lemaire MM, Sommereyns C, Warnier G, McKenzie A, et al. IL-9 promotes IL-13-dependent paneth cell hyperplasia and up-regulation of innate immunity mediators in intestinal mucosa. Journal of Immunology. 2009;**182**(8):4737-4743. Available from: http://www.ncbi.nlm.nih.gov/pubmed/19342650

[76] Omata J, Pierre JF, Heneghan AF, Tsao FHC, Sano Y, Jonker MA, et al. Parenteral nutrition suppresses the bactericidal response of the small intestine. Surgery. 2013;**153**(1):17-24. Available from: http://www.pubmedcentral.nih.gov/articlerender.fcgi?artid=3445757&tool=pmcentrez&rendertype=abstract

[77] Heneghan AF, Pierre JF, Gosain A, Kudsk KA. IL-25 improves luminal innate immunity and barrier function during parenteral nutrition. Annals of Surgery. 2014;**259**(2):394-400. Available from: http://www.pubmedcentral.nih.gov/articlerender.fcgi?artid=3661688&tool=pmcentrez&rendertype=abstract

[78] Busch RA, Jonker MA, Pierre JF, Heneghan AF, Kudsk KA. Innate mucosal immune system response of BALB/c vs C57BL/6 mice to injury in the setting of enteral and parenteral feeding. JPEN Journal of Parenteral and Enteral Nutrition. 2014;**40**(2):256-263. Available from: http://www.ncbi.nlm.nih.gov/pubmed/25403938

[79] Leone V, Gibbons SM, Martinez K, Hutchison AL, Huang EY, Cham CM, et al. Effects of diurnal variation of gut microbes and high-fat feeding on host circadian clock function and metabolism. Cell Host & Microbe. 2015;**17**(5):681-689. Available from: http://www.ncbi.nlm.nih.gov/pubmed/25891358

[80] Heneghan AF, Pierre JF, Kudsk KA. IL-25 improves IgA levels during parenteral nutrition through the JAK-STAT pathway. Annals of Surgery. 2013;**258**(6):1065-1071. Available from: http://www.pubmedcentral.nih.gov/articlerender.fcgi?artid=3587041&tool=pmcentrez&rendertype=abstract

[81] Pierre JF, Heneghan AF, Meudt JM, Shea MP, Krueger CG, Reed JD, et al. Parenteral nutrition increases susceptibility of ileum to invasion by *E coli*. The Journal of Surgical Research. 2013;**183**(2):583-591. Available from: http://www.pubmedcentral.nih.gov/articlerender.fcgi?artid=3840428&tool=pmcentrez&rendertype=abstract

[82] Kim YS, Ho SB. Intestinal goblet cells and mucins in health and disease: Recent insights and progress. Current Gastroenterology Reports. 2010;**12**(5):319-330. Available from: http://www.pubmedcentral.nih.gov/articlerender.fcgi?artid=2933006&tool=pmcentrez&rendertype=abstract

[83] Meyer-Hoffert U, Hornef MW, Henriques-Normark B, Axelsson L-G, Midtvedt T, Pütsep K, et al. Secreted enteric antimicrobial activity localises to the mucus surface layer. Gut. 2008;**57**(6):764-771. Available from: http://www.ncbi.nlm.nih.gov/pubmed/18250125

[84] Busch RA, Heneghan AF, Pierre JF, Neuman JC, Reimer CA, Wang X, et al. Bombesin preserves goblet cell resistin-like molecule β during parenteral nutrition but not other goblet cell products. JPEN Journal of Parenteral

and Enteral Nutrition. 2015;**40**(7):1042-1049. Available from: http://www.ncbi.nlm.nih.gov/pubmed/25934045

[85] Oeser K, Schwartz C, Voehringer D. Conditional IL-4/IL-13-deficient mice reveal a critical role of innate immune cells for protective immunity against gastrointestinal helminths. Mucosal Immunology. 2015;**8**(3):672-682. Available from: http://www.ncbi.nlm.nih.gov/pubmed/25336167

[86] Gunawardene AR, Corfe BM, Staton CA. Classification and functions of enteroendocrine cells of the lower gastrointestinal tract. International Journal of Experimental Pathology. 2011;**92**(4):219-231. Available from: http://www.pubmedcentral.nih.gov/articlerender.fcgi?artid=3144510&tool=pmcentrez&rendertype=abstract

[87] Selleri S, Palazzo M, Deola S, Wang E, Balsari A, Marincola FM, et al. Induction of pro-inflammatory programs in enteroendocrine cells by the Toll-like receptor agonists flagellin and bacterial LPS. International Immunology. 2008;**20**(8):961-970. Available from: http://www.ncbi.nlm.nih.gov/pubmed/18544573

[88] Palazzo M, Balsari A, Rossini A, Selleri S, Calcaterra C, Gariboldi S, et al. Activation of enteroendocrine cells via TLRs induces hormone, chemokine, and defensin secretion. Journal of Immunology. 2007;**178**(7):4296-4303. Available from: http://www.ncbi.nlm.nih.gov/pubmed/17371986

[89] Shreiner AB, Kao JY, Young VB. The gut microbiome in health and in disease. Current Opinion in Gastroenterology. 2015;**31**(1):69-75. Available from: http://www.ncbi.nlm.nih.gov/pubmed/25394236

[90] David LA, Maurice CF, Carmody RN, Gootenberg DB, Button JE, Wolfe BE, et al. Diet rapidly and reproducibly alters the human gut microbiome. Nature. 2014;**505**(7484):559-563. Available from: http://www.pubmedcentral.nih.gov/articlerender.fcgi?artid=3957428&tool=pmcentrez&rendertype=abstract

[91] Magnúsdóttir S, Ravcheev D, de Crécy-Lagard V, Thiele I. Systematic genome assessment of B-vitamin biosynthesis suggests co-operation among gut microbes. Frontiers in Genetics. 2015;**6**:148. Available from: http://www.ncbi.nlm.nih.gov/pubmed/25941533

[92] Heneghan AF, Pierre JF, Tandee K, Shanmuganayagam D, Wang X, Reed JD, et al. Parenteral nutrition decreases paneth cell function and intestinal bactericidal activity while increasing susceptibility to bacterial enteroinvasion. JPEN Journal of Parenteral and Enteral Nutrition. 2014;**38**(7):817-824. Available from: http://www.pubmedcentral.nih.gov/articlerender.fcgi?artid=4843109&tool=pmcentrez&rendertype=abstract

[93] Ralls MW, Demehri FR, Feng Y, Raskind S, Ruan C, Schintlmeister A, et al. Bacterial nutrient foraging in a mouse model of enteral nutrient deprivation: Insight into the gut origin of sepsis. American Journal of Physiology-Gastrointestinal and Liver Physiology. 2016 311 G734

[94] Miyasaka EA, Feng Y, Poroyko V, Falkowski NR, Erb-Downward J, Gillilland MG, et al. Total parenteral nutrition-associated lamina propria inflammation in mice is mediated by a MyD88-dependent mechanism. Journal of Immunology. 2013;**190**(12):6607-6615. Available from: http://www.pubmedcentral.nih.gov/articlerender.fcgi?artid=3679213&tool=pmcentrez&rendertype=abstract

[95] David R. Regulatory T cells: A helping hand from *Bacteroides fragilis*. Nature Reviews. Immunology. 2010;**10**(8):539. Available from: http://

www.ncbi.nlm.nih.gov/pubmed/20677358

[96] Romanowski K, Zaborin A, Valuckaite V, Rolfes RJ, Babrowski T, Bethel C, et al. Candida albicans isolates from the gut of critically ill patients respond to phosphate limitation by expressing filaments and a lethal phenotype. PLoS One. 2012;**7**(1):e30119. Available from: http://www.pubmedcentral.nih.gov/articlerender.fcgi?artid=3258262&tool=pmcentrez&rendertype=abstract

[97] Pappo I, Polacheck I, Zmora O, Feigin E, Freund HR. Altered gut barrier function to Candida during parenteral nutrition. Nutrition. 1994;**10**(2):151-154. Available from: http://www.ncbi.nlm.nih.gov/pubmed/8025369

[98] Ward MA, Pierre JF, Leal RF, Huang Y, Shogan BD, Dalal SR, et al. Insights into the pathogenesis of ulcerative colitis from a murine model of stasis-induced dysbiosis, colonic metaplasia, and genetic susceptibility. American Journal of Physiology. Gastrointestinal and Liver Physiology. 2016;**310**(11):G973. DOI: 10.1152/ajpgi.00017.2016. Available from: http://www.ncbi.nlm.nih.gov/pubmed/27079612

[99] Żalikowska-Gardocka M, Przybyłkowski A. Review of parenteral nutrition-associated liver disease. Clinical and Experimental Hepatology. 2020;**6**(2):65. Available from: https://pubmed.ncbi.nlm.nih.gov/32728621/

[100] Willis KA, Gomes CK, Rao P, Micic D, Moran ER, Stephenson E, et al. TGR5 signaling mitigates parenteral nutrition-associated liver disease. American Journal of Physiology-Gastrointestinal and Liver Physiology. 2020;**318**(2):G322-G335

[101] Buchman AL. Complications of long-term home total parenteral nutrition: Their identification, prevention and treatment. Digestive Diseases and Sciences. 2001;**46**(1):1-18. Available from: https://pubmed.ncbi.nlm.nih.gov/11270772/

[102] Nowak K. Parenteral nutrition-associated liver disease. Clinics in Liver Disease. 2020;**15**(2):59-62. Available from: https://pubmed.ncbi.nlm.nih.gov/32226616/

[103] Xu Z-W, Li YS. Pathogenesis and treatment of parenteral nutrition-associated liver disease. Hepatobiliary & Pancreatic Diseases International. 2012;**11**(6):586-593. Available from: https://pubmed.ncbi.nlm.nih.gov/23232629/

[104] Messing B, Bories C, Kunstlinger F, Bernier JJ. Does total parenteral nutrition induce gallbladder sludge formation and lithiasis? Gastroenterology. 1983;**84**(5 Pt 1):1012-1019

[105] Lappas BM, Patel D, Kumpf V, Adams DW, Seidner DL. Parenteral nutrition: Indications, access, and complications. Gastroenterology Clinics of North America. 2018;**47**(1):39-59. Available from: https://pubmed.ncbi.nlm.nih.gov/29413018/

[106] El Kasmi KC, Anderson AL, Devereaux MW, Vue PM, Zhang W, Kenneth DRS, et al. Phytosterols promote liver injury and Kupffer cell activation in parenteral nutrition-associated liver disease. Science Translational Medicine. 2013;**5**(206):1. Available from: https://pubmed.ncbi.nlm.nih.gov/24107776/

[107] Inagaki T, Moschetta A, Lee Y-K, Peng L, Zhao G, Downes M, et al. Regulation of antibacterial defense in the small intestine by the nuclear bile acid receptor. Proceedings of the National Academy of Sciences of the United States of America. 2006;**103**(10):3920-3925. Available

from: http://www.pubmedcentral.nih.gov/articlerender.fcgi?artid=1450165&tool=pmcentrez&rendertype=abstract

[108] Jain AK, Stoll B, Burrin DG, Holst JJ, Moore DD, Al-Mukhtar M, et al. Enteral bile acid treatment improves parenteral nutrition-related liver disease and intestinal mucosal atrophy in neonatal pigs. American Journal of Physiology. Gastrointestinal and Liver Physiology. 2012;**302**(2):G218-G224. Available from: http://www.ncbi.nlm.nih.gov/pubmed/22094603

[109] Modica S, Petruzzelli M, Bellafante E, Murzilli S, Salvatore L, Celli N, et al. Selective activation of nuclear bile acid receptor FXR in the intestine protects mice against cholestasis. Gastroenterology. 2012;**142**(2):355. Available from: https://pubmed.ncbi.nlm.nih.gov/22057115/

[110] Bharadwaj S, Gohel T, Deen OJ, DeChicco R, Shatnawei A. Fish oil-based lipid emulsion: Current updates on a promising novel therapy for the management of parenteral nutrition-associated liver disease. Gastroenterology Report. 2015;**3**(2):110-114. Available from: https://pubmed.ncbi.nlm.nih.gov/25858884/

[111] de Meijer VE, Gura KM, Meisel JA, Le HD, Puder M. Parenteral fish oil monotherapy in the management of patients with parenteral nutrition-associated liver disease. Archives of Surgery. 2010;**145**(6):547-551. Available from: https://pubmed.ncbi.nlm.nih.gov/20566974/

[112] Mundi MS, Salonen BR, Bonnes S. Home parenteral nutrition: Fat emulsions and potential complications. Nutrition in Clinical Practice. 2016;**31**(5):629-641. Available from: https://pubmed.ncbi.nlm.nih.gov/27533943/

[113] Kosters A, Karpen SJ. The role of inflammation in cholestasis: Clinical and basic aspects. Seminars in Liver Disease. 2010;**30**(2):186-194. Available from: https://pubmed.ncbi.nlm.nih.gov/20422500/

[114] Novak TE, Babcock TA, Jho DH, Scott Helton W, Joseph Espat N. NF-kappa B inhibition by omega-3 fatty acids modulates LPS-stimulated macrophage TNF-alpha transcription. American Journal of Physiology. Lung Cellular and Molecular Physiology. 2003;**284**(1):L84. Available from: https://pubmed.ncbi.nlm.nih.gov/12388359/

[115] Gura KM, Duggan CP, Collier SB, Jennings RW, Folkman J, Bistrian BR, et al. Reversal of parenteral nutrition-associated liver disease in two infants with short bowel syndrome using parenteral fish oil: Implications for future management. Pediatrics. 2006;**118**(1):197. Available from: https://pubmed.ncbi.nlm.nih.gov/16818533/

[116] Vlaardingerbroek H, Ng K, Stoll B, Benight N, Chacko S, Kluijtmans LAJ, et al. New generation lipid emulsions prevent PNALD in chronic parenterally fed preterm pigs. Journal of Lipid Research. 2014;**55**(3):466-477. Available from: https://pubmed.ncbi.nlm.nih.gov/24478031/

[117] Freund HR, Muggia-Sullam M, LaFrance R, Enrione EB, Popp MB, Bjornson HS. A possible beneficial effect of metronidazole in reducing TPN-associated liver function derangements. The Journal of Surgical Research. 1985;**38**(4):356-363. Available from: https://pubmed.ncbi.nlm.nih.gov/3923267/

[118] Lambert JR, Thomas SM. Metronidazole prevention of serum liver enzyme abnormalities during total parenteral nutrition. JPEN Journal of Parenteral and Enteral Nutrition. 1985;**9**(4):501-503. Available from: https://pubmed.ncbi.nlm.nih.gov/2863398/

[119] Grant JP, Synder PJ. Use of L-glutamine in total parenteral nutrition. The Journal of Surgical Research. 1988;**44**(5):506-513. Available from: https://pubmed.ncbi.nlm.nih.gov/3131588/

[120] Cooke RJ, Embleton ND. Feeding issues in preterm infants. Archives of Disease in Childhood. Fetal and Neonatal Edition. 2000;**83**(3):F215. Available from: https://pubmed.ncbi.nlm.nih.gov/11040172/

[121] Serenius F, Källén K, Blennow M, Ewald U, Fellman V, Holmström G, et al. Neurodevelopmental outcome in extremely preterm infants at 2.5 years after active perinatal care in Sweden. JAMA. 2013;**309**(17):1810-1820. Available from: https://pubmed.ncbi.nlm.nih.gov/23632725/

[122] Terrin G, Coscia A, Boscarino G, Faccioli F, Di Chiara M, Greco C, et al. Long-term effects on growth of an energy-enhanced parenteral nutrition in preterm newborn: A quasi-experimental study. PLoS One. 2020;**15**(7):1. Available from: https://pubmed.ncbi.nlm.nih.gov/32628715/

[123] Agostoni C, Guz-Mark A, Marderfeld L, Milani GP, Silano M, Shamir R. The long-term effects of dietary nutrient intakes during the first 2 years of life in healthy infants from developed countries: An umbrella review. Advances in Nutrition. 2019;**10**(3):489-501. Available from: https://pubmed.ncbi.nlm.nih.gov/30843039/

[124] Singhal A. Long-term adverse effects of early growth acceleration or catch-up growth. Annals of Nutrition & Metabolism. 2017;**70**(3):236-240. Available from: https://pubmed.ncbi.nlm.nih.gov/28301849/

[125] Reilly JJ, Armstrong J, Dorosty AR, Emmett PM, Ness A, Rogers I, et al. Early life risk factors for obesity in childhood: Cohort study. BMJ. 2005;**330**(7504):1357-1359. Available from: https://pubmed.ncbi.nlm.nih.gov/15908441/

[126] Clouchoux C, Guizard N, Evans AC, du Plessis AJ, Limperopoulos C. Normative fetal brain growth by quantitative in vivo magnetic resonance imaging. American Journal of Obstetrics and Gynecology. 2012;**206**(2):173.e1-173.e8. Available from: https://pubmed.ncbi.nlm.nih.gov/22055336/

[127] Volpe JJ. Brain injury in premature infants: A complex amalgam of destructive and developmental disturbances. Lancet Neurology. 2009;**8**(1):110-124. Available from: https://pubmed.ncbi.nlm.nih.gov/19081519/

[128] Rose J, Vassar R, Cahill-Rowley K, Guzman XS, Stevenson DK, Barnea-Goraly N. Brain microstructural development at near-term age in very-low-birth-weight preterm infants: An atlas-based diffusion imaging study. NeuroImage. 2014;**86**:244-256. Available from: https://pubmed.ncbi.nlm.nih.gov/24091089/

[129] Munakata S, Okada T, Okahashi A, Yoshikawa K, Usukura Y, Makimoto M, et al. Gray matter volumetric MRI differences late-preterm and term infants. Brain & Development. 2013;**35**(1):10-16. Available from: https://pubmed.ncbi.nlm.nih.gov/22285528/

[130] Borre YE, O'Keeffe GW, Clarke G, Stanton C, Dinan TG, Cryan JF. Microbiota and neurodevelopmental windows: Implications for brain disorders. Trends in Molecular Medicine. 2014;**20**(9):509-518. Available from: https://pubmed.ncbi.nlm.nih.gov/24956966/

[131] Craig-Schmidt MC, Stieh KE, Lien EL. Retinal fatty acids of piglets fed

docosahexaenoic and arachidonic acids from microbial sources. Lipids. 1996;**31**(1):53-59. Available from: https://pubmed.ncbi.nlm.nih.gov/8649234/

[132] de la Pressa-Owens S, Innis SM, Rioux FM. Addition of triglycerides with arachidonic acid or docosahexaenoic acid to infant formula has tissue- and lipid class-specific effects on fatty acids and hepatic desaturase activities in formula-fed piglets. The Journal of Nutrition. 1998;**128**(8):1376-1384. Available from: https://pubmed.ncbi.nlm.nih.gov/9687559/

[133] de la Pressa-Owens S, Innis SM. Diverse, region-specific effects of addition of arachidonic and docosahexanoic acids to formula with low or adequate linoleic and alpha-linolenic acids on piglet brain monoaminergic neurotransmitters. Pediatric Research. 2000;**48**(1):125-130. Available from: https://pubmed.ncbi.nlm.nih.gov/10879811/

[134] Wischmeyer PE. Glutamine: Role in critical illness and ongoing clinical trials. Current Opinion in Gastroenterology. 2008;**24**(2):190-197. Available from: http://www.ncbi.nlm.nih.gov/pubmed/18301270

[135] Pierre JF, Heneghan AF, Lawson CM, Wischmeyer PE, Kozar RA, Kudsk KA. Pharmaconutrition review: Physiological mechanisms. JPEN Journal of Parenteral and Enteral Nutrition. 2013;**37**(5 Suppl):51S-65S. Available from: http://www.ncbi.nlm.nih.gov/pubmed/24009249

[136] Erickson CS, Barlow AJ, Pierre JF, Heneghan AF, Epstein ML, Kudsk KA, et al. Colonic enteric nervous system analysis during parenteral nutrition. The Journal of Surgical Research. 2013;**184**(1):132-137. Available from: http://www.pubmedcentral.nih.gov/articlerender.fcgi?artid=3947919&tool=pmcentrez&rendertype=abstract

[137] Pierre JF, Heneghan AF, Wang X, Roenneburg DA, Groblewski GE, Kudsk KA. Bombesin improves adaptive immunity of the salivary gland during parenteral nutrition. JPEN Journal of Parenteral and Enteral Nutrition. 2015;**39**(2):190-199. Available from: http://www.pubmedcentral.nih.gov/articlerender.fcgi?artid=4105332&tool=pmcentrez&rendertype=abstract

[138] Zarzaur BL, Wu Y, Fukatsu K, Johnson CD, Kudsk KA. The neuropeptide bombesin improves IgA-mediated mucosal immunity with preservation of gut interleukin-4 in total parenteral nutrition-fed mice. Surgery. 2002;**131**(1):59-65. Available from: http://www.ncbi.nlm.nih.gov/pubmed/11812964

[139] Jonker MA, Hermsen JL, Sano Y, Heneghan AF, Lan J, Kudsk KA. Small intestine mucosal immune system response to injury and the impact of parenteral nutrition. Surgery. 2012;**151**(2):278-286. Available from: http://www.pubmedcentral.nih.gov/articlerender.fcgi?artid=3076529&tool=pmcentrez&rendertype=abstract

[140] Keith Hanna M, Zarzaur BL, Fukatsu K, Chance DeWitt R, Renegar KB, Sherrell C, et al. Individual neuropeptides regulate gut-associated lymphoid tissue integrity, intestinal immunoglobulin A levels, and respiratory antibacterial immunity. Journal of Parenteral and Enteral Nutrition. 2000;**24**(5):261-268; discussion 268-269. Available from: http://www.ncbi.nlm.nih.gov/pubmed/11011780

[141] Busch RA, Heneghan AF, Pierre JF, Wang X, Kudsk KA. The enteric nervous system neuropeptide, bombesin, reverses innate immune impairments during parenteral nutrition. Annals of Surgery. 2014;**260**(3):432-443;

discussion 443-444. Available from: http://www.pubmedcentral.nih.gov/articlerender.fcgi?artid=4152867&tool=pmcentrez&rendertype=abstract

[142] Pierre JF, Neuman JC, Brill AL, Brar HK, Thompson MF, Cadena MT, et al. The gastrin-releasing peptide analog bombesin preserves exocrine and endocrine pancreas morphology and function during parenteral nutrition. American Journal of Physiology. Gastrointestinal and Liver Physiology. 2015;**309**(6):G431-G442. Available from: http://www.ncbi.nlm.nih.gov/pubmed/26185331

[143] Qiu J, Heller JJ, Guo X, Chen ZE, Fish K, Fu Y-X, et al. The aryl hydrocarbon receptor regulates gut immunity through modulation of innate lymphoid cells. Immunity. 2012;**36**(1):92-104

[144] Tanaka G, Kanaji S, Hirano A, Arima K, Shinagawa A, Goda C, et al. Induction and activation of the aryl hydrocarbon receptor by IL-4 in B cells. International Immunology. 2005;**17**(6):797-805. Available from: http://www.ncbi.nlm.nih.gov/pubmed/15899923

[145] Lu H, Crawford RB, Suarez-Martinez JE, Kaplan BLF, Kaminski NE. Induction of the aryl hydrocarbon receptor-responsive genes and modulation of the immunoglobulin M response by 2, 3, 7, 8-tetrachlorodibenzo-p-dioxin in primary human B cells. Toxicological Sciences. 2010;**118**(1):86-97. Available from: http://www.ncbi.nlm.nih.gov/pubmed/20702590

[146] Kim M, Qie Y, Park J, Kim CH. Gut microbial metabolites fuel host antibody responses. Cell Host & Microbe. 2016;**20**(2):202-214. Available from: http://linkinghub.elsevier.com/retrieve/pii/S1931312816302992

[147] Singh N, Gurav A, Sivaprakasam S, Brady E, Padia R, Shi H, et al. Activation of Gpr109a, receptor for niacin and the commensal metabolite butyrate, suppresses colonic inflammation and carcinogenesis. Immunity. 2014;**40**(1):128-139. Available from: http://linkinghub.elsevier.com/retrieve/pii/S1074761313005645

[148] Willemsen LEM, Koetsier MA, van Deventer SJH, van Tol EAF. Short chain fatty acids stimulate epithelial mucin 2 expression through differential effects on prostaglandin E(1) and E(2) production by intestinal myofibroblasts. Gut. 2003;**52**(10):1442-1447. Available from: http://www.ncbi.nlm.nih.gov/pubmed/12970137

[149] Gaudier E, Jarry A, Blottière HM, de Coppet P, Buisine MP, Aubert JP, et al. Butyrate specifically modulates MUC gene expression in intestinal epithelial goblet cells deprived of glucose. American Journal of Physiology. Gastrointestinal and Liver Physiology. 2004;**287**(6):G1168-G1174. Available from: http://ajpgi.physiology.org/cgi/doi/10.1152/ajpgi.00219.2004

[150] den Besten G, Bleeker A, Gerding A, van Eunen K, Havinga R, van Dijk TH, et al. Short-chain fatty acids protect against high-fat diet-induced obesity via a PPARγ-dependent switch from lipogenesis to fat oxidation. Diabetes. 2015;**64**(7):2398-2408. Available from: https://pubmed.ncbi.nlm.nih.gov/25695945/

[151] Shimizu H, Masujima Y, Ushiroda C, Mizushima R, Taira S, Ohue-Kitano R, et al. Dietary short-chain fatty acid intake improves the hepatic metabolic condition via FFAR3. Scientific Reports. 2019;**9**(1):1. Available from: https://pubmed.ncbi.nlm.nih.gov/31719611/

[152] Silva YP, A Bernardi A, Frozza RL. The role of short-chain fatty acids from gut microbiota in gut-brain communication. Frontiers in Endocrinology (Lausanne). 2020;**11**:1.

Available from: https://pubmed.ncbi.nlm.nih.gov/32082260/

[153] Erny D, de Angelis ALH, Jaitin D, Wieghofer P, Staszewski O, David E, et al. Host microbiota constantly control maturation and function of microglia in the CNS. Nature Neuroscience. 2015;**18**(7):965-977. Available from: https://pubmed.ncbi.nlm.nih.gov/26030851/

[154] Lin HV, Frassetto A, Kowalik Jr EJ, Nawrocki AR, Lu MM, Kosinski JR, et al. Butyrate and propionate protect against diet-induced obesity and regulate gut hormones via free fatty acid receptor 3-independent mechanisms. PLoS One. 2012;7(4):1. Available from: https://pubmed.ncbi.nlm.nih.gov/22506074/

[155] Löser C, Eisel A, Harms D, Fölsch UR. Dietary polyamines are essential luminal growth factors for small intestinal and colonic mucosal growth and development. Gut. 1999;**44**(1):12-6. Available from: http://www.ncbi.nlm.nih.gov/pubmed/9862820

[156] Chen J, Rao JN, Zou T, Liu L, Marasa BS, Xiao L, et al. Polyamines are required for expression of Toll-like receptor 2 modulating intestinal epithelial barrier integrity. American Journal of Physiology. Gastrointestinal and Liver Physiology. 2007;**293**(3):G568-G576. Available from: http://ajpgi.physiology.org/cgi/doi/10.1152/ajpgi.00201.2007

[157] Liu L, Guo X, Rao JN, Zou T, Xiao L, Yu T, et al. Polyamines regulate E-cadherin transcription through c-Myc modulating intestinal epithelial barrier function. American Journal of Physiology-Cell Physiology. 2009;**296**(4):C801-C810. Available from: http://www.ncbi.nlm.nih.gov/pubmed/19176757

[158] Dufour C, Dandrifosse G, Forget P, Vermesse F, Romain N, Lepoint P. Spermine and spermidine induce intestinal maturation in the rat. Gastroenterology. 1988;**95**(1):112-116. Available from: http://www.ncbi.nlm.nih.gov/pubmed/3371606

[159] Pérez-Cano FJ, González-Castro A, Castellote C, Franch A, Castell M. Influence of breast milk polyamines on suckling rat immune system maturation. Developmental and Comparative Immunology. 2010;**34**(2):210-218. Available from: http://linkinghub.elsevier.com/retrieve/pii/S0145305X09002158

[160] Chiang JYL, Ferrell JM. Bile acids as metabolic regulators and nutrient sensors. Annual Review of Nutrition. 2019;**39**:175-200. Available from: https://pubmed.ncbi.nlm.nih.gov/31018107/

[161] Goodwin B, Jones SA, Price RR, Watson MA, McKee DD, Moore LB, et al. A regulatory cascade of the nuclear receptors FXR, SHP-1, and LRH-1 represses bile acid biosynthesis. Molecular Cell. 2000;**6**(3):517-526. Available from: https://pubmed.ncbi.nlm.nih.gov/11030332/

[162] Porex G, Prawitt J, Gross B, Staels B. Bile acid receptors as targets for the treatment of dyslipidemia and cardiovascular disease. Journal of Lipid Research. 2012;**53**(9):1723-1737. Available from: https://pubmed.ncbi.nlm.nih.gov/22550135/

[163] Pathak P, Liu H, Boehme S, Xie C, Krausz KW, Gonzalez F, et al. Farnesoid X receptor induces Takeda G-protein receptor 5 cross-talk to regulate bile acid synthesis and hepatic metabolism. The Journal of Biological Chemistry. 2017;**292**(26):11055-11069. Available from: https://pubmed.ncbi.nlm.nih.gov/28478385/

[164] Inagaki T, Choi M, Moschetta A, Peng L, Cummins CL, McDonald JG, et al. Fibroblast growth factor 15 functions

as an enterohepatic signal to regulate bile acid homeostasis. Cell Metabolism. 2005;**2**(4):217-225. Available from: https://pubmed.ncbi.nlm.nih.gov/16213224/

[165] Song KH, Li T, Owsley E, Strom S, Chiang JY. Bile acids activate fibroblast growth factor 19 signaling in human hepatocytes to inhibit cholesterol 7alpha-hydroxylase gene expression. Hepatology. 2009;**49**(1):297-305. Available from: https://pubmed.ncbi.nlm.nih.gov/19085950/

[166] de Oliveira MC, Gilglioni EH, de Boer BA, Runge JH, de Waart DR, Salguiero CL, et al. Bile acid receptor agonists INT747 and INT777 decrease oestrogen deficiency-related postmenopausal obesity and hepatic steatosis in mice. Biochimica et Biophysica Acta. 2016;**1862**(11):2054-2062. Available from: https://pubmed.ncbi.nlm.nih.gov/27475255/

[167] Baghdasaryan A, Claudel T, Gumhold J, Silbert D, Adorini L, Roda A, et al. Dual farnesoid X receptor/TGR5 agonist INT-767 reduces liver injury in the Mdr2-/- (Abcb4-/-) mouse cholangiopathy model by promoting biliary HCO_3^- output. Hepatology. 2011;**54**(4):1303-1312. Available from: https://pubmed.ncbi.nlm.nih.gov/22006858/

[168] Raman M, Almutairdi A, Mulesa L, Alberda C, Beattie C, Gramlich L. Parenteral nutrition and lipids. Nutrients. 2017;**9**(4):1. Available from: https://pubmed.ncbi.nlm.nih.gov/28420095/

[169] Itzhaki MH, Singer P. Advances in medical nutrition therapy: Parenteral Nutrition. Nutrients. 2020;**12**(3):1. Available from: https://pubmed.ncbi.nlm.nih.gov/32182654/

[170] Feng S, Wang L, Shao P, Sun P, Yang CS. A review on chemical and physical modifications of phytosterols and their influence on bioavailability and safety. Critical Reviews in Food Science and Nutrition. 2021:1-20. Available from: https://pubmed.ncbi.nlm.nih.gov/33612007/

[171] Feng S, Belwal T, Li L, Limwachiranon J, Liu X, Luo Z. Phytosterols and their derivatives: Potential health-promoting uses against lipid metabolism and associated diseases, mechanism, and safety issues. Comprehensive Reviews in Food Science and Food Safety. 2020;**19**(4):1243-1267. Available from: https://pubmed.ncbi.nlm.nih.gov/33337101/

[172] Bolia R, Srivastava A. Fish oil based lipid emulsions for the treatment of intestinal failure associated liver disease: Nothing fishy about it! Indian Journal of Pediatrics. 2019;**86**(6):494-495. Available from: https://pubmed.ncbi.nlm.nih.gov/30972700/

[173] Skouroliakou M, Konstantinou D, Agakidis C, Delikou N, Koutri K, Antoniadi M, et al. Cholestasis, bronchopulmonary dysplasia, and lipid profile in preterm infants receiving MCT/ω-3-PUFA-containing or soybean-based lipid emulsions. Nutrition in Clinical Practice. 2012;**27**(6):817-824. Available from: https://pubmed.ncbi.nlm.nih.gov/22878361/

[174] Park HW, Lee NM, Kim JH, Kim KS, Kim SN. Parenteral fish oil-containing lipid emulsions may reverse parenteral nutrition-associated cholestasis in neonates: A systematic review and meta-analysis. The Journal of Nutrition. 2015;**145**(2):277-283. Available from: https://pubmed.ncbi.nlm.nih.gov/25644348/

[175] Venick RS, Calkins K. The impact of intravenous fish oil emulsions on pediatric intestinal failure-associated liver disease. Current Opinion in Organ Transplantation. 2011;**16**(3):306-311. Available from: https://pubmed.ncbi.nlm.nih.gov/21505340/

[176] Yoshikawa T, Shimano H, Yahagi N, Ide T, Amemiya-Kudo M, Matsuzaka T, et al. Polyunsaturated fatty acids suppress sterol regulatory element-binding protein 1c promoter activity by inhibition of liver X receptor (LXR) binding to LXR response elements. The Journal of Biological Chemistry. 2002;**277**(3):1705-1711. Available from: https://pubmed.ncbi.nlm.nih.gov/11694526/

[177] Binder C, Giordano V, Thanhaeuser M, Kreissl A, Huber-Dangl M, Longford N, et al. A mixed lipid emulsion containing fish oil and its effect on electrophysiological brain maturation in infants of extremely low birth weight: A secondary analysis of a randomized clinical trial. The Journal of Pediatrics. 2019;**211**:46-53.e2. Available from: https://pubmed.ncbi.nlm.nih.gov/31030946/

[178] Dai Y-J, Sun L-L, Li M-Y, Ding C-L, Su Y-C, Sun L-J, et al. Comparison of formulas based on lipid emulsions of olive oil, soybean oil, or several oils for parenteral nutrition: A systematic review and meta-analysis. Advances in Nutrition. 2016;**7**(2):279-286. Available from: https://pubmed.ncbi.nlm.nih.gov/26980811/

[179] Jensen AR, Goldin AB, Koopmeiners JS, Stevens J, Waldhausen JHT, Kim SS. The association of cyclic parenteral nutrition and decreased incidence of cholestatic liver disease in patients with gastroschisis. Journal of Pediatric Surgery. 2009;**44**(1):183-189. Available from: https://pubmed.ncbi.nlm.nih.gov/19159741/

[180] Villafranca JJA, Guindo MN, Álvaro Sanz EA, Santamaria MM, Siles MG, Abilés J. Effects of cyclic parenteral nutrition on parenteral-associated liver dysfunction parameters. Nutrition Journal. 2017;**16**(1):1. Available from: https://pubmed.ncbi.nlm.nih.gov/28978317/

Chapter 3

Gut Feeding the Brain: *Drosophila* Gut an Animal Model for Medicine to Understand Mechanisms Mediating Food Preferences

Zoha Sadaqat, Shivam Kaushik and Pinky Kain

Abstract

Fruit fly, *Drosophila melanogaster* is a most powerful animal model for exploring fundamental biological processes and modeling molecular and cellular aspects of human diseases. It provides the flexibility and tool box with which scientists can experimentally manipulate and study behavior as well as gene expression in specific, defined population of cells in their normal tissue contexts. The utility and increasing value of a sophisticated genetic system of flies, the tool box available for studying physiological function, functional imaging, neural circuitry from gut to brain, taste receptors expression and controlling gene expression by determining the specific cells in the intestine, makes fly gut the most useful tissue for studying the regulation of feeding behavior under changing internal state. To understand the intestine and its connectivity with the brain, *Drosophila* has proved an ideal model organism for studying gut brain axis aspects of human metabolic diseases. Various markers and fly lines are available to characterize the expression of transgenes in the intestine. The newly generated genetic tools aim to streamline the design of experiments to target specific cells in intestine for genetic manipulations based on their type and location within physiologically specialized intestinal regions. This chapter will be useful for understanding post-ingestive sensing system that mediate food preferences and to investigate fundamental biological processes and model human diseases at the level of single cells in the fly gut. Furthermore, the utility of adult fly gut can be extended to the study of dietary and environmental factors relevant to health and disease by screening for cells and micro circuits stimulated by internal state or the consumption of various nutrients.

Keywords: gut brain axis, *Drosophila*, taste receptors, enterocytes, enteroendocrine cells

1. Introduction

Mammalian central nervous system (CNS) consists of brain and spinal cord. The neuronal network extends from the brain to all over the body and various neurotransmitters help transmit the message to target cells in different tissues. The part of the nervous system located in our gut is called the enteric nervous system (ENS). In all animals, gut brain axis is a lesser known nervous system so far. Our gut or "second brain" (ENS) chemically connects with the brain through neurons, secreted chemicals like hormones and neurotransmitters that send messages to the brain. The enteric nervous system's network of neurons and neurotransmitters extends along the entire digestive tract – it starts from the esophagus to the stomach and intestines, and down to the anus. The "gut microbiome" comprises of microorganisms living in the gut (bacteria, viruses, and fungi) that can affect the chemical messages that pass between the gut and the brain. Microorganisms residing in the gut help regulate the body's immune response. Since, the brain and the gastrointestinal (GI) system are intimately connected, therefore, they play key roles in certain diseases and to maintain our overall health to regulate cognitive and digestive behavior. The bidirectional communication between the brain and digestive system hence, are opening up avenues to think about diseases considering this angle.

Gut has recently become a subject of research in medical sciences wherein subjects with depressive symptoms, Parkinson's and Alzheimer's disease, autism, amyotrophic lateral sclerosis, multiple sclerosis, pain, anxiety and other neurodegenerative conditions are beginning to be looked to see what is going on in the gut. Effects of conditions like ulcers, constipation, and other GI problems have been a focus of research on aspects of brain functioning. The enteric microbiota impacts the gut brain axis (GBA), interacts locally with the intestinal cells and ENS as well as with the CNS through neuroendocrine and metabolic pathways. These studies suggest that GBA plays a vital role in maintaining mental health and can affect the feeding behavior when nutrient detection or absorption does not function properly as in case of metabolic conditions.

To ensure stability in the internal environment of body and drive adaptive changes, control mechanisms are key to animal's survival. Recently GI has been recognized as a major source of signals modulating feeding behaviors, food intake, metabolism, insulin secretion and energy balance. Through its interaction with microbiota, it can shape our physiology and behavior in complex and sometimes unexpected ways. A growing scientific community has exploited the genetic amenability of *Drosophila* gut in great and resourceful ways. In this chapter, we are shedding some light on a broad range of biological questions revolving around gut-brain axis, neural connectivity and its role in regulating food preferences by using inter-organ signaling and disease state, especially metabolic and neurodegenerative diseases. Despite being a relatively new research area for fly biologist, many of the mechanisms active in the intestine of flies have already been shown to be more widely applicable to gastrointestinal systems of higher system and humans, and may therefore become relevant in the context of human pathologies such as metabolic disorders, neurodegenerative diseases, gastrointestinal cancers, aging, or bowel disorders. This chapter will be summarizing our current understanding and knowledge of function of the adult *Drosophila* digestive tract with a major focus on gut-brain neural connectivity and role in digestive/absorptive functions.

2. *Drosophila* as an emerging model system for studying gut: comparison of human and fly gut

Easy genetic manipulation and effortless genetic tools make flies an insect of choice to study inter organ neuronal signaling including gut-brain axis neuronal connectivity. To understand human metabolic diseases and how a GI play a key role there is a recent focus of research. Some progressive studies also draw a link between neurodegenerative disorders and gut microbiota of humans and other insects. *Drosophila's* assistance for studying these and metabolic diseases with respect to its gut will be covered in this chapter.

Fruit flies have a simple and similar to humans- gut system (**Figure 1**). In mammals including humans, the esophagus (*Drosophila* foregut) passes the consumed food to the stomach (crop in flies), where food stores and digestion proceeds. Nutrient absorption takes place in the small intestine (anterior midgut in flies). Later nutrient, water and electrolyte absorption commences in the large intestine (fly hindgut). Finally, it reaches the rectum and anus for excretion (**Figure 1**) [1, 2]. In flies, after food passes through the middle midgut (a region of low pH, contains the iron and copper cells), it transits through the posterior midgut for further absorption and through the hindgut and rectum to exchange water and electrolytes and finally reaches the anus for excretion. Malpighian tubules (renal-like structures) are tubular excretory organs in flies connected to the midgut-hindgut junction and they absorb solutes, water and waste from the surrounding hemolymph, and release them in the gut in the form of solid nitrogenous compounds (**Figure 1**) [3]. Though the malpighian tubules are drastically different from human kidneys, similarities have been seen in function and development.

The adult *Drosophila* gut is like a tube structure lined by an epithelial monolayer comprising of four cell types: intestinal stem cells (ISCs), absorptive enterocytes (ECs), secretory enteroendocrine (EE) cells, and enteroblasts (EBs) (**Figures 1** and **2**). Ectodermally derived foregut consists of esophagus, crop, and cardia (**Figures 1** and **2**). The crop is a diverticulated structure unique to Diptera. A complex array of valves and sphincters ensure passage of intestinal matter in and

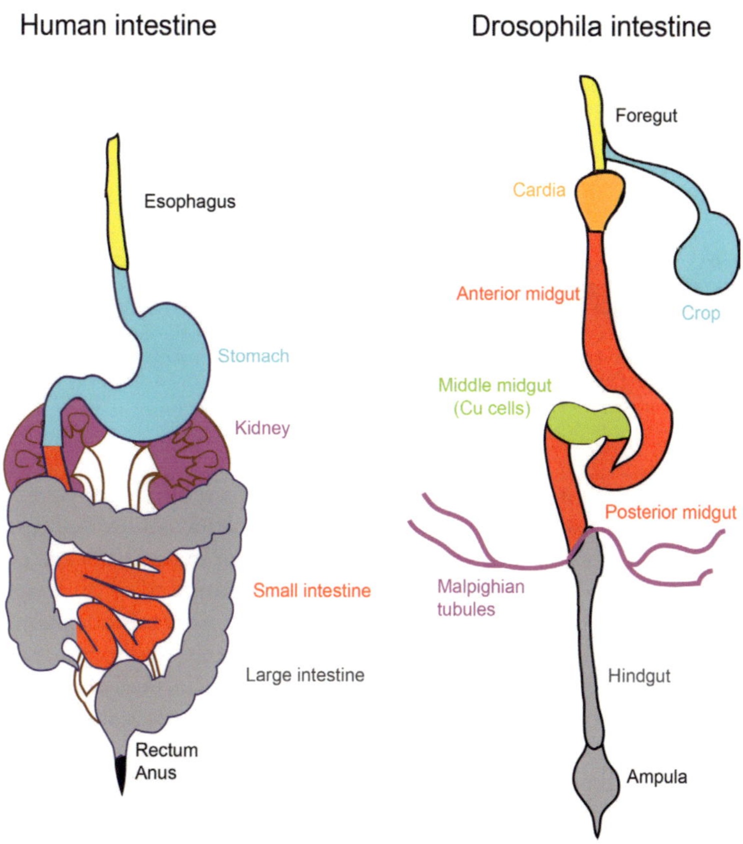

Figure 1.
Comparison between human and Drosophila gut. Organs with similar functions are coded with same colors. Drosophila contains many tissues/organs that functionally resemble to most essential human gastrointestinal system: Esophagus (foregut), midgut (small intestine) and large intestine (hindgut), stomach (crop), kidneys (malpighian tubules).

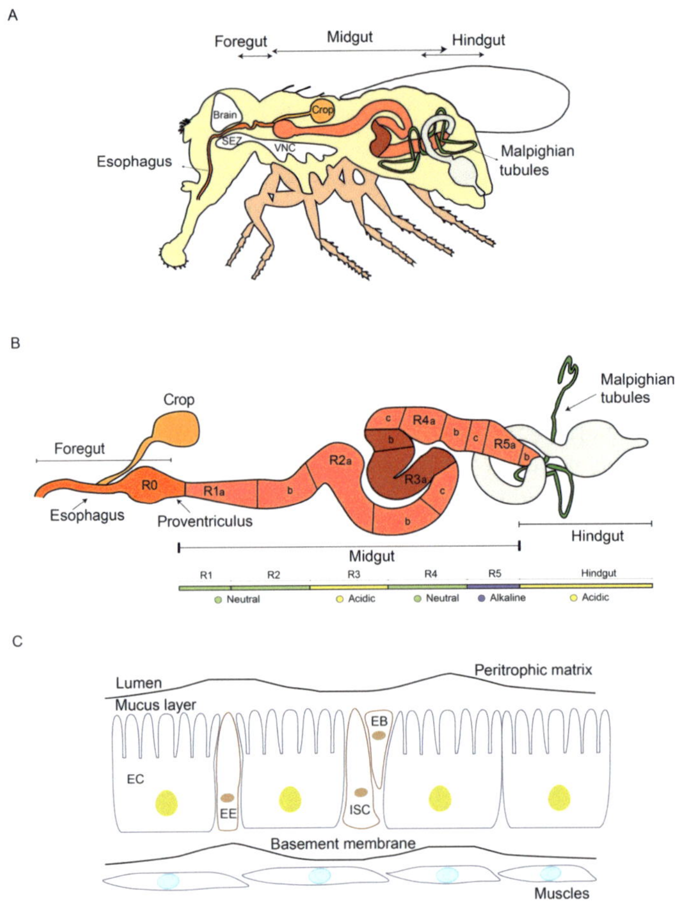

Figure 2.
Fly gut anatomy. (A) the Drosophila gut-brain axis consists of central nervous system (brain and ventral nerve cord-VNC; shown in white), gastrointestinal system (foregut, midgut and hindgut), crop and malpighian tubules. (B) the whole fly gut is divided into foregut (esophagus, crop and proventriculus), midgut (R1-R5), and hindgut (gray). pH divisions are also observed in midgut. (C) In Drosophila gut epithelia, the epithelium is protected by the peritrophic matrix and thin mucus layer apically and is covered in a basal lamina and visceral muscle cells. The fly midgut is composed of absorptive enterocytes (ECs) and secretory enteroendocrine cells (EE) that stand up from differentiation of the basally embedded intestinal stem cells (ISCs). Enteroblasts (EBs) are transient progenitors destined to differentiate into ECs.

out of the crop into the main alimentary canal. Crop function is poorly determined, its function in processes like early digestion, detoxification, microbial control, and food storage in flies has been speculated from other insects [4]. The cardia (or proventriculus) is a complex bulb-shaped structure composed of three epithelial layers. It makes the peritrophic matrix (site of antimicrobial peptide production) [5, 6] which may act as a valve, regulating the entry of ingested food into the midgut (**Figures 1, 2B** and **C**). Posterior to the cardia is endodermally derived midgut (with average length of 6 mm in adult flies), the main digestive/absorptive portion [7, 8] (**Figures 1, 2A** and **B**). It has been found that fly midgut epithelial cells have an opposite arrangement of junctions, with occluding junctions above *adherens* junctions, as in mammals [9]. The visceral muscle surrounds the epithelium. It is protected toward the lumen by secreted mucus and, posterior to the foregut, by a chitinous layer (peritrophic matrix) [10] (**Figure 2C**).

The fly midgut has been segmented into the anterior, middle and the posterior midgut (**Figures 1, 2A** and **B**). It has been further subdivided morphologically and molecularly into 10–14 regions (**Figure 2B**) [11–13]. Midgut regionalization has been seen in the muscles, trachea and neurons that surround it [12–15]. Physical properties (*e.g.*, luminal pH), histological and cellular features (villi size, lumen width), stem cell proliferation rates, and gene expression profiles [11–13, 16, 17] have been used to characterized all midgut regions. The middle midgut (R3) contains a copper cell region in R3ab, which produces gastric acid, followed by a large flat cell region (R3c) with uncertain role (**Figure 2B**). Two boundaries flanking this region are inflection points where the midgut folds stereotypically inside the body cavity.

The Malpighian tubules release at the junction between the midgut and hindgut (**Figures 1,2A** and **B**). The water/ion exchange occurs in the hindgut which consist of pylorus (a second valve-like structure), ileum, and rectum [7, 8]. The muscles that surround the epithelium in flies are striated, as opposed to the smooth muscles found in mammalian intestines [18]. An outer layer of longitudinal muscles found surrounding the midgut. Circular muscles are found to be present throughout the fly tract. Physiology of the intestine is maintained and regulated by autonomic innervation and by hormones. The tracheal system forms a branched structure surrounding the gut during development [15] and may influence epithelial regeneration in the adult. Owning to similarity of flies and human gut, we will be discussing further how gut of the flies is handled and controlled to understand about neural circuitry drawing it closer to the brain and diseases related to intestinal illnesses.

2.1 Intestinal anatomy of *Drosophila* and human

Both humans and fly intestines share similar tissue, anatomy and physiological function [19, 20]. Their gut are of endothelial origin in nature [21, 22] and comprise of an epithelial monolayer of columnar or cuboidal ECs. A series of sequential depressions called the crypts of Lieberkühn, along the small and large intestine, and protruding villi along the internal surface of the small intestine in mammalian intestinal epithelium maximize its surface area [23]. Extensive folding has not been reported in the *Drosophila* intestine. Cytoplasmic extensions (microvilli) of the apical side of ECs and ISCs [24] do increase the cellular surface area facing the gut lumen in both flies and mammals. Microvilli spread parallel to each other toward the lumen to form the brush border [24–26]. A layer of mucus present above the brush border protects the host from intestinal microbes. The peritrophic matrix in *Drosophila* gut helps to sequester microbes from coming in contact with the midgut and hindgut [27, 28] (**Figure 2C**).

In both flies and mammals, the epithelial monolayer is associated on its basal side on an extracellular collagenous matrix (known as basement membrane) [29]. A checkerboard of innervated and trachea-oxygenated longitudinal and circular muscles tissue underneath the basement membrane in flies drive the peristaltic movements [30] (**Figure 2C**). Mammalian intestine has a similar organization of intestinal external musculature in the outer layers where musculature is also innervated and oxygenated by a plexus of vasculature [31, 32]. Layers including, the submucosa, (a dense layer of connective tissue containing nerves and lymphatic and blood vessels); muscularis mucosae (an additional muscle layer); and the lamina propria underling the intestinal epithelium and contains connective tissue, lymph nodes (Peyer's patches), immune cells (leukocytes, and dendritic and mast cells), vessels and myofibroblasts [33], fill the space between the outer musculature and the basement membrane in mammals.

2.2 ISCs, ECs, and EE cells of fly gut

About 65% of human-disease causing genes are shared as a functional homolog in fruit flies. This shows conservation of genes and function at an evolutionary level. Fundamental processes such as digestion is also conserved from flies to humans. *Drosophila* intestine is composed of many cell types of heterogeneous developmental origin. Adult multipotent ISCs are present in both fly and mammalian guts [34–37]. ISCs differentiate throughout to self-renew and form new specialized cells namely absorptive type ECs and secretory type EE cells (**Figure 2C**) [38]. ECs and EE cells are found in both mammals and flies. ECs help in absorbing nutrients. EE cells release hormones for gut mobility and function. They also have antimicrobial purposes which are fulfilled by analogous cells in humans such as goblet and Paneth cells [39, 40]. *Drosophila* intestine produce both mucus and AMPs, but secretory cells (mucus-producing goblet cells) and the AMP-producing Paneth cells of mammalian gut have not been found in *Drosophila* midgut [28, 41]. Mammalian ECs and secretory cells are located at the bottom of the crypts and specifically express Lgr5 and/or Bmi1 (stem cell markers). Both of these cell types can give rise to all lineages of intestinal cells, including the transient amplifying (TA) cells that lie immediately above ISCs. TA gradually move upwards while maturing to eventually reach complete maturation close to the opening of the crypts. There is a continuous turnover of TA cells, which are either shed or become apoptotic upon maturation [23, 42].

The lineage of fly posterior midgut with only one type of mature absorptive cell and one main type of secretory cell is very simple. Although asymmetric ISC divisions in the fly midgut produce transient cells (EBs), these cells do not undergo further cell division and remain close to the ISCs before maturation. Fly midgut ISCs are situated basally and are broadly dispersed in the intestinal epithelium. The cellular composition and regeneration in *Drosophila* hindgut are interestingly similar to mammals. As in mammals, the ISCs of the hindgut are specified anteriorly and move posteriorly, as TA cells do, before their further differentiation in the posterior hindgut [37]. Nonetheless fly hindgut has not been examined as extensively as the midgut which has served as the prototype *Drosophila* tissue for the study of intestinal pathology [43–45].

2.3 The fly intestine functions

Like the regional specialization of digestive functions, the expression of digestive enzymes has also been found to confined to specific segments of the digestive tract in flies [12, 46, 47]. In addition to its roles in nutrient extraction and utilization, the digestive tract responds to the food and bacteria in its lumen. Digestion takes place in fly midgut [48] which can be further modulated by various factors like temperature, redox potential, pH, and intestinal transit [8, 48]. It has been shown that the expression and activity of digestive enzymes are tightly regulated in many insects like enzymes involved in the breakdown of sugars in flies are enriched in anterior (R1/R3) portions of the adult midgut and Peptidase genes express more posteriorly [47].

The enzymatic activity of the intestine is a key factor determining availability of certain nutrients. A substantial reduction of intestinal digestive enzyme activities (trypsin, chymotrypsin, aminopeptidase, and acetate esterase) has been reported in flies lacking EE cells [49]. Though not extensively investigated in *Drosophila,* modulation by nutrient quality and quantity, neuronal activity, and endocrine signals has been described in many insects [8, 50, 51]. Models suggesting role of ECs in integrating information about sugar uptake (sensed intrinsically in the intestine by Mondo-Bigmax) and the carbohydrate status of the fat body (relayed by TGF-β/Activin signaling) to modulate expression of the carbohydrate digestive enzymes have been proposed. Repression mechanism involving the TGF-β/Activin ligand Dawdle (Daw) which, upon refeeding with nutritious sugars (but not non-nutritious sugars) after a period of starvation, reduces the expression of carbohydrate digestive enzymes in the adult ECs [52]. Activation of the intracellular sugar sensor complex Mondo-Bigmax promotes the expression of both Daw and the transcription factor *sugarbabe (sug)* [53]. Sug further repress the expression of amylases. Low cholesterol in the diet upregulate expression of the Hr96 nuclear receptor (homologous to the vertebrate LXR receptor involved in regulated cholesterol homeostasis) [54]. Hr96 binds cholesterol and promotes the expression of genes involved in cholesterol homeostasis and lipid breakdown including Magro (Mag) [54–56]. Mag plays a dual role in breaking down intestinal cholesterol esters to maintain cholesterol homeostasis. It also enables triacylglyceride (TAG) breakdown, required for intestinal lipid absorption and peripheral fat accumulation [56, 57]. It has been suggested that intestinal mag expression can also repressed by a sugar-rich diet in a foxo-dependent manner [58]. Such a mechanism becomes chronically active in the aging intestine due to disrupting lipid homeostasis and activation of JNK pathway affecting the metabolic homeostasis [58].

2.3.1 Role in nutrients absorption

Carbohydrates: A diverse array of transporters internalizes simple sugars into the ECs for further digestion and absorption [59] in insects like Glucose transporters, the GLUT/Slc2 family of facilitative glucose transporters and the SGLT/Slc5 family of Na^{+}-glucose symporters [60–64]. GLUT-like gene has been described in flies [65]. *Drosophila* genome harbors homologs of other glucose transporters including a homolog of SWEET family of sugar transporters [66, 67] a disaccharide transporter Slc45–1 [68]; trehalose transporters (Tret1–1 and Tret1–2) [69] and Slc45–1 (can transport sucrose) [68, 70]. The possible intestinal activity of many of these transporters deserves further investigation.

Proteins: A mixture of amino acids, di- and tri-peptides are products of protein break down. This chemical diversity is handled by a broad range of apical and basolateral transport systems (many are homologous to known mammalian transporter systems) [59, 71]. *Drosophila* homologs of cationic amino acid transporters [72], ion-dependent and independent amino acid transporters for neutral amino acids [73–76] and oligopeptide transporters [77, 78] are some examples. Intestinal expression of amino acid transporters Pathetic [74] has also been reported. Minidiscs [73], NAT1 and other Slc6 family members [75, 79], and the oligopeptide transporters Yin and CG2930, with enriched expression in proventriculus/hindgut and midgut [77, 78] has been shown. The nature, physiological modulation, and significance of many of these amino acid/oligopeptide transporters remains to be investigated.

Lipids and sterols: Intestinal lipid transport in *Drosophila* is still undetermined. Intestinal cells absorb free fatty acids, glycerol, mono- and diacylglycerols, and phospholipid derivatives (products of lipid digestion) along with dietary sterols. Diffusion and emulsification have been proposed for absorption [80]. Vertebrates emulsify by covering lipids with bile salts, but in insects emulsification is achieved by forming fatty acid-amino acid and glycolipid complexes, as well as fatty acids and lysophospholipid micelles [80]. In ECs, the products of lipid breakdown are used to resynthesize diacylglycerols and TAG. They get packaged together with cholesterol and fat body-derived carrier proteins to form lipoprotein particles and trafficked throughout the body [81] ensuring that the products of lipid breakdown are kept at low concentrations inside the ECs, which may facilitate diffusion. Mutants in which lipoprotein secretion from the fat body is compromised has revealed both anterior and posterior midgut regions as sites of lipid efflux [81]. The absorption of sterols is crucial to insects as they cannot synthesize sterols and require a dietary source of sterol for the synthesis of the steroid molting hormone ecdysone. In *Drosophila*

Niemann-Pick Chomologs-Npc1a and Npc2a are broadly required for intracellular sterol trafficking [82], whereas Npc1b is expressed in the midgut and is required for intestinal sterol absorption [83].

Changes in the expression of p38 kinase or the Atf3 and Foxo transcription factors cause accumulation of neutral lipid in ECs [58, 84]. It has been shown that neutral lipid increase following depletion of the EE hormone Tk [85], or in sterile female flies after mating [86]. It has been suggested that activation of intestinal lipogenesis is key to survival in diet-restricted flies. Indeed, nutrient scarcity induces expression of the sugar sensor transcription factor *sug* in the intestine which, in turn, promotes intestinal lipogenesis. Internal nutritional challenges may be equally dependent on deployment of these intestinal adaptations [86].

2.3.2 Intestinal pH

Many animals generate localized regions of low pH inside the intestinal lumen to facilitate protein breakdown, absorption of minerals and metals, and limit the survival of ingested microbes. While mammalian digestion takes place in acidic conditions, insect digestion occurs at neutral or basic pH including *Drosophila* (neutral or mildly alkaline). Luminal pH does, however, display consistent transitions along the length of the intestine and becomes strongly acidic (pH 2–4) in the copper cell region of both larvae and adults [24, 87, 88]. Posterior to this region, the midgut lumen becomes mildly alkaline again (pH 7–9), but is again acidified in the hindgut (pH 5), partly as a result of discharges from the malpighian tubules. Diet affects the acidity of rectal ampulla where final pH adjustments may take place [14]. Copper cells are specialized ECs with a highly invaginated apical membrane, similar to the mammalian gastric parietal cells [89]. During aging in adult flies, genetic interference with copper cell identity or their progressive loss are associated with loss of gut acidity [90].

The contribution of five ion transporters enriched in the acidic region have been studied [88]. These include: the potassium/chloride symporter Kazachoc (Kcc), a member the Slc12 family of electroneutral cation-chloride transporters (express in intestine) [91, 92]; the Slowpoke pore-forming subunit of a calcium-activated K^+ channel (express in neurons, muscles, tracheal cells, and two types of midgut ECs in the copper and iron cell regions) [93]; the ligand-gated chloride channel pHCL-2 which, in addition to regulating fluid secretion in malpighian tubules (express in the copper cell, iron, and large flat cell regions of the midgut) [94, 95]; the carbonic anhydrase CAH1; and the bicarbonate/chloride exchanger CG8177, belonging to the Slc4a1–3 subfamily of anion exchangers (express in a specific midgut pattern similar to that of pHCl-2) [96]. Collectively, these findings suggest that the transport of H^+, Cl^-, K^+, and $HCO3^-$ contributes to acid generation in the *Drosophila* midgut.

2.3.3 Water and osmolytes

Flies extract water from their diet to maintain hydration and ionic balance. This compensates for substantial water loss resulting from metabolic and physiological processes. Although malpighian tubules are important for this process, but intestine also contributes. Water absorption from the food occurs in the insect midgut and in rectal pads of rectum [8]. The rectal pads are also the crucial site for reabsorption of ions. Ions and water can cross the intestinal epithelium through or between cells and their transport play an important role in the maintenance of ion gradients that sustain active transport in the intestinal epithelium. The scanning ion-selective electrode technique (SIET) provides a way to probe intestinal gradients for ions such as K^+, Na^+, H^+, or Cl^- [24, 97]. K^+ and Na^+ absorption occur largely in the large flat cell and posterior regions of the midgut and, also in the anterior hindgut in the case of Na^+ [97]. The two *Drosophila* Nha members express in intestine epithelia and their ubiquitous knockdown decrease survival, especially under Na^+ stress [12, 98–100]. Including kcc, four different genes encoding homologs of the cation-Cl^- Slc12 cotransporters express in osmoregulatory organs (gut, anal pads, and Malpighian tubules) [91, 92].

2.3.4 Metal ions

Metal ions such as copper, iron and zinc are essential micronutrients required for the correct folding and activity of a broad range of enzymes. The contribution of the intestine to metal homeostasis has not been extensively investigated but midgut regions, the Cu cell and Fe regions, are the most proposed sites of metal ion absorption. The Cu cell region turns bright luminescent orange upon Cu ingestion due to the fixation of copper by metallothionein [101, 102], and appears to be an important site of accumulation of ingested radioactively labeled Cu [101, 103]. The Fe cell region in R4a stains by Prussian blue and also accumulates exogenously administered radioactive Fe [101, 104]. Many studies have confirmed the roles for the Cu/Fe regions by exploring the molecular machinery involved in the intestinal uptake, intracellular trafficking, and efflux of metal ions.

2.3.5 Transit and excretion

Nutrient extraction and utilization may get affected by the passage of food along the alimentary canal and by its subsequent excretion. Transport of food to travel the entire length of the digestive tract takes less than 1 hour [105] in flies. As suggested, the amount of food retained in the crop is much larger in starved flies then refed flies than in flies fed *ad libitum* [2, 105]. Starvation also lowers defecation rate long before the gut is emptied [14]. Chronic food deprivation during the larval life has been shown to subsequently increase excretion in adult flies [106]. The hindgut may contribute to the pH adjustment of excreta, which may help offset the excess acid produced [14]. Changes in intestinal fluid retention are likely to involve the distal part of the hindgut (rectum and/or rectal glands), as known for its role in water reabsorption in other insects [8], and may help maximize absorption at a time of high nutritional demand. Such a mechanism is partly mediated by the sex peptide transferred by males during copulation [14, 107], affecting the HGN1 (Hindgut Neuron1) subset of hindgut-innervating neurons [14]. Further investigations are required to clarify the connections between intestinal fluid retention, absorption, peristalsis, and excretion where crop may prove to be a key organ, given that its differential peristalsis and engorgement can determine whether food is temporarily stored or released into the midgut for digestion and absorption [4]. Apart from affecting the nervous system, mutations in the *drop-dead* gene are also associated with increased crop size, reduced transfer of ingested food from the crop to the midgut, and reduced defecation [108, 109].

3. ENS and GBA

The ENS in humans, equivalent to GBA in flies is a part of the peripheral nervous system (PNS) that governs the running of the neurons which influence the GI. It is exploited nowadays in flies to understand more about how the two organs affect one another and lead to decisions regarding appetite, feeding mechanisms, taste preference and how to deal with hunger and satiety. How taste receptors detect different nutrients in the gut remains to be explored.

3.1 Gustatory receptors in gut

3.1.1 Humans

In humans, G-protein coupled receptors (GPCR) are involved in detection of five common tastes- sweet, salty, bitter, sour and umami. T1R family of taste receptors determine sweet and umami flavor. T2R family includes the bitter receptors [110]. Sweet taste receptors (T1R family) are found in intestinal tract as well as EE cells [111]. T1R1, T1R2, T1R3 and α-gustducin are expressed in the stomach, intestine and colon of humans and mice [112]. Cells of duodenal villi show co-localization of T1R1, T1R3 and α-gustuducin. Mammalian Gustducin protein is involved in bitter and sweet taste signaling and detection [113, 114]. α-subunit of gustducin is expressed in gastric cells and may play a role in nutrient detection [115–117] in rats and mice. Present in the mucosal lining of mammals and taste cells of the epithelium suggesting its possible role in taste uncovering on exposure to luminal contents [118]. Expression of T2R receptors in mouse GI tract including mT2R119 and mT2R108 has been looked into. mT2R119 expression is found in gastric and intestinal tissues, tongue and liver [115] like mT2R134 [118]. mT2R108, mT2R138 are present in the fundus, antrum, duodenum and tongue (not in liver) [119].

It has been found that sweet taste receptors stimulated in rat intestine influence and increase glucose absorption [120] through GLUT (glucose transporter) [121]. Presence of sugar in the diet galvanizes ECs into action to release hormones which in turn activate SGLT (Na^+ / glucose cotransporter) [122, 123]. Similar results are shown in sheep where sugar receptor / sensor present on the luminal membrane stimulates SGLT1 via cAMP and G-protein dependent pathway [124]. Equine T1R2 (homologous to cows and pigs) is expressed on the luminal membrane of EE cells in the small intestine. In response to increased sugars, T1R2 along with T1R3, stimulates SGLT1 and enhances the ability of gut to absorb more glucose [125]. Analysis of in vitro line of ECs suggest that T1R2 and T1R3 detect sweet taste and exposure to sucralose increases release of hormones such as GIP (Gastric Inhibitory Polypeptide) and GLP (Glucagon like peptide) which further activate glucose activation and metabolism. An inhibitor of these receptors inhibits glucose metabolism suggesting these receptors present in the gut alter feeding mechanisms and post-ingestion decisions [120, 121].

3.1.2 Flies

Gustatory system in *Drosophila* includes the taste receptors spread all over its body including proboscis, legs, wings and ovipositor. These receptors help in detecting the appropriate nutrient rich food, and avoid toxic chemicals. Because of the similarities in structure and functioning of mammalian intestine and flies' gut, the expression of gustatory receptors (Grs) in flies gut has been investigated. Using Gal4/UAS system, 15 Grs (*Gr28b.e, Gr33a, Gr36c, Gr39a.a, Gr39a.b, Gr43a, Gr64a, Gr93a, Gr28a, Gr59a, Gr28b.a, Gr28b.b, Gr28b.c, Gr28b.d, Gr58c*) are found to be expressed in gut, but only 12 of these Grs labeled EE cells in the midgut of fly [126]. Different nutrient sources to monitor the activation of EE cells in midgut have been used. With minimal sucrose, EE cells show high activation in middle midgut [127]. Other than sugar, protein cues also leads to the activation of EE cells but in posterior midgut, suggesting a role in the detection of nutrients in the diet including amino acids specifically. These cells do not get activated by carbohydrates per se and only react to proteins and amino acids. This subset of EE cells also co-expresses neuropeptides such as Diuretic hormone 31 (*DH31*) and Tachykinin (*Tk*). These brain-gut peptides get involved in feeding pathways and nutrient sensing mechanism

[85, 127, 128]. In other organisms such as rat, it has been shown that Gq-coupled calcium sensing receptor such as CaSR, expressed in EE cells is involved in amino acid sensing [129]. Taste cells or EE cells in mammals also produce several peptides which have roles in feeding, satiety, hunger as well as metabolism. They include Glucagon, Neuropeptide Y, Peptide YY and some others [130]. *Drosophila* has homologous proteins for these and other peptides which points toward obvious conservation of these peptides and their functions.

3.2 Gut-brain Neural Circuits

3.2.1 Humans

Nutrient signaling and sensing are fundamental processes that animals including humans and flies undergo [131]. Proper coordination and communication between gut and brain is necessary to regulate metabolic homeostasis and physiology in all animals. In this regard, many research groups have shown the role of enteric neurons and endocrine signals as important mediators of these processes. The way the enteric nervous system communicates to the brain via neural circuits is a multifaceted question and poorly explored. In mammals such as humans, alterations in neuropeptides and brain – gut hormone levels can derail people otherwise on the path to a healthy life. These changes can also lead to diseases such as neurodegenerative diseases, metabolic syndrome and diabetes [132].

Gluconeogenesis is a biochemical pathway by which animals make sugars from non-carbohydrate precursors and sources [133]. It is used to regulate homeostasis and a stable internal state in post – fed state [134]. Studies in rats showed that stimulation of intestinal gluconeogenesis (IGN) sends a signal from sodium – glucose co- transporters present at the intestinal mucosa to the brain, initiating a neural gut – brain axis [135–137]. Diets rich in protein [138–140] and fiber [141] promote IGN stressing on the importance of nutrient sensing for initiating several gut – brain axis [137]. It has been found that μ – opoid receptors (MOR) regulate IGN. These receptors (present in the nerves in the portal vein wall) react to neuropeptides to stimulate a gut – brain neural circuit that affects IGN, hunger and satiety mechanisms [141]. Further analysis of MOR deficient mice shows the role of MORs in regulating food intake, referred as "reward" system [142, 143]. Analyses of MOR-knockouts (MOR-KO) demonstrate how they play a role in managing satiety effects of alimentary proteins, through a neural gut-brain circuit [140].

Vagus nerve (VN; pneumogastric nerve) is the longest cranial nerve [144] in humans which runs from the medulla oblongata in brain to colon in GI [145]. It innervates other structures as well such as larynx, pharynx, heart and lungs thus affects digestive, cardiovascular and respiratory system – all at one [146]. Vagal efferent send down signals from the brain to gut, which accounts for about 10% – 20% of all the nerve fibers. Remaining 80% is accounted for by the vagal afferents carrying information from the gut to the brain [147]. Vagal sensory neurons in the GI keep an eye on stomach volume and luminal contents through different neural circuits [148]. VN contains and branches into several sensory neurons (~2300 in mouse) that further innervate and render support and supply to other internal organs. A variety of sensory neurons, one side facing the brainstem and the terminal one facing the organ such as GI [149] have been revealed. Free terminals of vagal afferents are rooted within lamina propria of intestinal villi [148]. Some mammalian models like in cat and rat, it has been shown how these sensory neurons detect different nutrients in diets with the help of unambiguous and explicit fibers [150–152]. Vagal afferent endings in the intestine express several mechanosensitive as well as chemical receptors [153]. Glucagon- like peptide 1 (GLP1) is a gut hormone receptor that intercedes the nutrient sensing mechanism via VN [154]. GLP1R (GLP1 receptor) is present in many cells [155]. Agonists for GLP1R show how it affects brain further proving its presence in both, gut and brain [156]. Another receptor of vagal afferents, GPR65 near the intestinal villi, plays a role in nutrient detection drawing attention to how these sensory neurons are a part of the gut – brain axis [157, 158]. It detects serotonin and impact gut motility [147]. Such receptors detect several hormones present in the gut, like choleocystokinin (CKK), ghrelin and leptin which play a role in the regulation of hunger and satiety [159–161]. Because of its role in gut motility and mobility, VN and its afferent neurons present in the gut play a role in Intestinal Bowel Syndrome (IBS) [162] and new treatment plans around the same are being looked at in rat [162] and mice [158] models.

To take the findings in vagal nerves forward, nerves allowing communication of cNST (caudal nucleus of the solitary tract) with gut were focused on. Information about sugar detection to cNST via gut – brain axis is a topic of research nowadays. In live mice, it is noticed that glucose detection by cNST is robust and VN transaction silences that activation [163]. Nodose ganglion of vagus nerve when silenced prevents the sugar preference of cNST [163] suggesting the presence of a physical gut – brain axis. It has been shown that inactivation of sugar-activated cSNT prevents the mice to choose sugar from water or an artificial sweetener [163]. This study specifically calls attention to how organisms have paths for detecting nutrient signals, sensing them in the diet and also have circuitries to carry forward the signals and communicate with the rest of the body, purposely the brain.

3.2.2 *Drosophila*

With the help of several markers and reporter genes, it is found that *Drosophila* intestine is innervated by neurons- efferent and sensory [14]. Other studies have stated that fly's gut receives innervations from three regions – stomato-gastric nervous system [164–167]; the *corpora cardiaca*, neurosecretory structures [168]; and neurons located in the CNS extending their axons toward three different portions of the digestive tract [14, 169–172]. The expression of Ret receptor tyrosine kinase in gut innervating neurons in adult fly has recently been shown to contribute to the development of stomato- gastric ganglia in flies [173, 174]. In contrast to mammalian gastrointestinal tracts which are profusely innervated throughout their entire length, the innervation of the fly's digestive tract is restricted to only three different portions. The first is the anterior-most slice comprising the pharynx, esophagus, crop and anterior midgut. The second is midgut/hindgut junction and third is the posterior hindgut [14, 164, 167, 172]. Muscle valves present in all three regions support and regulate peristaltic regulation and intestinal transit functions of gut-innervating neurons. Most neurites terminate on the visceral muscles and some reach the underlying epithelium, particularly in the esophagus, proventriculus, pyloric valve, and rectal ampulla [14, 175] suggesting neuronal regulation of epithelial properties such as secretion or absorption. In flies, not all innervation is efferent. Gustatory neuron afferents from the pharynx send their axons to the suboesophageal zone (SEZ, the primary taste center of the fly brain), where they target a distinct domain adjacent to the projections of other (leg/labellum) gustatory receptor neurons [176–179]. Dendrites of peripheral sensory neurons can be seen in the anterior and posterior-most regions of the digestive tract [14], and appear most abundant in the esophagus and anterior midgut.

In the anterior portion of adult and larval midgut, serotonin positive neurites and various neuropeptides including Akh, Dh44, Myosuppressin, and possibly Allatostatin C and FMRFamide (or an FMRFamide-like peptide such as the NPY-like neuropeptide short neuropeptide F [sNPF]) [131, 168, 172, 180–182] have been described suggesting chemical diversity of enteric innervation. Four serotonergic neurons are found to innervate the enteric nervous system in fly larva. These neurons project from the antennal nerve (AN) near the SEZ and extend throughout the ENs [14]. These projections end at the anterior region of the midgut and are primarily around the proventriculus region and the foregut. These innervations are considered structurally analogous to the mammalian VN because of similar projections from the brain to the different structures of the foregut. It is yet to be seen if there are functional similarities as well [172].

Pigment- dispersing factor (Pdf), Ion transport peptide, and Proctolin positive neurites have been reported in the larval and adult hindgut [169, 183–186]. All three innervated regions receive insulinergic innervation from the CNS; the *pars intercerebralis* (PI) insulin-producing cells extend axons beyond the ring gland that innervate the anterior midgut and crop in adult flies (**Figure 3**), and the insulin-like peptide 7 (Ilp7)-producing neurons of the abdominal ganglion innervate the midgut/hindgut junction and the rectal ampulla [170, 187]. Interestingly, putative dendritic termini of both kinds of insulin-producing neurons have been found in very close proximity in the CNS. This data suggests the release of different insulins to the different portions of the digestive tract may be co-regulated centrally [14].

Functional studies of insect innervation have primarily focused on the control of peristalsis and peptide hormone secretion so far. Studies of peristaltic regulation in flies have primarily concerned the effects of neuropeptides (Allatostatins, Myosuppressin, or Drosulfakinins) on *ex vivo* intestinal preparations [188–191] ascribing distinct roles for these peptides in the modulation of crop or anterior midgut contractions in adults. Both intestinal and non-intestinal roles of Pdf-expressing neurons in the regulation of muscle peristalsis for a set of hindgut-innervating neurons located in the abdominal ganglion of the CNS have been demonstrated [171, 192]. It is found that this neural source of Pdf (a neuropeptide related to mammalian vasoactive intestinal polypeptides, known for its roles in the central circadian clock) promotes peristalsis of hindgut muscles and sustains the defecation cycle in larvae [192]. Pdf can also promote contractions of the muscles of the ureters, the proximal part of the malpighian tubules [171]. Hence, the digestive tract is used by some enteric neurons as a docking site to exert their functions on other internal organs at some distance.

Recently epithelial roles for gut-innervating neurons e.g. role in the control of fluid balance have been revealed by a semi-automated analysis of defecation behavior in adult flies, providing quantitative readouts for food intake, fluid/ion balance, and intestinal transit [14, 193]. The HGN1 neurons (2–5 CNS neurons located in the posterior segments of the abdominal ganglion) innervate the hindgut and the rectum (**Figure 3**), with a subset of their neurites projecting through the visceral muscles to reach the underlying epithelium [14]. HGN1 neuronal silencing experiments resulted in increased defecation rate. These neurons are shown to be required for the post-mating changes in intestinal fluid retention due to their epithelial innervation. It has been established that HGN1 neurons and the Pdf hindgut-innervating neurons have their direct action on the hindgut and anal sphincter muscles [192]. A role for gut-innervating neurons in the maintenance of epithelial turnover has also been suggested by the finding of anatomical proximity between enteric neurites in the posterior midgut and adult somatic intestinal progenitors, and the reduced ISC to EC differentiation resulting from downregulating Hedgehog (Hh) signaling (albeit pan-neuronally) [194]. The more anterior innervation of the proventriculus may also play a role in maintaining gut permeability. This is inferred from the finding that inactivation of a relatively broad subset of neurons, including a subset of anterior midgut-innervating neurons results in an abnormal

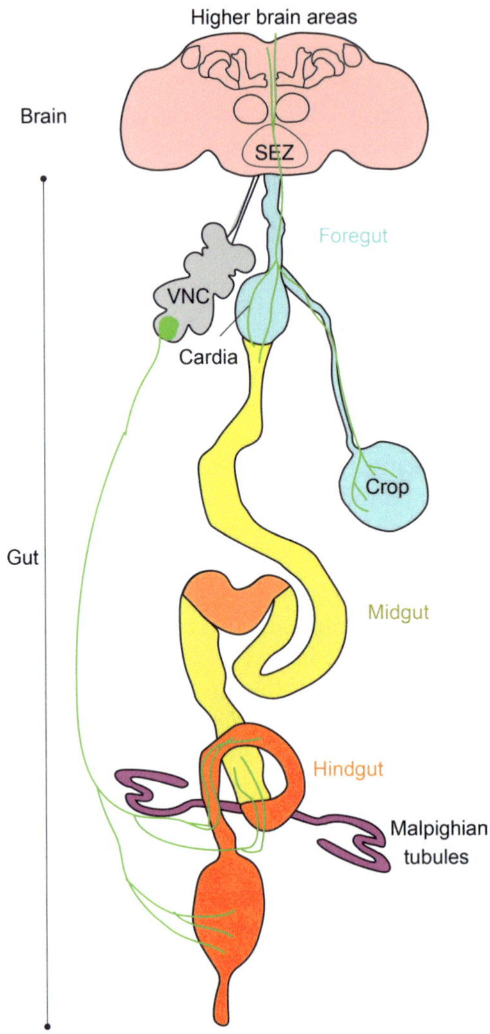

Figure 3.
Innervation of adult Drosophila intestine. Enteric innervation (shown in green) along Drosophila gut-brain axis (central nervous system and gastrointestinal system). Neurons from brain and enteric ganglia innervate anterior portion of gut. Neurons from ventral nerve cord send axons in the hindgut which also extend anteriorly along the posterior midgut. Adopted from Miguel-Aliaga et al., 2018.

proventricular structure, increased permeability of the epithelial barrier, and increased susceptibility to oral bacterial infection: all suggestive of defects in the production of peritrophic matrix [175].

In adult flies, inactivation of insulin-producing neurons results in contrasting effects on the hyperphagic response triggered by nutrient scarcity. Silencing of the insulin-producing cells of the brain PI that innervates the anterior midgut lowered this response, whereas silencing of the hindgut-innervating Ilp7 neurons increased it, and also resulted in higher circulating glucose [14, 195]. Not much is known about the importance of sparse sensory innervation of the intestine. One remarkable exception are the pharyngeal taste neurons. *Pox-neuro* (*poxn*) mutant flies lack gustatory function in the legs and labial palps but retain expression of sweet taste receptors in their pharynx and a preference for sweet compounds, highlighting the pharyngeal contribution to sugar detection [196, 197]. Further understanding of the taste circuit relaying this pharyngeal sensory signal is provided by IN1 neurons (subset of interneurons) receiving input from the pharyngeal sensory neurons.

The activity of IN1 neurons is exquisitely dependent on the amount and duration of feeding [198]. Posterior to the pharynx, in the gastrointestinal tract, the contribution of sensory innervation to nutritional homeostasis remains to be investigated.

Post-ingestive sensory feedback from the gut has been assumed to inhibit feeding based on work in other insects for example severing the recurrent nerve or the medial abdominal nerve, which transmit information from the gut to the brain, results in overconsumption in blowflies [199]. Work done in flies lends support to this idea; whereas severing the medial abdominal nerve did not disturb food consumption, severing the recurrent nerve elevated consumption of sucrose but not water or bitter tasting solutions [200]. The existence of neuronal stretch receptors on the gut that monitor the volume of ingested food is supported by both neurophysiological and anatomical data in numerous other insects [4, 80, 199, 201]. However, the existence and molecular nature of these receptors in *Drosophila* remains to be established. Interestingly, six peripheral neurons on the proventriculus have been shown to express the gustatory receptor Gr43a (function as fructose receptor), which is also expressed by some pharyngeal neurons [202–204]. These proventricular neurons extend dendritic processes into the foregut lumen, and a subset of their axons innervate the midgut, whereas another subset extends along the esophagus, forming a nerve bundle with axons of gustatory receptor neurons projecting toward SEZ. Hence, they may relay nutritional information back to central/more anterior neurons or act locally on the gut. Establishing their roles will require genetic tools able to target the enteric subset without affecting the central or peripheral Gr43a-expressing neurons.

4. Enteroendocrine hormones, neuropeptides and signals

4.1 Humans

The gut–brain transmission systems involve both circulation-based endocrine-like and neuronal communication routes [205]. Neuropeptides (transmitters or neurosecretory) act as messenger molecules of enteric, sensory, autonomic and central neurons. Several peptide families have been found in both brain and gut. They act as neuropeptides and/or gut hormones and have significantly contributed to the understanding of gut brain interaction. Central and peripheral neurons together with EE cells in the GI tract and other endocrinologically active cells produce variety of peptides [206–211] including hormones peptide YY (PYY) and pancreatic polypeptide (PP); neuropeptide Y (NPY), on the other hand [212]. These and other peptide families represented by glucagon-like peptide (GLP), ghrelin, cholecystokinin (CCK), corticotropin-releasing factor (CRF), leptin, osteocalcin and insulin (the last three are extra intestinal endocrine peptides) act on specific and genetically related groups of receptors that are expressed by distinct cells in the periphery and CNS. For their functional roles, endocrine peptides and neuropeptides are relevant for the regulation of digestion, control of food intake, metabolic homeostasis, and the impact of GI signals on sensation, emotion, affect, and cognition. Disturbances of the gut microbiota–brain axis result in changes of the expression and activity of many neuropeptides and their receptors in the CNS. Neuropeptides are therefore important secondary messengers of gut microbes in cerebral neuro circuitries that mediate the alterations in brain function and behavior that take place in response to changes in the GI microbial community [212]. Together it is emerging that neuropeptide systems such as NPY, CRF, ghrelin, and brain-derived neurotrophic factor (BDNF) play a particular role in the cerebral manifestations of gut microbiota perturbations.

In rats, choleocystokinin and glutamate neuro-epithelial circuit makes the communication between the brain and intestinal lumen possible stressing on the importance of a physical gut – brain axis [213]. It has been proposed that the physical connection between vagal nodose neurons and EE cells is present in rats which leads to regulation of gastrointestinal functions [213]. Intragastric nutrient infusion and optical readings of AgRP (Agouti-related protein) neurons in live and awake mice [214] suggest AgRP neurons affect long term homesostasis and energy balance of the body and do not get altered by minute changes in nutrient levels [215]. AgRP neurons get inhibited by high levels of satiation signals such as CCK and PYY (peptide YY). Receptors for both CCK and PYY are expressed by vagal afferent neurons' terminals that innervate GI [159] suggesting a possibility of a physical connection between the gut and brain carrying the message from one point to another [216].

4.2 *Drosophila* hormones and neuropeptides

Apart from using neurons, fly intestine can also communicate with other organs through systemic signals. Intestinal physiology is modulated by both extrinsic hormonal signals (emanating from endocrine glands, neuroendocrine structures, or organs such as the fat body) and by its own peptide hormones, produced by EE cells. In turn, gut-derived signals such as EE cell-derived peptide hormones can have long-range effects on other internal organs. EE cells accounts for 5–10% of midgut epithelial cells in flies compared to 0.4–0.6% in the mammalian small intestine [217–219]. Majority of them express peptide hormones, often more than one and with regional stereotypy [219–222]. The developmental program of EE cells shares similarities with that of neurons, probably reflecting a common phylogenetic origin [223–225]. Consistent with this idea, all known EE peptide hormones (exception insect CCHamides) [226] are also produced by the brain. Acting through these hormones, EE cells may play "neural-like" roles in regulating intestinal physiology and conveying intestinal as well as nutritional state to other cell types or organs. These roles are particularly prominent in the midgut given the relatively sparse innervation of midgut region. *Scute* mutant flies lacks all EE cells and show normal food intake and fertility, but are short-lived and display abnormal intestinal homeostasis [49].

A role for EE cells on muscle peristalsis has been suggested by the finding that ablation of Diuretic hormone 31 (Dh31)-expressing EE cells or Dh31 downregulation both reduce muscle peristalsis in the larval anterior midgut, which may function as a valve to minimize mixing of acidified and non-acidified food in the acidic region of the midgut [227]. Adult EE cells produce Bursicon. Signaling through the Bursicon/DLGR2 receptor in visceral muscle, represses the production of the visceral muscle-derived mitogen Vein and, consequently, ISC proliferation. Another study found in *scute* mutants, depletion on EE cells compromised the nutrient-dependent midgut growth that occurs post-eclosion [49] partly by the lack of EE cell-derived Tk, which normally promotes expression of the visceral muscle-derived Ilp3 insulin-like peptide shown to sustain ISC proliferation and nutrient-dependent midgut growth [49, 228]. A recent comparative fly–mouse–human study has pointed to neurotensin-like signaling from EE cells to ECs in flies, with effects on lipid metabolism and AMPK activation. Indeed, expression of mouse neurotensin from *Drosophila* EE cells (and possibly also peripheral sensory neurons) promoted lipid accumulation in both standard and high-fat diets in the midgut, fat body, and oenocytes, and also decreased gut AMPK activation [229]. The effect was dependent on expression of the Pyrokinin 1 receptor in ECs, but did not seem to be mediated by EE cell-derived Pyrokinin 1, pointing to an involvement of a different ligand [229].

A high-sugar diet leads to increased midgut EE cell number and enhanced production of EE-derived Activin ligand (Activin-β not Daw) [230] suggesting systemic roles for EE-derived peptide hormones. Mirroring the activin-mediated fat-to-gut signaling involved in sucrose repression, midgut-derived Activin-β binds to the TGF-β receptor Baboon in fat cells which, in turn, leads to enhancement of Akh signaling it the fat body and consequent hyperglycemia [230]. CCHamides are insect hormones [231, 232] and their expression is promoted by nutrient availability and sites of expression include the gut EE cells, a subset of central neurons and, possibly, the fat body [226, 233, 234]. Their receptors are expressed in the nervous system including the insulin-producing neurons, and are absent from the gut [226, 234]. Although not strictly gut-derived, a new peptide hormone produced not by EE cells, but by an adjacent secretory gland may have provided the most compelling example to date of gut-to-brain communication. Indeed, Limostatin (Lst) peptide is produced by the *corpus cardiacum*: the Akh-producing gland which, in the adult, is found adjacent to the hypocerebral ganglion on the gastrointestinal tract, at the junction between the esophagus and anterior midgut. Lst is released in response to nutrient restriction and suppresses insulin production by the insulin-producing cells of the brain PI. *Lst* mutant flies accumulate excess fat and display phenotypes associated with insulin excess [235].

In animals with a vascular system, peptides secreted from EE cells can enter the bloodstream and reach tissues at a considerable distance, ranging from other cells in the digestive tract to brain centers regulating appetite [236]. Nutrient availability can also affect the number of EE cells; signaling through the nuclear hormone receptor Hr96, dietary lipids control EE differentiation during the first few days of adult life, providing another way to couple nutrient availability with tissue architecture and physiology [237]. Modulation of intestinal physiology by systemic signals has also been looked into [220, 221]. Control of epithelial turnover by insulin-like peptides or JH (juvenile hormone), and the coupling of dietary availability of sugars with EC digestive enzyme production via the fat body-derived Activin ligand Daw are some examples. The actions of the diuretic peptide Leucokinin (Lk), secreted into the circulation from CNS-derived nerves that terminate at the abdominal wall [14, 238, 239] is an another example. Downregulation of either this peptide or its receptor leads to abnormal excreta and extreme fluid retention that can rupture the abdominal wall [14]. Finally, a link between energy balance, intestinal permeability, and immunity has been suggested by the finding that sNPF is a target of the Crtc/CREB energy sensing pathway, and functions to maintain epithelial barrier integrity acting through its receptor in ECs [240]. Although the precise source of sNPF remains to be established, tissue-specific genetic and expression data points to roles in neurosecretory cells [240], consistent with roles as a neuroendocrine hormone or in gut-innervating neurons. Gut can also produce long-range signals to affect the physiology of other organs, for example by production of the signaling protein Hh by larval EC. Circulating Hh regulates developmental timing by controlling ecdysteroid production in the prothoracic gland, and is required for mobilization of fat body TAG stores during starvation [241].

Other functions of brain-gut peptides and hormones include detection and utilization of nutrients during hunger, stress or normal conditions. Diuretic hormone 44 (Dh44), a homolog of the mammalian corticotropin –releasing -hormone (CRH) activate by nutritive sugars. Disturbed activity of Dh44 neurons leads to fail to select nutritive sugars [131]. These neurons localized to PI in adult brain, counterpart of mammalian hypothalamus [242] are filled with neurosecretory cells [131]. Dh44 conveys information from Dh44 neurons to Dh44 receptor R1 neurons in the brain and R2 cells in the gut suggesting requirement for nutrient selection. Artificial activation of these neurons causes rapid PER and it has been suggested that Dh44 is necessary and sufficient for gut motility and excretion in flies [131]. Both Dh44 neurons and the gut-innervating insulin-producing neurons of the PI are innervated by Hugin-producing neurons that suppress food intake and induce locomotion, providing a possible link between food-related behaviors and intestinal physiology [243]. It is seen later that Dh44+ neurons rapidly activate during amino acid feeding and are a direct sensor of dietary amino acids [244].

Fly gut peptide Dromyosuppressin [181] expresses in the number of cells in central nervous system (CNS) in adult stage, extending into the rectum, near the anus; part of the adult gut. Their immunoreactive fibers also project into the crop and show expression of Dromyosuppressin [172] and crop abundantly expresses Dromyosuppressin receptors (Dromyosuppressin receptor I) [220]. The effects of neuropeptide on neural regulation of crop motility and contractions have been shown [245]. Serotonergic neurons have also been shown to regulate insulin producing cells (IPC) located in the PI of the adult brain of the fly [246]. DILP2, 3 and 5 express particularly in midgut [187, 220, 247] and extend their axons to proventriculus, crop and corpora cardiaca [248]. DILP2 is particularly involved in carbohydrate metabolism [249]. Decreased levels of DILP2 affects stored trehalose as well [248]. IPC knockdown flies show increased glycogen storage, high levels of circulating triglycerides and extended lifespan [248].

Mammalian neuropeptide NPY (Neuropeptide – Y- precursor) has an invertebrate homologous peptide called NPF due to characteristic C- terminal F residue [250]. NPF has been shown to co- localize within midgut cells in *Drosophila* and in brain and it plays a role of co- transmitter in many neural circuits [251, 252]. Its receptors are expressed primarily in the malpighian tubules but also hindgut and midgut [253]. There are some regulatory peptides found in both gut and brain. Small neuropeptide-F (sNPF) is found in the neurons in the hypocerebral ganglion innervating the midgut as well. sNPF gene encodes four kinds of sNPFs and is predominantly found in the central nervous system suggesting it might be directly involved in several neural circuits that affect hunger and feeding mechanisms [254]. The receptor for sNPF is further identified and found to be expressed in the crop, Malpighian tubules, hindgut, and the midgut [253]. Over expression or knockdown of sNPF leads to an increase or decrease in adult feeding respectively [255]. sNPF also directly affects and alters DILPs levels in larval and adult IPCs [254]. RFAmides are a class of different neuropeptides, all containing a common C-terminal RFamide sequence [256]. Using antisera to recognize the gene products of the five genes in *Drosophila* genome encoding for RFAmides, endocrine cells in anterior, middle and posterior midgut are labeled [220], axons in the midgut and crop as well as hypocerebral ganglion. RFAmides also play a key role in food intake, sensing and feeding mechanisms pointing toward conservation in these pathways from insects to mammals [257].

Other neuropeptides include Allatostatin characterized into three kinds namely Allatostatin A/B/C [258–260]. The endocrine cells producing Allatostatin are found in the posterior midgut and is innervated by axons from thoracico-abdominal ganglion [220]. Its receptors, DAR1 and DAR2 are predominantly located in the central nervous system and gastrointestinal tract (including crop, midgut and hindgut) respectively [261, 262]. Allatostain is also present throughout midgut. Another major peptide is PDF. It is expressed in central nervous system [263] and its neurons are also found in thoracico-abdominal ganglion [184]. Axons from these neurons innervate midgut and hindgut and in the crop. These neuropeptides are closely associated to circadian rhythm [264] and locomotor activity as well.

5. *Drosophila* gut brain axis: role in health and disease

Various studies have suggested that intestinal health has a significant impact on neurodegeneration. Specifically, dysregulation of GBA cross talk has been associated with metabolic syndrome [265, 266] and psychiatric disorders. GBA is largely mediated by CNS, ENS and intestinal microbiota. With its much simpler gut microbiota (1–30 taxa) as opposed to vertebrates intestine (1–500 taxa) [267], *Drosophila* intestine provides an experimental tools where whole microbiota can be removed in its entirety to perform screens to probe the relation between gut flora and the brain disorders.

5.1 Metabolic disorders

Most genes and pathways that play crucial roles in metabolic diseases are conserved between flies and humans [268]. Diet-induced obesity in flies is associated with many of the pathophysiological consequences found in humans, including hyperglycemia, insulin resistance, cardiac arrhythmia and fibrosis, reduced longevity [269, 270] and nephrosis [271]. The gut is crucial for peripheral body fat storage and serves as a major site of dietary lipid absorption and absorbs other dietary macronutrients (sugars, proteins and fats). It also metabolizes both glucose and lipids into metabolic intermediates, which after loading into hemolymph get used in other tissues and organs. In flies, lipoprotein complexes containing apolipophorins carry sterols and diacylglycerols from the gut to other tissues [81]. Fly lipoproteins also contain Hh, a cholesterol-linked, gut-derived ligand that binds the transmembrane receptor Patched on fat body target cells to promote lipolysis during larval starvation [241, 272]. The human anti-obesity drug orlistat, a gastric lipase inhibitor, has been shown to reduce body fat accumulation in adult flies [56]. Supporting a crucial role for lipolysis, midgut lipid accumulation and global fat storage are reduced by the insulin signaling pathway inhibitor Foxo in enterocytes, via reducing the expression of *magro* as flies age [58]. Excessive lipid accumulation in the fly gut and fat body is also a feature of 'humanized' flies upon cross-species expression of the human peptide neurotensin in *Drosophila* midgut EE cells. Obesity in these flies is triggered by an evolutionarily conserved mechanism acting via the cellular energy sensor 5′ adenosine monophosphate (AMP)-activated protein kinase [229]. Additionally, the acidic pH of the gastric lumen may be important for fly obesity given that both global vacuolar-type H^+-adenosine triphosphatase (ATPase) mutants and flies treated with pharmacological inhibitors of alimentary acidity store extra fat [273]. This effect could be mediated via the gut microbiome, which both shapes and depends upon the acidity of the gut [88]. Collectively, these data emphasize the importance of gut physiology for fat homeostasis in *Drosophila* and highlight the intricate interaction between the gut epithelium and the gut microbiome.

The gut microbiota and its metabolism plays an important role in modulation of fat storage in the fly. As seen in humans, fly gut is enriched in *Lactobacillus* and *Acetobacter* species. Adult axenic flies overstore fats under various dietary conditions compared with natural gut microbiota flies [274]. *Lactobacillus* sp. abundance supports co-colonization by *Acetobacter* sp. in the adult gut, which in turn negatively correlates with the fat storage level of the fly [275]. The diet of a fly impacts the composition of the gut microbiota as a high-sugar diet shifts the gut microbiome to uracil-producing species, which promote fat storage and growth in *Drosophila* larvae [276]. The availability of dietary glucose to the adult fly depends on the microbiome because flies with commensal *Acetobacter tropicalis* eat more than axenic flies but store less TAG owing to the consumption of dietary sugar by the bacteria [277].

5.2 Neurodegenerative diseases

Alzheimer's disease (AD): AD is a progressive neurodegenerative disease characterized by senile plaques consisting of misfolded β-amyloid (Aβ) fibrils and oligomers [278]. Presence of hyper phosphorylated tau protein in the various regions of the brain including cerebral cortex, locus coeruleus, and hippocampus [279] has also been suggested. Microbial dysbiosis [280], dietary changes [281], probiotics [282], or a variety of other disease conditions [283, 284] results in involvement of the GBA in the pathophysiology of neurodegenerative diseases. Multiple studies have shown an association between gut microbiome dysbiosis and the aggregation of Aβ peptides in intestinal epithelial cells [285, 286] and the CNS [287, 288] after high-fat diet feeding. Many neurodegenerative diseases exhibit accumulation of fibrillary, misfolded proteins similar to the propagation of prion-opathies in the CNS [289]. Prionopathy also involves the GBA and the local immune system, where prions accumulate in dendritic cells in the Peyer's patches and other lymphoid follicles once entering the intestinal epithelium layer [290]. Senescence-accelerated mouse model studies have identified systemic senile amyloid proteins in Peyer's patches [291]. By interacting with dendritic cells, the misfolded protein may transport to the ENS, and ultimately spread to the CNS compartment [290]. Gut bacteria can affect peripheral nerve functions through the production of neuromodulatory metabolites such as short-chain fatty acid (SCFAs) [292]. It has been suggested that Lactobacillus probiotics, given orally through feeding, showed improvement in the rough-eye phenotype, famous of the AD flies [293] and reduces *Wolbachia's* presence in the gut, which is known to be associated to neurodegenerative disorders. These studies emphasize on the relation between gut microbiota, GBA and the disorder. Pharmaceutical companies are hence targeting these probiotics and prebiotics in order to treat the disorder.

Parkinson's disease (PD): PD is a progressive brain disorder like other neurodegenerative diseases affects thinking, mobility, walking, balance and coordination. Research on PD using *Drosophila* has revealed links between gut microbiota composition and PD to one of the major genes *parkin*, which in an autosomal recessive fashion causes this disease [294, 295]. Both *Parkin* and *PINK1* genes disturb mitochondrial function and integration in PD patients. *Parkin* mutants shows steep rise in gut microbiota in comparison to control flies. Also *PINK1* mutants did not show much of a difference suggesting that gut microbiome gets affected independently in both autosomal recessive genes [294]. It is also found that *parkin* gene in ECs is required to maintain the microbial load. It has been seen that the microbial composition in *parkin* mutants is drastically different from those of wild-type flies.

Autism spectrum disorder (ASD): ASD is a developmental brain disorder characterized by impaired social behavior and disrupted communication and language. Loss of function mutants of histone demethylase KDM5 in *Drosophila* show how change in the abundance and composition of gut microbiota leads to impairment of social behavior, characteristic of ASD. Decreased levels of KDM5 cause intestinal epithelium disruption. As opposed to the control flies, the presences of gases produced by the overgrowth of bacteria cause bubble formation in the midgut in mutants [296]. It is found that KDM5 mutant flies has different composition of gut flora than controls [296]. The administered of *Lactobacillus plantarum* to KDM5 mutant flies rescued social behavior and other intestinal defects. Flies supplemented with *L. plantarum* also shows 2.3 fold increase approximately in longevity [296]. $kdm5^{JmjC^*}$, another kind of KDM5 mutant displayed impaired gut permeability, intestinal epithelium and microbiota. In this case as well, administration of *L. plantarum* rescued gut permeability, the defective social interaction and communication. These studies have helped establishing a link between gut microbiota and ASD. The probiotics that rescued ASD flies are good candidates for pharmaceutical companies to be sold as therapeutic. These results can be used for drug discovery and in treatment of these otherwise, untreatable disorders.

5.3 Intestinal dysbiosis and infections

Drosophila and its microbiome has provided invaluable information in understanding intestinal dysbiosis and chronic inflammatory infections. Two pathways that are present in *Drosophila* innate immune system to act against microbiota are immune deficiency (IMD) pathway (homologous to human NFκB pathway) and dual oxidase (DUOX) pathway. IMD pathway leads to anti-microbial peptide (AMP) synthesis whereas DUOX pathway leads to the formation of reactive oxygen species (ROS). Intestinal AMP overproduction changes the microbial community structure. This change is dysbiotic in nature because it leads to cell apoptosis of host cells [297]. IMD pathway over-activation leads to an increase in dysbiotic community structure and IMD inactivation leads to over-proliferation of community members in general [44]. Inflammatory bowel disorders also involve apoptosis of intestinal cells in humans which shows a link between the intestinal pathogenesis in both mammals and flies [297]. DUOX knockdown (DUOX-KD) flies show a high mortality rate after gut infections, which indicates DUOX-dependent ROS formation. These flies show huge amounts of microbial cells in the gut as opposed to wild-type flies. DUOX-KD flies survive normally in a GF environment. Inactivation of this pathway leads to host infections [298] whereas over-activation induces oxidative stress in host [299]. Extensive research in *Drosophila* midgut shows that intestinal epithelium damage induces inflammatory signals and growth factors to lead to ISC proliferation and tumor proliferation.

5.4 Gut-cancer model

Drosophila is an important tool in medicine to explore the details of cancer. There are a wide range of cancers where *Drosophila* is taken into consideration – from brain, gut to thyroid and lung. The loss of Adenomatous polyposis coli gene (*APC*, tumor suppressor gene) in flies leads to an increase in ISC proliferation in the gut [300]. This resembles the condition seen in intestinal adenomas (benign tumor of epithelial tissue). JNK-Wg signaling controls the number of ISCs found in the gut. Injured or damaged ECs lead to an increase in JNK signaling and increase in Wg ligands in (EB). This in turn activates JAK STAT ligands - Upd2 and Upd3, which further increase ISCs' non-autonomous over proliferation [301]. Loss of *Apc* in ISCs increases JAK–STAT pathway as well, which in turn affects ISCs proliferation. This helps in establishing the conservation of pathways that regulate ISC proliferation and gut homeostasis [302]. In some studies, it is also shown that *Apc* and RAS control growth of cells in gut by interacting with one another. Non-receptor tyrosine kinase c-Src is associated to quite a few forms of cancer including colorectal cancer (CRC). In wildtype *Drosophila*, orthologous forms of c-Src act exactly how they would in mammals. Activation in c-Src leads to ISC proliferation and decrease or inactivation in c-Src inhibits further ISC proliferation [303]. These results show beyond doubt how ISC proliferation is directly involved with cancer formation and these genes and mechanisms are conserved from flies to mammals. Few studies have looked into hindgut (equivalent of mammalian colon) as a model for cancer. Oncogenes in the hindgut synergize with innate immunity system to stimulate tumor cell invasion. After bacterial infection, ISCs proliferate but less in hindgut as opposed to midgut. RAS oncogene, RAS^{v12} induces cell invasion and dissemination of ECs into the abdominal cavity. Upon RAS^{v12}expression, hindgut shows cancer-like phenotype. It activates JNK signaling pathway which in turn increases ISC proliferation and hence, tumor growth [304].

6. Conclusion and outlook

Recently *Drosophila* has emerged as a model to study intestinal infection and pathology because of conservation between *Drosophila* and mammalian intestinal pathophysiology, regeneration, and signaling pathways that control them. Real time and other *Drosophila* assays provide the complex cellular composition of a real intestine and opportunities to assess toxicity in a whole organism at a relatively low cost compared to mammalian system. Its simpler cellular structure, flexibility to doing screening, availability of molecular markers and other genetic tools adds up to its value as an ideal model system to study intestine. Also, it has been shown that human intestinal pathogens can cause intestinal pathology in flies as well.

In the recent past, data from the intestinal mechanisms found in flies have been shown to be active in mammals, and may therefore become relevant in the context of human pathologies including diabetes, obesity, neurodegenerative diseases, gastrointestinal cancers, or aging. Parallel findings of communication between gut and brain via neuropeptides in *Drosophila* and humans highlight on the importance of GBA in maintaining health. Identification of neural circuitries is of prime importance to apprehend more about the link between the gut and brain and their link with metabolic and neurodegenerative diseases. Greater understanding of gut-brain feeding circuits, paracrine signaling of peptides and physical communication via neural circuitries will establish their functioning in several metabolic disorders, neurological syndromes, aging and cardiovascular diseases. Research using flies on specific gut regions, cell types during various developmental stages and on stem cell biology and aging have been conducted so far. Other functions including role of unidentified taste receptors in the gut, their connection with the brain mediating nutrient digestion and transport, or organs such as the crop and the proventiculus, remain poorly characterized. Deeper understanding is required on the function of gut brain neural connectivity and to investigate what may be their key role in human or insect (patho)physiology concerning feeding behavior and appetitive learning. Techniques like *in vivo* CRISPR transcriptional activation (CRISPRa) and interference (CRISPRi) approaches [288, 305], to allow tightly regulated and reversible promoter activation and blocking in fly gut can be fruitful for future studies.

Developing new techniques and behavioral assays can help us explore physiological drives: what is the gut function to maintain the overall health of the animal. It would be interesting to find out the key intestinal sensors. How the physical association between gut and brain via neural micro circuits regulate decisions regarding nutrition, hunger and satiety is under question. Better "holistic" and quantitative methods, integration of spatial and temporal information about genetic events more comprehensively are required, so that cause and effect can be uncoupled in a physiological context [306]. We anticipate and hope that fly models of intestinal pathology, in addition to uncovering newly identified genes (chemosensory and others) and basic biology mechanisms will emphasize the most conserved aspects of human intestinal biology. As a result, fly will contribute to translational research investigating drug effects, and microbial and host genetic component analyses, leading to biological findings that are broadly applicable to human health and disease.

Funding declaration

This work is supported by Wellcome Trust/DBT India Alliance Fellowship (grant number IA/I/15/2/502074) awarded to PK.

Conflict of interest

The authors declare no conflict of interest.

Criteria for authorship

ZS, SK and PK all substantially contributed to the conception and design of the work. Everybody participated in drafting and revising the work, made the figures, wrote the chapter and approved the final version for publication.

Abbreviations

ENS	Enteric nervous system
GI	Gastrointestinal
GBA	Gut brain axis
CNS	Central nervous system
ISCs	Intestinal stem cells
ECs	Enterocytes
EE	Enteroendocrine
EBs	Enteroblasts
TA	Transient amplifying
AMP-5′	Adenosine monophosphate
AMPK- 5′	AMP activated kinase
TAG	Triacylglyceride
Sug	*Sugarbabe*
CD36	Cluster of differentiation 36
Npc1	Niemann-Pick C1
SREBPs	Sterol regulatory element-binding proteins
Akh	Adipokinetic hormone
RNAi	RNA interference
Kcc	Kazachoc
SIET	Scanning ion-selective electrode technique
Dh44	Diuretic hormone 44
GPCR	G-protein coupled receptors
PNS	Peripheral nervous system
GLUT	Glucose transporter
SGLT	Na^+/glucose cotransporter
GIP	Gastric inhibitory polypeptide
GLP	Glucagon like peptide
TK	Tachykinin
MOR	μ – opoid receptors
IGN	Intestinal gluconeogenesis
MOR-KO	MOR-knockouts
cNST	Caudal nucleus of the solitary tract
GLP1	Glucagon- like peptide 1

sNPF	Short neuropeptide F
AN	Antennal nerve
Ilp7	Insulin-like peptide 7
VN	Vagus nerve
IBS	Intestinal bowel syndrome
HGN1	Hindgut neuron1
Hh	Hedgehog
Poxn	*Pox-neuro*
Dh31	Diuretic hormone 31
Lst	Limostatin
Lk	Leucokinin
JH	Juvenile hormone
Crtc/CREB	cAMP-regulated transcriptional co-activator/ cyclic AMP-responsive element-binding protein
SEZ	Suboesophageal zone
CRH	Corticotropin –releasing -hormone
PI	Pars intercerebralis
IPC	Insulin producing cells
DILP	*Drosophila* insulin- like- peptide
$5\text{-}HT_{1A}$-5	Hydroxy tryptamine /serotonin
AKH	Adipokinetic hormone
PYY	Peptide YY
AgRP	Agouti-related protein
CCK	Choleocystokinin
PP	Pancreatic polypeptide
NPY	Neuropeptide Y
PDF	Pigment- dispersing factor
CRF	Corticotropin-releasing factor
BDNF	Brain-derived neurotrophic factor
SCFAs	Short-chain fatty acid
AMP	Anti-microbial peptide
ROS	Reactive oxygen species
DUOX	Dual oxidase
IMD	Immune deficiency
APC	Adenomatous polyposis coli gene
CRC	Colorectal cancer

Author details

Zoha Sadaqat, Shivam Kaushik and Pinky Kain*
Regional Centre for Biotechnology, NCR Biotech Science Cluster, Faridabad, Haryana, India

*Address all correspondence to: pinkykain@gmail.com; pksharma@rcb.res.in

References

[1] Thompson DG, Malagelada JR. Guts and their motions (gastrointestinal motility in health and disease). J Clin Gastroenterol. 1981;3 Suppl 1:81-87.

[2] Edgecomb RS, Harth CE, Schneiderman AM. Regulation of feeding behavior in adult *Drosophila melanogaster* varies with feeding regime and nutritional state. J Exp Biol. 1994;197:215-35.

[3] Demerec M. Biology of *Drosophila*. Cold Spring Harbor, NY: Cold Spring Harbor Laboratory Press. 1994:425-41.

[4] Stoffolano JG, Jr., Haselton AT. The adult Dipteran crop: a unique and overlooked organ. Annu Rev Entomol. 2013;58:205-25.

[5] King DG. Cellular organization and peritrophic membrane formation in the cardia (proventriculus) of *Drosophila melanogaster*. J Morphol. 1988;196(3):253-82.

[6] Tzou P, Ohresser S, Ferrandon D, Capovilla M, Reichhart JM, Lemaitre B, et al. Tissue-specific inducible expression of antimicrobial peptide genes in *Drosophila* surface epithelia. Immunity. 2000;13(5):737-48.

[7] Demerec M. (Editor). Biology of *Drosophila*. John Wiley & Sons, Inc, New York. 1950.

[8] Douglas A. E. ebCRF, Simpson S. J., Douglas A. E. The alimentary canal in The Insects: Structure and Function. Cambridge University Press, Cambridge. 2013:46-80.

[9] Chen J, Sayadian AC, Lowe N, Lovegrove HE, St Johnston D. An alternative mode of epithelial polarity in the *Drosophila* midgut. PLoS Biol. 2018;16(10):e3000041.

[10] Hegedus D, Erlandson M, Gillott C, Toprak U. New insights into peritrophic matrix synthesis, architecture, and function. Annu Rev Entomol. 2009;54:285-302.

[11] Murakami R, Shigenaga A, Matsumoto A, Yamaoka I, Tanimura T. Novel tissue units of regional differentiation in the gut epithelium of Drosopbila, as revealed by P-element-mediated detection of enhancer. Rouxs Arch Dev Biol. 1994;203(5): 243-9.

[12] Buchon N, Osman D, David FP, Fang HY, Boquete JP, Deplancke B, et al. Morphological and molecular characterization of adult midgut compartmentalization in *Drosophila*. Cell Rep. 2013;3(5):1725-38.

[13] Marianes A, Spradling AC. Physiological and stem cell compartmentalization within the *Drosophila* midgut. Elife. 2013;2:e00886.

[14] Cognigni P, Bailey AP, Miguel-Aliaga I. Enteric neurons and systemic signals couple nutritional and reproductive status with intestinal homeostasis. Cell Metab. 2011;13(1):92-104.

[15] Linneweber GA, Jacobson J, Busch KE, Hudry B, Christov CP, Dormann D, et al. Neuronal control of metabolism through nutrient-dependent modulation of tracheal branching. Cell. 2014;156(1-2):69-83.

[16] Strand M, Micchelli CA. Quiescent gastric stem cells maintain the adult *Drosophila* stomach. Proc Natl Acad Sci U S A. 2011;108(43):17696-701.

[17] Strand M, Micchelli CA. Regional control of *Drosophila* gut stem cell proliferation: EGF establishes GSSC proliferative set point & controls emergence from quiescence. PLoS One. 2013;8(11):e80608.

[18] Sandborn EB, Duclos S, Messier PE, Roberge JJ. Atypical intestinal striated muscle in *Drosophila melanogaster*. J Ultrastruct Res. 1967;18(5):695-702.

[19] Pitsouli C, Apidianakis Y, Perrimon N. Homeostasis in infected epithelia: stem cells take the lead. Cell Host Microbe. 2009;6(4):301-7.

[20] Rubin DC. Intestinal morphogenesis. Curr Opin Gastroenterol. 2007;23(2):111-4.

[21] Kedinger M, Simon-Assmann P, Haffen K. Growth and differentiation of intestinal endodermal cells in a coculture system. Gut. 1987;28 Suppl:237-41.

[22] Tepass U, Hartenstein V. Epithelium formation in the *Drosophila* midgut depends on the interaction of endoderm and mesoderm. Development. 1994;120(3):579-90.

[23] Crosnier C, Stamataki D, Lewis J. Organizing cell renewal in the intestine: stem cells, signals and combinatorial control. Nat Rev Genet. 2006;7(5):349-59.

[24] Shanbhag S, Tripathi S. Epithelial ultrastructure and cellular mechanisms of acid and base transport in the *Drosophila* midgut. J Exp Biol. 2009;212(Pt 11):1731-44.

[25] Baumann O. Posterior midgut epithelial cells differ in their organization of the membrane skeleton from other *drosophila* epithelia. Exp Cell Res. 2001;270(2):176-87.

[26] Gartner LP. Submicroscopic morphology of the adult *drosophila* midgut. J Baltimore Coll Dent Surg. 1970;25(2):64-76.

[27] Gooday GW. Aggressive and defensive roles for chitinases. EXS. 1999;87:157-69.

[28] Vodovar N, Vinals M, Liehl P, Basset A, Degrouard J, Spellman P, et al. *Drosophila* host defense after oral infection by an entomopathogenic Pseudomonas species. Proc Natl Acad Sci U S A. 2005;102(32):11414-9.

[29] Sengupta N, MacDonald TT. The role of matrix metalloproteinases in stromal/epithelial interactions in the gut. Physiology (Bethesda). 2007;22:401-9.

[30] Jiang H, Edgar BA. EGFR signaling regulates the proliferation of *Drosophila* adult midgut progenitors. Development. 2009;136(3):483-93.

[31] Kvietys PR, Granger DN. Physiology and pathophysiology of the colonic circulation. Clin Gastroenterol. 1986;15(4):967-83.

[32] Rhee SH, Pothoulakis C, Mayer EA. Principles and clinical implications of the brain-gut-enteric microbiota axis. Nat Rev Gastroenterol Hepatol. 2009;6(5):306-14.

[33] Komuro T, Hashimoto Y. Three-dimensional structure of the rat intestinal wall (mucosa and submucosa). Arch Histol Cytol. 1990;53(1):1-21.

[34] Barker N, van de Wetering M, Clevers H. The intestinal stem cell. Genes Dev. 2008;22(14):1856-64.

[35] Barker N, van Es JH, Kuipers J, Kujala P, van den Born M, Cozijnsen M, et al. Identification of stem cells in small intestine and colon by marker gene Lgr5. Nature. 2007;449(7165):1003-7.

[36] Ohlstein B, Spradling A. The adult *Drosophila* posterior midgut is maintained by pluripotent stem cells. Nature. 2006;439(7075):470-4.

[37] Takashima S, Mkrtchyan M, Younossi-Hartenstein A, Merriam JR, Hartenstein V. The behaviour of

Drosophila adult hindgut stem cells is controlled by Wnt and Hh signalling. Nature. 2008;454(7204):651-5.

[38] Apidianakis Y, Rahme LG. *Drosophila* melanogaster as a model for human intestinal infection and pathology. Dis Model Mech. 2011;4(1):21-30.

[39] Martini E, Krug SM, Siegmund B, Neurath MF, Becker C. Mend Your Fences: The Epithelial Barrier and its Relationship With Mucosal Immunity in Inflammatory Bowel Disease. Cell Mol Gastroenterol Hepatol. 2017;4(1):33-46.

[40] Kopp ZA, Jain U, Van Limbergen J, Stadnyk AW. Do antimicrobial peptides and complement collaborate in the intestinal mucosa? Front Immunol. 2015;6:17.

[41] Buchon N, Broderick NA, Poidevin M, Pradervand S, Lemaitre B. *Drosophila* intestinal response to bacterial infection: activation of host defense and stem cell proliferation. Cell Host Microbe. 2009;5(2):200-11.

[42] Scoville DH, Sato T, He XC, Li L. Current view: intestinal stem cells and signaling. Gastroenterology. 2008;134(3):849-64.

[43] Amcheslavsky A, Jiang J, Ip YT. Tissue damage-induced intestinal stem cell division in *Drosophila*. Cell Stem Cell. 2009;4(1):49-61.

[44] Buchon N, Broderick NA, Chakrabarti S, Lemaitre B. Invasive and indigenous microbiota impact intestinal stem cell activity through multiple pathways in *Drosophila*. Genes Dev. 2009;23(19):2333-44.

[45] Cronin SJ, Nehme NT, Limmer S, Liegeois S, Pospisilik JA, Schramek D, et al. Genome-wide RNAi screen identifies genes involved in intestinal pathogenic bacterial infection. Science. 2009;325(5938):340-3.

[46] Abraham I, Doane WW. Genetic regulation of tissue-specific expression of amylase structural genes in *Drosophila melanogaster*. Proc Natl Acad Sci U S A. 1978;75(9):4446-50.

[47] Dutta D, Buchon N, Xiang J, Edgar BA. Regional Cell Specific RNA Expression Profiling of FACS Isolated *Drosophila* Intestinal Cell Populations. Curr Protoc Stem Cell Biol. 2015;34:2F 1-2F 14.

[48] Lehane M. J. BPF. Biology of the Insect Midgut. Chapman & Hall, London. 1996.

[49] Amcheslavsky A, Song W, Li Q, Nie Y, Bragatto I, Ferrandon D, et al. Enteroendocrine cells support intestinal stem-cell-mediated homeostasis in *Drosophila*. Cell Rep. 2014;9(1):32-9.

[50] Wigglesworth V. B. The Principles of Insect Physiology. Chapman and Hall Ltd, London. 1972.

[51] Clissold FJ, Tedder BJ, Conigrave AD, Simpson SJ. The gastrointestinal tract as a nutrient balancing organ. Proc Biol Sci. 2010;277(1688):1751-9.

[52] Chng WA, Sleiman MSB, Schupfer F, Lemaitre B. Transforming growth factor beta/activin signaling functions as a sugar-sensing feedback loop to regulate digestive enzyme expression. Cell Rep. 2014;9(1):336-48.

[53] Mattila J, Havula E, Suominen E, Teesalu M, Surakka I, Hynynen R, et al. Mondo-Mlx Mediates Organismal Sugar Sensing through the Gli-Similar Transcription Factor Sugarbabe. Cell Rep. 2015;13(2):350-64.

[54] Bujold M, Gopalakrishnan A, Nally E, King-Jones K. Nuclear receptor DHR96 acts as a sentinel for low cholesterol concentrations in *Drosophila melanogaster*. Mol Cell Biol. 2010;30(3):793-805.

[55] Horner MA, Pardee K, Liu S, King-Jones K, Lajoie G, Edwards A, et al. The *Drosophila* DHR96 nuclear receptor binds cholesterol and regulates cholesterol homeostasis. Genes Dev. 2009;23(23):2711-6.

[56] Sieber MH, Thummel CS. The DHR96 nuclear receptor controls triacylglycerol homeostasis in *Drosophila*. Cell Metab. 2009;10(6):481-90.

[57] Sieber MH, Thummel CS. Coordination of triacylglycerol and cholesterol homeostasis by DHR96 and the *Drosophila* LipA homolog magro. Cell Metab. 2012;15(1):122-7.

[58] Karpac J, Biteau B, Jasper H. Misregulation of an adaptive metabolic response contributes to the age-related disruption of lipid homeostasis in *Drosophila*. Cell Rep. 2013;4(6): 1250-61.

[59] Miguel-Aliaga I. Nerveless and gutsy: intestinal nutrient sensing from invertebrates to humans. Semin Cell Dev Biol. 2012;23(6):614-20.

[60] Caccia S, Leonardi MG, Casartelli M, Grimaldi A, de Eguileor M, Pennacchio F, et al. Nutrient absorption by Aphidius ervi larvae. J Insect Physiol. 2005;51(11):1183-92.

[61] Caccia S, Casartelli M, Grimaldi A, Losa E, de Eguileor M, Pennacchio F, et al. Unexpected similarity of intestinal sugar absorption by SGLT1 and apical GLUT2 in an insect (Aphidius ervi, Hymenoptera) and mammals. Am J Physiol Regul Integr Comp Physiol. 2007;292(6):R2284-91.

[62] Price DR, Wilkinson HS, Gatehouse JA. Functional expression and characterisation of a gut facilitative glucose transporter, NlHT1, from the phloem-feeding insect *Nilaparvata lugens* (rice brown planthopper). Insect Biochem Mol Biol. 2007;37(11):1138-48.

[63] Price DR, Tibbles K, Shigenobu S, Smertenko A, Russell CW, Douglas AE, et al. Sugar transporters of the major facilitator superfamily in aphids; from gene prediction to functional characterization. Insect Mol Biol. 2010;19 Suppl 2:97-112.

[64] Bifano TD, Alegria TG, Terra WR. Transporters involved in glucose and water absorption in the *Dysdercus peruvianus* (Hemiptera: Pyrrhocoridae) anterior midgut. Comp Biochem Physiol B Biochem Mol Biol. 2010;157(1):1-9.

[65] Escher SA, Rasmuson-Lestander A. The *Drosophila* glucose transporter gene: cDNA sequence, phylogenetic comparisons, analysis of functional sites and secondary structures. Hereditas. 1999;130(2):95-103.

[66] Artero RD, Terol-Alcayde J, Paricio N, Ring J, Bargues M, Torres A, et al. saliva, a new *Drosophila* gene expressed in the embryonic salivary glands with homologues in plants and vertebrates. Mech Dev. 1998;75(1-2):159-62.

[67] Baker RF, Leach KA, Braun DM. SWEET as sugar: new sucrose effluxers in plants. Mol Plant. 2012;5(4):766-8.

[68] Meyer H, Vitavska O, Wieczorek H. Identification of an animal sucrose transporter. J Cell Sci. 2011;124(Pt 12): 1984-91.

[69] Kanamori Y, Saito A, Hagiwara-Komoda Y, Tanaka D, Mitsumasu K, Kikuta S, et al. The trehalose transporter 1 gene sequence is conserved in insects and encodes proteins with different kinetic properties involved in trehalose import into peripheral tissues. Insect Biochem Mol Biol. 2010;40(1):30-7.

[70] Vitavska O, Wieczorek H. The SLC45 gene family of putative sugar

transporters. Mol Aspects Med. 2013;34(2-3):655-60.

[71] Boudko DY. Molecular basis of essential amino acid transport from studies of insect nutrient amino acid transporters of the SLC6 family (NAT-SLC6). J Insect Physiol. 2012;58(4):433-49.

[72] Colombani J, Raisin S, Pantalacci S, Radimerski T, Montagne J, Leopold P. A nutrient sensor mechanism controls *Drosophila* growth. Cell. 2003;114(6):739-49.

[73] Martin JF, Hersperger E, Simcox A, Shearn A. minidiscs encodes a putative amino acid transporter subunit required non-autonomously for imaginal cell proliferation. Mech Dev. 2000;92(2):155-67.

[74] Goberdhan DC, Meredith D, Boyd CA, Wilson C. PAT-related amino acid transporters regulate growth via a novel mechanism that does not require bulk transport of amino acids. Development. 2005;132(10):2365-75.

[75] Miller MM, Popova LB, Meleshkevitch EA, Tran PV, Boudko DY. The invertebrate B(0) system transporter, *D. melanogaster* NAT1, has unique d-amino acid affinity and mediates gut and brain functions. Insect Biochem Mol Biol. 2008;38(10):923-31.

[76] Reynolds B, Roversi P, Laynes R, Kazi S, Boyd CA, Goberdhan DC. *Drosophila* expresses a CD98 transporter with an evolutionarily conserved structure and amino acid-transport properties. Biochem J. 2009;420(3):363-72.

[77] Roman G, Meller V, Wu KH, Davis RL. The opt1 gene of *Drosophila melanogaster* encodes a proton-dependent dipeptide transporter. Am J Physiol. 1998;275(3):C857-69.

[78] Capo F, Chaduli D, Viallat-Lieutaud A, Charroux B, Royet J. Oligopeptide Transporters of the SLC15 Family Are Dispensable for Peptidoglycan Sensing and Transport in *Drosophila*. J Innate Immun. 2017;9(5):483-92.

[79] Thimgan MS, Berg JS, Stuart AE. Comparative sequence analysis and tissue localization of members of the SLC6 family of transporters in adult *Drosophila melanogaster*. J Exp Biol. 2006;209(Pt 17):3383-404.

[80] Chapman R. F. The Insects. Structure and Function. Cambridge University Press, New York. 2013.

[81] Palm W, Sampaio JL, Brankatschk M, Carvalho M, Mahmoud A, Shevchenko A, et al. Lipoproteins in *Drosophila melanogaster*--assembly, function, and influence on tissue lipid composition. PLoS Genet. 2012;8(7):e1002828.

[82] Huang X, Warren JT, Buchanan J, Gilbert LI, Scott MP. *Drosophila* Niemann-Pick type C-2 genes control sterol homeostasis and steroid biosynthesis: a model of human neurodegenerative disease. Development. 2007;134(20):3733-42.

[83] Voght SP, Fluegel ML, Andrews LA, Pallanck LJ. *Drosophila* NPC1b promotes an early step in sterol absorption from the midgut epithelium. Cell Metab. 2007;5(3):195-205.

[84] Chakrabarti S, Poidevin M, Lemaitre B. The *Drosophila* MAPK p38c regulates oxidative stress and lipid homeostasis in the intestine. PLoS Genet. 2014;10(9):e1004659.

[85] Song W, Veenstra JA, Perrimon N. Control of lipid metabolism by tachykinin in *Drosophila*. Cell Rep. 2014;9(1):40-7.

[86] Reiff T, Jacobson J, Cognigni P, Antonello Z, Ballesta E, Tan KJ, et al. Endocrine remodelling of the adult

intestine sustains reproduction in *Drosophila*. Elife. 2015;4:e06930.

[87] Dubreuil RR, Frankel J, Wang P, Howrylak J, Kappil M, Grushko TA. Mutations of alpha spectrin and labial block cuprophilic cell differentiation and acid secretion in the middle midgut of *Drosophila* larvae. Dev Biol. 1998;194(1):1-11.

[88] Overend G, Luo Y, Henderson L, Douglas AE, Davies SA, Dow JA. Molecular mechanism and functional significance of acid generation in the *Drosophila* midgut. Sci Rep. 2016;6:27242.

[89] Dubreuil RR. Copper cells and stomach acid secretion in the *Drosophila* midgut. Int J Biochem Cell Biol. 2004;36(5):745-52.

[90] Li H, Qi Y, Jasper H. Preventing Age-Related Decline of Gut Compartmentalization Limits Microbiota Dysbiosis and Extends Lifespan. Cell Host Microbe. 2016;19(2):240-53.

[91] Filippov V, Aimanova K, Gill SS. Expression of an *Aedes aegypti* cation-chloride cotransporter and its *Drosophila* homologues. Insect Mol Biol. 2003;12(4):319-31.

[92] Sun Q, Tian E, Turner RJ, Ten Hagen KG. Developmental and functional studies of the SLC12 gene family members from *Drosophila melanogaster*. Am J Physiol Cell Physiol. 2010;298(1):C26-37.

[93] Brenner R, Atkinson NS. Calcium-activated potassium channel gene expression in the midgut of *Drosophila*. Comp Biochem Physiol B Biochem Mol Biol. 1997;118(2):411-20.

[94] Feingold D, Starc T, O'Donnell MJ, Nilson L, Dent JA. The orphan pentameric ligand-gated ion channel pHCl-2 is gated by pH and regulates fluid secretion in *Drosophila* Malpighian tubules. J Exp Biol. 2016;219(Pt 17): 2629-38.

[95] Remnant EJ, Williams A, Lumb C, Yang YT, Chan J, Duchene S, et al. Evolution, Expression, and Function of Nonneuronal Ligand-Gated Chloride Channels in *Drosophila melanogaster*. G3 (Bethesda). 2016;6(7):2003-12.

[96] Dubreuil RR, Das A, Base C, Mazock GH. The *Drosophila* Anion Exchanger (DAE) lacks a detectable interaction with the spectrin cytoskeleton. J Negat Results Biomed. 2010;9:5.

[97] Naikkhwah W, O'Donnell MJ. Phenotypic plasticity in response to dietary salt stress: Na+ and K+ transport by the gut of *Drosophila melanogaster* larvae. J Exp Biol. 2012;215(Pt 3): 461-70.

[98] Chintapalli VR, Wang J, Dow JA. Using FlyAtlas to identify better *Drosophila melanogaster* models of human disease. Nat Genet. 2007;39(6):715-20.

[99] Chintapalli VR, Kato A, Henderson L, Hirata T, Woods DJ, Overend G, et al. Transport proteins NHA1 and NHA2 are essential for survival, but have distinct transport modalities. Proc Natl Acad Sci U S A. 2015;112(37):11720-5.

[100] Day JP, Wan S, Allan AK, Kean L, Davies SA, Gray JV, et al. Identification of two partners from the bacterial Kef exchanger family for the apical plasma membrane V-ATPase of Metazoa. J Cell Sci. 2008;121(Pt 15):2612-9.

[101] Poulson D. F. BLE. Organization and function of the inorganic constituents of nuclei. Exp Cell Res. 1952;2:161-80.

[102] McNulty M, Puljung M, Jefford G, Dubreuil RR. Evidence that

a copper-metallothionein complex is responsible for fluorescence in acid-secreting cells of the *Drosophila* stomach. Cell Tissue Res. 2001;304(3):383-9.

[103] Lauverjat S, Ballan-Dufrancais C, Wegnez M. Detoxification of cadmium. Ultrastructural study and electron-probe microanalysis of the midgut in a cadmium-resistant strain of *Drosophila melanogaster*. Biol Met. 1989;2(2):97-107.

[104] Missirlis F, Kosmidis S, Brody T, Mavrakis M, Holmberg S, Odenwald WF, et al. Homeostatic mechanisms for iron storage revealed by genetic manipulations and live imaging of *Drosophila* ferritin. Genetics. 2007;177(1):89-100.

[105] Wong R, Piper MDW, Blanc E, Partridge L. Pitfalls of measuring feeding rate in the fruit fly *Drosophila melanogaster*. Nat Methods. 2008;5(3):214-5.

[106] Urquhart-Cronish M, Sokolowski MB. Gene-environment interplay in *Drosophila melanogaster*: chronic nutritional deprivation in larval life affects adult fecal output. J Insect Physiol. 2014;69:95-100.

[107] Apger-McGlaughon J, Wolfner MF. Post-mating change in excretion by mated *Drosophila melanogaster* females is a long-term response that depends on sex peptide and sperm. J Insect Physiol. 2013;59(10):1024-30.

[108] Buchanan RL, Benzer S. Defective glia in the *Drosophila* brain degeneration mutant drop-dead. Neuron. 1993;10(5):839-50.

[109] Peller CR, Bacon EM, Bucheger JA, Blumenthal EM. Defective gut function in drop-dead mutant *Drosophila*. J Insect Physiol. 2009;55(9):834-9.

[110] Li X, Staszewski L, Xu H, Durick K, Zoller M, Adler E. Human receptors for sweet and umami taste. Proc Natl Acad Sci U S A. 2002;99(7):4692-6.

[111] Dyer J, Salmon KS, Zibrik L, Shirazi-Beechey SP. Expression of sweet taste receptors of the T1R family in the intestinal tract and enteroendocrine cells. Biochem Soc Trans. 2005;33 (Pt 1):302-5.

[112] Bezencon C, le Coutre J, Damak S. Taste-signaling proteins are coexpressed in solitary intestinal epithelial cells. Chem Senses. 2007;32(1):41-9.

[113] Wong GT, Gannon KS, Margolskee RF. Transduction of bitter and sweet taste by gustducin. Nature. 1996;381(6585):796-800.

[114] Ueda T, Ugawa S, Yamamura H, Imaizumi Y, Shimada S. Functional interaction between T2R taste receptors and G-protein alpha subunits expressed in taste receptor cells. J Neurosci. 2003;23(19):7376-80.

[115] Wu SV, Rozengurt N, Yang M, Young SH, Sinnett-Smith J, Rozengurt E. Expression of bitter taste receptors of the T2R family in the gastrointestinal tract and enteroendocrine STC-1 cells. Proc Natl Acad Sci U S A. 2002;99(4):2392-7.

[116] Hofer D, Puschel B, Drenckhahn D. Taste receptor-like cells in the rat gut identified by expression of alpha-gustducin. Proc Natl Acad Sci U S A. 1996;93(13):6631-4.

[117] Hofer D, Drenckhahn D. Identification of the taste cell G-protein, alpha-gustducin, in brush cells of the rat pancreatic duct system. Histochem Cell Biol. 1998;110(3):303-9.

[118] Wu SV, Chen MC, Rozengurt E. Genomic organization, expression, and function of bitter taste receptors (T2R) in mouse and rat. Physiol Genomics. 2005;22(2):139-49.

[119] Rozengurt E. Taste receptors in the gastrointestinal tract. I. Bitter taste receptors and alpha-gustducin in the mammalian gut. Am J Physiol Gastrointest Liver Physiol. 2006;291(2):G171-7.

[120] Mace OJ, Affleck J, Patel N, Kellett GL. Sweet taste receptors in rat small intestine stimulate glucose absorption through apical GLUT2. J Physiol. 2007;582(Pt 1):379-92.

[121] Egan JM, Margolskee RF. Taste cells of the gut and gastrointestinal chemosensation. Mol Interv. 2008;8(2):78-81.

[122] Margolskee RF, Dyer J, Kokrashvili Z, Salmon KS, Ilegems E, Daly K, et al. T1R3 and gustducin in gut sense sugars to regulate expression of Na+−glucose cotransporter 1. Proc Natl Acad Sci U S A. 2007;104(38): 15075-80.

[123] Au A, Gupta A, Schembri P, Cheeseman CI. Rapid insertion of GLUT2 into the rat jejunal brush-border membrane promoted by glucagon-like peptide 2. Biochem J. 2002;367(Pt 1):247-54.

[124] Dyer J, Vayro S, King TP, Shirazi-Beechey SP. Glucose sensing in the intestinal epithelium. Eur J Biochem. 2003;270(16):3377-88.

[125] Daly K, Al-Rammahi M, Arora DK, Moran AW, Proudman CJ, Ninomiya Y, et al. Expression of sweet receptor components in equine small intestine: relevance to intestinal glucose transport. Am J Physiol Regul Integr Comp Physiol. 2012;303(2):R199-208.

[126] Park JH, Kwon JY. Heterogeneous expression of *Drosophila* gustatory receptors in enteroendocrine cells. PLoS One. 2011;6(12):e29022.

[127] Park JH, Chen J, Jang S, Ahn TJ, Kang K, Choi MS, et al. A subset of enteroendocrine cells is activated by amino acids in the *Drosophila* midgut. FEBS Lett. 2016;590(4):493-500.

[128] Palamiuc L, Noble T, Witham E, Ratanpal H, Vaughan M, Srinivasan S. A tachykinin-like neuroendocrine signalling axis couples central serotonin action and nutrient sensing with peripheral lipid metabolism. Nat Commun. 2017;8:14237.

[129] Mace OJ, Schindler M, Patel S. The regulation of K- and L-cell activity by GLUT2 and the calcium-sensing receptor CasR in rat small intestine. J Physiol. 2012;590(12):2917-36.

[130] Depoortere I. Taste receptors of the gut: emerging roles in health and disease. Gut. 2014;63(1):179-90.

[131] Dus M, Lai JS, Gunapala KM, Min S, Tayler TD, Hergarden AC, et al. Nutrient Sensor in the Brain Directs the Action of the Brain-Gut Axis in *Drosophila*. Neuron. 2015;87(1):139-51.

[132] Sandoval D, Cota D, Seeley RJ. The integrative role of CNS fuel-sensing mechanisms in energy balance and glucose regulation. Annu Rev Physiol. 2008;70:513-35.

[133] Miyamoto T, Amrein H. Gluconeogenesis: An ancient biochemical pathway with a new twist. Fly (Austin). 2017;11(3):218-23.

[134] Mithieux G, Andreelli F, Magnan C. Intestinal gluconeogenesis: key signal of central control of energy and glucose homeostasis. Curr Opin Clin Nutr Metab Care. 2009;12(4):419-23.

[135] Delaere F, Duchampt A, Mounien L, Seyer P, Duraffourd C, Zitoun C, et al. The role of sodium-coupled glucose co-transporter 3 in the satiety effect of portal glucose sensing. Mol Metab. 2012;2(1):47-53.

[136] Delaere F, Akaoka H, De Vadder F, Duchampt A, Mithieux G. Portal glucose influences the sensory, cortical and reward systems in rats. Eur J Neurosci. 2013;38(10):3476-86.

[137] Soty M, Penhoat A, Amigo-Correig M, Vinera J, Sardella A, Vullin-Bouilloux F, et al. A gut-brain neural circuit controlled by intestinal gluconeogenesis is crucial in metabolic health. Mol Metab. 2015;4(2):106-17.

[138] Mithieux G, Misery P, Magnan C, Pillot B, Gautier-Stein A, Bernard C, et al. Portal sensing of intestinal gluconeogenesis is a mechanistic link in the diminution of food intake induced by diet protein. Cell Metab. 2005;2(5):321-9.

[139] Pillot B, Soty M, Gautier-Stein A, Zitoun C, Mithieux G. Protein feeding promotes redistribution of endogenous glucose production to the kidney and potentiates its suppression by insulin. Endocrinology. 2009;150(2):616-24.

[140] Duraffourd C, De Vadder F, Goncalves D, Delaere F, Penhoat A, Brusset B, et al. Mu-opioid receptors and dietary protein stimulate a gut-brain neural circuitry limiting food intake. Cell. 2012;150(2):377-88.

[141] De Vadder F, Kovatcheva-Datchary P, Goncalves D, Vinera J, Zitoun C, Duchampt A, et al. Microbiota-generated metabolites promote metabolic benefits via gut-brain neural circuits. Cell. 2014;156(1-2):84-96.

[142] Glass MJ, Billington CJ, Levine AS. Opioids and food intake: distributed functional neural pathways? Neuropeptides. 1999;33(5):360-8.

[143] Shin AC, Pistell PJ, Phifer CB, Berthoud HR. Reversible suppression of food reward behavior by chronic mu-opioid receptor antagonism in the nucleus accumbens. Neuroscience. 2010;170(2):580-8.

[144] Howland RH. Vagus Nerve Stimulation. Curr Behav Neurosci Rep. 2014;1(2):64-73.

[145] Krahl SE. Vagus nerve stimulation for epilepsy: A review of the peripheral mechanisms. Surg Neurol Int. 2012;3(Suppl 1):S47-52.

[146] George MS, Sackeim HA, Rush AJ, Marangell LB, Nahas Z, Husain MM, et al. Vagus nerve stimulation: a new tool for brain research and therapy. Biol Psychiatry. 2000;47(4):287-95.

[147] Breit S, Kupferberg A, Rogler G, Hasler G. Vagus Nerve as Modulator of the Brain-Gut Axis in Psychiatric and Inflammatory Disorders. Front Psychiatry. 2018;9:44.

[148] Brookes SJ, Spencer NJ, Costa M, Zagorodnyuk VP. Extrinsic primary afferent signalling in the gut. Nat Rev Gastroenterol Hepatol. 2013;10(5):286-96.

[149] Berthoud HR, Blackshaw LA, Brookes SJ, Grundy D. Neuroanatomy of extrinsic afferents supplying the gastrointestinal tract. Neurogastroenterol Motil. 2004;16 Suppl 1:28-33.

[150] Mei N. Vagal glucoreceptors in the small intestine of the cat. J Physiol. 1978;282:485-506.

[151] Jeanningros R. Vagal unitary responses to intestinal amino acid infusions in the anesthetized cat: a putative signal for protein induced satiety. Physiol Behav. 1982;28(1):9-21.

[152] Lal S, Kirkup AJ, Brunsden AM, Thompson DG, Grundy D. Vagal afferent responses to fatty acids of different chain length in the rat. Am J Physiol Gastrointest Liver Physiol. 2001;281(4):G907-15.

[153] Berthoud HR. Vagal and hormonal gut-brain communication: from satiation to satisfaction.

Neurogastroenterol Motil. 2008;20 Suppl 1:64-72.

[154] Holst JJ. The physiology of glucagon-like peptide 1. Physiol Rev. 2007;87(4):1409-39.

[155] Thorens B. Expression cloning of the pancreatic beta cell receptor for the gluco-incretin hormone glucagon-like peptide 1. Proc Natl Acad Sci U S A. 1992;89(18):8641-5.

[156] Hayes MR, De Jonghe BC, Kanoski SE. Role of the glucagon-like-peptide-1 receptor in the control of energy balance. Physiol Behav. 2010;100(5):503-10.

[157] Williams EK, Chang RB, Strochlic DE, Umans BD, Lowell BB, Liberles SD. Sensory Neurons that Detect Stretch and Nutrients in the Digestive System. Cell. 2016;166(1):209-21.

[158] Bonaz B, Bazin T, Pellissier S. The Vagus Nerve at the Interface of the Microbiota-Gut-Brain Axis. Front Neurosci. 2018;12:49.

[159] Berthoud HR. The vagus nerve, food intake and obesity. Regul Pept. 2008;149(1-3):15-25.

[160] Badman MK, Flier JS. The gut and energy balance: visceral allies in the obesity wars. Science. 2005;307(5717):1909-14.

[161] Owyang C, Heldsinger A. Vagal control of satiety and hormonal regulation of appetite. J Neurogastroenterol Motil. 2011;17(4):338-48.

[162] Zurowski D, Nowak L, Wordliczek J, Dobrogowski J, Thor PJ. Effects of vagus nerve stimulation in visceral pain model. Folia Med Cracov. 2012;52(1-2):57-69.

[163] Tan HE, Sisti AC, Jin H, Vignovich M, Villavicencio M, Tsang KS, et al. The gut-brain axis mediates sugar preference. Nature. 2020;580(7804):511-6.

[164] Hartenstein V, Tepass U, Gruszynski-Defeo E. Embryonic development of the stomatogastric nervous system in *Drosophila*. J Comp Neurol. 1994;350(3):367-81.

[165] Gonzalez-Gaitan M, Jackle H. Invagination centers within the *Drosophila* stomatogastric nervous system anlage are positioned by Notch-mediated signaling which is spatially controlled through wingless. Development. 1995;121(8):2313-25.

[166] Pankratz MJ, Hoch M. Control of epithelial morphogenesis by cell signaling and integrin molecules in the *Drosophila* foregut. Development. 1995;121(6):1885-98.

[167] Spiess R, Schoofs A, Heinzel HG. Anatomy of the stomatogastric nervous system associated with the foregut in *Drosophila melanogaster* and *Calliphora vicina* third instar larvae. J Morphol. 2008;269(3):272-82.

[168] Lee G, Park JH. Hemolymph sugar homeostasis and starvation-induced hyperactivity affected by genetic manipulations of the adipokinetic hormone-encoding gene in *Drosophila melanogaster*. Genetics. 2004;167(1):311-23.

[169] Miguel-Aliaga I, Thor S. Segment-specific prevention of pioneer neuron apoptosis by cell-autonomous, postmitotic Hox gene activity. Development. 2004;131(24):6093-105.

[170] Miguel-Aliaga I, Thor S, Gould AP. Postmitotic specification of *Drosophila* insulinergic neurons from pioneer neurons. PLoS Biol. 2008;6(3):e58.

[171] Talsma AD, Christov CP, Terriente-Felix A, Linneweber GA, Perea D,

Wayland M, et al. Remote control of renal physiology by the intestinal neuropeptide pigment-dispersing factor in *Drosophila*. Proc Natl Acad Sci U S A. 2012;109(30):12177-82.

[172] Schoofs A, Huckesfeld S, Surendran S, Pankratz MJ. Serotonergic pathways in the *Drosophila* larval enteric nervous system. J Insect Physiol. 2014;69:118-25.

[173] Myers L, Perera H, Alvarado MG, Kidd T. The *Drosophila* Ret gene functions in the stomatogastric nervous system with the Maverick TGFbeta ligand and the Gfrl co-receptor. Development. 2018;145(3).

[174] Perea D, Guiu J, Hudry B, Konstantinidou C, Milona A, Hadjieconomou D, et al. Ret receptor tyrosine kinase sustains proliferation and tissue maturation in intestinal epithelia. EMBO J. 2017;36(20): 3029-45.

[175] Kenmoku H, Ishikawa H, Ote M, Kuraishi T, Kurata S. A subset of neurons controls the permeability of the peritrophic matrix and midgut structure in *Drosophila* adults. J Exp Biol. 2016;219(Pt 15):2331-9.

[176] Stocker RF. The organization of the chemosensory system in *Drosophila melanogaster*: a review. Cell Tissue Res. 1994;275(1):3-26.

[177] Wang Z, Singhvi A, Kong P, Scott K. Taste representations in the *Drosophila* brain. Cell. 2004;117(7):981-91.

[178] Marella S, Fischler W, Kong P, Asgarian S, Rueckert E, Scott K. Imaging taste responses in the fly brain reveals a functional map of taste category and behavior. Neuron. 2006;49(2):285-95.

[179] Ito K, Shinomiya K, Ito M, Armstrong JD, Boyan G, Hartenstein V, et al. A systematic nomenclature for the insect brain. Neuron. 2014;81(4):755-65.

[180] Budnik V, Wu CF, White K. Altered branching of serotonin-containing neurons in *Drosophila* mutants unable to synthesize serotonin and dopamine. J Neurosci. 1989;9(8):2866-77.

[181] McCormick J, Nichols R. Spatial and temporal expression identify dromyosuppressin as a brain-gut peptide in *Drosophila melanogaster*. J Comp Neurol. 1993;338(2):278-88.

[182] Nichols R, Bendena WG, Tobe SS. Myotropic peptides in *Drosophila melanogaster* and the genes that encode them. J Neurogenet. 2002;16(1):1-28.

[183] Anderson MS, Halpern ME, Keshishian H. Identification of the neuropeptide transmitter proctolin in *Drosophila* larvae: characterization of muscle fiber-specific neuromuscular endings. J Neurosci. 1988;8(1):242-55.

[184] Nassel DR, Shiga S, Mohrherr CJ, Rao KR. Pigment-dispersing hormone-like peptide in the nervous system of the flies Phormia and *Drosophila*: immunocytochemistry and partial characterization. J Comp Neurol. 1993;331(2):183-98.

[185] Dircksen H, Tesfai LK, Albus C, Nassel DR. Ion transport peptide splice forms in central and peripheral neurons throughout postembryogenesis of *Drosophila melanogaster*. J Comp Neurol. 2008;509(1):23-41.

[186] Dircksen H. Insect ion transport peptides are derived from alternatively spliced genes and differentially expressed in the central and peripheral nervous system. J Exp Biol. 2009;212 (Pt 3):401-12.

[187] Cao C, Brown MR. Localization of an insulin-like peptide in brains of two flies. Cell Tissue Res. 2001;304(2):317-21.

[188] Kaminski S, Orlowski E, Berry K, Nichols R. The effects of three *Drosophila melanogaster* myotropins on the frequency of foregut contractions differ. J Neurogenet. 2002;16(2):125-34.

[189] Price MD, Merte J, Nichols R, Koladich PM, Tobe SS, Bendena WG. *Drosophila* melanogaster flatline encodes a myotropin orthologue to Manduca sexta allatostatin. Peptides. 2002;23(4):787-94.

[190] Palmer GC, Tran T, Duttlinger A, Nichols R. The drosulfakinin 0 (DSK 0) peptide encoded in the conserved Dsk gene affects adult *Drosophila melanogaster* crop contractions. J Insect Physiol. 2007;53(11):1125-33.

[191] Vanderveken M, O'Donnell MJ. Effects of diuretic hormone 31, drosokinin, and allatostatin A on transepithelial K(+) transport and contraction frequency in the midgut and hindgut of larval *Drosophila melanogaster*. Arch Insect Biochem Physiol. 2014;85(2):76-93.

[192] Zhang W, Yan Z, Li B, Jan LY, Jan YN. Identification of motor neurons and a mechanosensitive sensory neuron in the defecation circuitry of *Drosophila* larvae. Elife. 2014;3.

[193] Wayland MT, Defaye A, Rocha J, Jayaram SA, Royet J, Miguel-Aliaga I, et al. Spotting the differences: probing host/microbiota interactions with a dedicated software tool for the analysis of faecal outputs in *Drosophila*. J Insect Physiol. 2014;69:126-35.

[194] Han H, Pan C, Liu C, Lv X, Yang X, Xiong Y, et al. Gut-neuron interaction via Hh signaling regulates intestinal progenitor cell differentiation in *Drosophila*. Cell Discov. 2015;1:15006.

[195] Olds WH, Xu T. Regulation of food intake by mechanosensory ion channels in enteric neurons. Elife. 2014;3.

[196] Galindo K, Smith DP. A large family of divergent *Drosophila* odorant-binding proteins expressed in gustatory and olfactory sensilla. Genetics. 2001;159(3):1059-72.

[197] LeDue EE, Chen YC, Jung AY, Dahanukar A, Gordon MD. Pharyngeal sense organs drive robust sugar consumption in *Drosophila*. Nat Commun. 2015;6:6667.

[198] Yapici N, Cohn R, Schusterreiter C, Ruta V, Vosshall LB. A Taste Circuit that Regulates Ingestion by Integrating Food and Hunger Signals. Cell. 2016;165(3):715-29.

[199] Dethier V. G. GA, 1967 HyperphagiaintheblowflyJExpBiol

[200] Pool AH, Kvello P, Mann K, Cheung SK, Gordon MD, Wang L, et al. Four GABAergic interneurons impose feeding restraint in *Drosophila*. Neuron. 2014;83(1):164-77.

[201] Belzer W. R. Recurrent nerve inhibition of protein feeding in the blowfly *Phormia regina*. Physiol Entomol. 1978;3:259-63.

[202] Miyamoto T, Slone J, Song X, Amrein H. A fructose receptor functions as a nutrient sensor in the *Drosophila* brain. Cell. 2012;151(5):1113-25.

[203] Mishra D, Miyamoto T, Rezenom YH, Broussard A, Yavuz A, Slone J, et al. The molecular basis of sugar sensing in *Drosophila* larvae. Curr Biol. 2013;23(15):1466-71.

[204] Miyamoto T, Amrein H. Diverse roles for the *Drosophila* fructose sensor Gr43a. Fly (Austin). 2014;8(1):19-25.

[205] Holzer P, Farzi A, Hassan AM, Zenz G, Jacan A, Reichmann F. Visceral Inflammation and Immune Activation Stress the Brain. Front Immunol. 2017;8:1613.

[206] Burbach JP. Neuropeptides from concept to online database www.neuropeptides.nl. Eur J Pharmacol. 2010;626(1):27-48.

[207] Dockray GJ. Gastrointestinal hormones and the dialogue between gut and brain. J Physiol. 2014;592(14):2927-41.

[208] Holzer P, Farzi A. Neuropeptides and the microbiota-gut-brain axis. Adv Exp Med Biol. 2014;817:195-219.

[209] Kastin AJ. Handbook of biologically active peptides (2nd ed.). New York, NY: Academic Press. 2013.

[210] Lach G, Schellekens H, Dinan TG, Cryan JF. Anxiety, Depression, and the Microbiome: A Role for Gut Peptides. Neurotherapeutics. 2018;15(1):36-59.

[211] Strand FL. Neuropeptides: Regulators of physiological processes. Cambridge, MA: MIT Press1999

[212] Holzer P. Neuropeptides, Microbiota, and Behavior. Int Rev Neurobiol. 2016;131:67-89.

[213] Kaelberer MM, Buchanan KL, Klein ME, Barth BB, Montoya MM, Shen X, et al. A gut-brain neural circuit for nutrient sensory transduction. Science. 2018;361(6408).

[214] Beutler LR, Chen Y, Ahn JS, Lin YC, Essner RA, Knight ZA. Dynamics of Gut-Brain Communication Underlying Hunger. Neuron. 2017;96(2):461-75 e5.

[215] Cummings DE, Overduin J. Gastrointestinal regulation of food intake. J Clin Invest. 2007;117(1):13-23.

[216] Koda S, Date Y, Murakami N, Shimbara T, Hanada T, Toshinai K, et al. The role of the vagal nerve in peripheral PYY3-36-induced feeding reduction in rats. Endocrinology. 2005;146(5):2369-75.

[217] Cheng H, Leblond CP. Origin, differentiation and renewal of the four main epithelial cell types in the mouse small intestine. III. Entero-endocrine cells. Am J Anat. 1974;141(4):503-19.

[218] Micchelli CA, Perrimon N. Evidence that stem cells reside in the adult *Drosophila* midgut epithelium. Nature. 2006;439(7075):475-9.

[219] Beehler-Evans R, Micchelli CA. Generation of enteroendocrine cell diversity in midgut stem cell lineages. Development. 2015;142(4):654-64.

[220] Veenstra JA, Agricola HJ, Sellami A. Regulatory peptides in fruit fly midgut. Cell Tissue Res. 2008;334(3):499-516.

[221] Veenstra JA. Peptidergic paracrine and endocrine cells in the midgut of the fruit fly maggot. Cell Tissue Res. 2009;336(2):309-23.

[222] Reiher W, Shirras C, Kahnt J, Baumeister S, Isaac RE, Wegener C. Peptidomics and peptide hormone processing in the *Drosophila* midgut. J Proteome Res. 2011;10(4):1881-92.

[223] Hartenstein V. The neuroendocrine system of invertebrates: a developmental and evolutionary perspective. J Endocrinol. 2006;190(3):555-70.

[224] Hartenstein V, Takashima S, Adams KL. Conserved genetic pathways controlling the development of the diffuse endocrine system in vertebrates and *Drosophila*. Gen Comp Endocrinol. 2010;166(3):462-9.

[225] Hartenstein V, Takashima S, Hartenstein P, Asanad S, Asanad K. bHLH proneural genes as cell fate determinants of entero-endocrine cells, an evolutionarily conserved lineage sharing a common root with sensory neurons. Dev Biol. 2017;431(1):36-47.

[226] Li S, Torre-Muruzabal T, Sogaard KC, Ren GR, Hauser F, Engelsen SM, et al. Expression patterns of the *Drosophila* neuropeptide CCHamide-2 and its receptor may suggest hormonal signaling from the gut to the brain. PLoS One. 2013;8(10):e76131.

[227] LaJeunesse DR, Johnson B, Presnell JS, Catignas KK, Zapotoczny G. Peristalsis in the junction region of the *Drosophila* larval midgut is modulated by DH31 expressing enteroendocrine cells. BMC Physiol. 2010;10:14.

[228] O'Brien LE, Soliman SS, Li X, Bilder D. Altered modes of stem cell division drive adaptive intestinal growth. Cell. 2011;147(3):603-14.

[229] Li J, Song J, Zaytseva YY, Liu Y, Rychahou P, Jiang K, et al. An obligatory role for neurotensin in high-fat-diet-induced obesity. Nature. 2016;533(7603):411-5.

[230] Song W, Cheng D, Hong S, Sappe B, Hu Y, Wei N, et al. Midgut-Derived Activin Regulates Glucagon-like Action in the Fat Body and Glycemic Control. Cell Metab. 2017;25(2):386-99.

[231] Roller L, Yamanaka N, Watanabe K, Daubnerova I, Zitnan D, Kataoka H, et al. The unique evolution of neuropeptide genes in the silkworm *Bombyx mori*. Insect Biochem Mol Biol. 2008;38(12):1147-57.

[232] Hansen KK, Hauser F, Williamson M, Weber SB, Grimmelikhuijzen CJ. The *Drosophila* genes CG14593 and CG30106 code for G-protein-coupled receptors specifically activated by the neuropeptides CCHamide-1 and CCHamide-2. Biochem Biophys Res Commun. 2011;404(1):184-9.

[233] Ren GR, Hauser F, Rewitz KF, Kondo S, Engelbrecht AF, Didriksen AK, et al. CCHamide-2 Is an Orexigenic Brain-Gut Peptide in *Drosophila*. PLoS One. 2015;10(7):e0133017.

[234] Sano H, Nakamura A, Texada MJ, Truman JW, Ishimoto H, Kamikouchi A, et al. The Nutrient-Responsive Hormone CCHamide-2 Controls Growth by Regulating Insulin-like Peptides in the Brain of *Drosophila melanogaster*. PLoS Genet. 2015;11(5):e1005209.

[235] Alfa RW, Park S, Skelly KR, Poffenberger G, Jain N, Gu X, et al. Suppression of insulin production and secretion by a decretin hormone. Cell Metab. 2015;21(2):323-34.

[236] Clemmensen C, Muller TD, Woods SC, Berthoud HR, Seeley RJ, Tschop MH. Gut-Brain Cross-Talk in Metabolic Control. Cell. 2017;168(5):758-74.

[237] Obniski R, Sieber M, Spradling AC. Dietary Lipids Modulate Notch Signaling and Influence Adult Intestinal Development and Metabolism in *Drosophila*. Dev Cell. 2018;47(1):98-111 e5.

[238] O'Donnell MJ, Dow JA, Huesmann GR, Tublitz NJ, Maddrell SH. Separate control of anion and cation transport in malpighian tubules of *Drosophila melanogaster*. J Exp Biol. 1996;199(Pt 5):1163-75.

[239] Radford JC, Davies SA, Dow JA. Systematic G-protein-coupled receptor analysis in *Drosophila melanogaster* identifies a leucokinin receptor with novel roles. J Biol Chem. 2002;277(41):38810-7.

[240] Shen R, Wang B, Giribaldi MG, Ayres J, Thomas JB, Montminy M. Neuronal energy-sensing pathway promotes energy balance by modulating disease tolerance. Proc Natl Acad Sci U S A. 2016;113(23):E3307-14.

[241] Rodenfels J, Lavrynenko O, Ayciriex S, Sampaio JL, Carvalho M,

Shevchenko A, et al. Production of systemically circulating Hedgehog by the intestine couples nutrition to growth and development. Genes Dev. 2014;28(23):2636-51.

[242] de Velasco B, Erclik T, Shy D, Sclafani J, Lipshitz H, McInnes R, et al. Specification and development of the pars intercerebralis and pars lateralis, neuroendocrine command centers in the *Drosophila* brain. Dev Biol. 2007;302(1):309-23.

[243] Schoofs A, Huckesfeld S, Schlegel P, Miroschnikow A, Peters M, Zeymer M, et al. Selection of motor programs for suppressing food intake and inducing locomotion in the *Drosophila* brain. PLoS Biol. 2014;12(6):e1001893.

[244] Yang Z, Huang R, Fu X, Wang G, Qi W, Mao D, et al. A post-ingestive amino acid sensor promotes food consumption in *Drosophila*. Cell Res. 2018;28(10):1013-25.

[245] Richer S, Stoffolano JG, Jr., Yin CM, Nichols R. Innervation of dromyosuppressin (DMS) immunoreactive processes and effect of DMS and benzethonium chloride on the *Phormia regina* (Meigen) crop. J Comp Neurol. 2000;421(1):136-42.

[246] Luo J, Lushchak OV, Goergen P, Williams MJ, Nassel DR. *Drosophila* insulin-producing cells are differentially modulated by serotonin and octopamine receptors and affect social behavior. PLoS One. 2014;9(6):e99732.

[247] Ikeya T, Galic M, Belawat P, Nairz K, Hafen E. Nutrient-dependent expression of insulin-like peptides from neuroendocrine cells in the CNS contributes to growth regulation in *Drosophila*. Curr Biol. 2002;12(15):1293-300.

[248] Nassel DR, Kubrak OI, Liu Y, Luo J, Lushchak OV. Factors that regulate insulin producing cells and their output in *Drosophila*. Front Physiol. 2013;4:252.

[249] Kannan K, Fridell YW. Functional implications of *Drosophila* insulin-like peptides in metabolism, aging, and dietary restriction. Front Physiol. 2013;4:288.

[250] Brown MR, Crim JW, Arata RC, Cai HN, Chun C, Shen P. Identification of a *Drosophila* brain-gut peptide related to the neuropeptide Y family. Peptides. 1999;20(9):1035-42.

[251] Fadda M, Hasakiogullari I, Temmerman L, Beets I, Zels S, Schoofs L. Regulation of Feeding and Metabolism by Neuropeptide F and Short Neuropeptide F in Invertebrates. Front Endocrinol (Lausanne). 2019;10:64.

[252] Nassel DR, Wegener C. A comparative review of short and long neuropeptide F signaling in invertebrates: Any similarities to vertebrate neuropeptide Y signaling? Peptides. 2011;32(6):1335-55.

[253] Mertens I, Meeusen T, Huybrechts R, De Loof A, Schoofs L. Characterization of the short neuropeptide F receptor from *Drosophila melanogaster*. Biochem Biophys Res Commun. 2002;297(5):1140-8.

[254] Lee KS, Kwon OY, Lee JH, Kwon K, Min KJ, Jung SA, et al. *Drosophila* short neuropeptide F signalling regulates growth by ERK-mediated insulin signalling. Nat Cell Biol. 2008;10(4):468-75.

[255] Lee KS, You KH, Choo JK, Han YM, Yu K. *Drosophila* short neuropeptide F regulates food intake and body size. J Biol Chem. 2004;279(49):50781-9.

[256] Findeisen M, Rathmann D, Beck-Sickinger AG. Structure-activity studies of RFamide peptides reveal

subtype-selective activation of neuropeptide FF1 and FF2 receptors. ChemMedChem. 2011;6(6):1081-93.

[257] Bechtold DA, Luckman SM. The role of RFamide peptides in feeding. J Endocrinol. 2007;192(1):3-15.

[258] Woodhead AP, Stay B, Seidel SL, Khan MA, Tobe SS. Primary structure of four allatostatins: neuropeptide inhibitors of juvenile hormone synthesis. Proc Natl Acad Sci U S A. 1989;86(15):5997-6001.

[259] Lorenz MW, Kellner R, Hoffmann KH. A family of neuropeptides that inhibit juvenile hormone biosynthesis in the cricket, Gryllus bimaculatus. J Biol Chem. 1995;270(36):21103-8.

[260] Kramer SJ, Toschi A, Miller CA, Kataoka H, Quistad GB, Li JP, et al. Identification of an allatostatin from the tobacco hornworm Manduca sexta. Proc Natl Acad Sci U S A. 1991;88(21):9458-62.

[261] Birgul N, Weise C, Kreienkamp HJ, Richter D. Reverse physiology in *drosophila*: identification of a novel allatostatin-like neuropeptide and its cognate receptor structurally related to the mammalian somatostatin/galanin/opioid receptor family. EMBO J. 1999;18(21):5892-900.

[262] Lenz C, Williamson M, Grimmelikhuijzen CJ. Molecular cloning and genomic organization of an allatostatin preprohormone from *Drosophila melanogaster*. Biochem Biophys Res Commun. 2000;273(3):1126-31.

[263] Renn SC, Park JH, Rosbash M, Hall JC, Taghert PH. A pdf neuropeptide gene mutation and ablation of PDF neurons each cause severe abnormalities of behavioral circadian rhythms in *Drosophila*. Cell. 1999;99(7):791-802.

[264] Shafer OT, Yao Z. Pigment-Dispersing Factor Signaling and Circadian Rhythms in Insect Locomotor Activity. Curr Opin Insect Sci. 2014;1:73-80.

[265] de Lartigue G, de La Serre CB, Raybould HE. Vagal afferent neurons in high fat diet-induced obesity; intestinal microflora, gut inflammation and cholecystokinin. Physiol Behav. 2011;105(1):100-5.

[266] Grasset E, Puel A, Charpentier J, Collet X, Christensen JE, Terce F, et al. A Specific Gut Microbiota Dysbiosis of Type 2 Diabetic Mice Induces GLP-1 Resistance through an Enteric NO-Dependent and Gut-Brain Axis Mechanism. Cell Metab. 2017;25(5):1075-90 e5.

[267] Broderick NA, Lemaitre B. Gut-associated microbes of *Drosophila melanogaster*. Gut Microbes. 2012;3(4):307-21.

[268] Reiter LT, Potocki L, Chien S, Gribskov M, Bier E. A systematic analysis of human disease-associated gene sequences in *Drosophila melanogaster*. Genome Res. 2001;11(6):1114-25.

[269] Birse RT, Choi J, Reardon K, Rodriguez J, Graham S, Diop S, et al. High-fat-diet-induced obesity and heart dysfunction are regulated by the TOR pathway in *Drosophila*. Cell Metab. 2010;12(5):533-44.

[270] Na J, Musselman LP, Pendse J, Baranski TJ, Bodmer R, Ocorr K, et al. A *Drosophila* model of high sugar diet-induced cardiomyopathy. PLoS Genet. 2013;9(1):e1003175.

[271] Na J, Sweetwyne MT, Park AS, Susztak K, Cagan RL. Diet-Induced Podocyte Dysfunction in *Drosophila* and Mammals. Cell Rep. 2015;12(4):636-47.

[272] Palm W, Swierczynska MM, Kumari V, Ehrhart-Bornstein M, Bornstein SR, Eaton S. Secretion and signaling activities of lipoprotein-associated hedgehog and non-sterol-modified hedgehog in flies and mammals. PLoS Biol. 2013;11(3):e1001505.

[273] Lin WS, Huang CW, Song YS, Yen JH, Kuo PC, Yeh SR, et al. Reduced Gut Acidity Induces an Obese-Like Phenotype in *Drosophila melanogaster* and in Mice. PLoS One. 2015;10(10):e0139722.

[274] Wong AC, Dobson AJ, Douglas AE. Gut microbiota dictates the metabolic response of *Drosophila* to diet. J Exp Biol. 2014;217(Pt 11):1894-901.

[275] Newell PD, Douglas AE. Interspecies interactions determine the impact of the gut microbiota on nutrient allocation in *Drosophila melanogaster*. Appl Environ Microbiol. 2014;80(2):788-96.

[276] Whon TW, Shin NR, Jung MJ, Hyun DW, Kim HS, Kim PS, et al. Conditionally Pathogenic Gut Microbes Promote Larval Growth by Increasing Redox-Dependent Fat Storage in High-Sugar Diet-Fed *Drosophila*. Antioxid Redox Signal. 2017;27(16):1361-80.

[277] Huang JH, Douglas AE. Consumption of dietary sugar by gut bacteria determines *Drosophila* lipid content. Biol Lett. 2015;11(9):20150469.

[278] Iadanza MG, Jackson MP, Hewitt EW, Ranson NA, Radford SE. A new era for understanding amyloid structures and disease. Nat Rev Mol Cell Biol. 2018;19(12):755-73.

[279] Llorens F, Thune K, Andres-Benito P, Tahir W, Ansoleaga B, Hernandez-Ortega K, et al. MicroRNA Expression in the Locus Coeruleus, Entorhinal Cortex, and Hippocampus at Early and Middle Stages of Braak Neurofibrillary Tangle Pathology. J Mol Neurosci. 2017;63(2):206-15.

[280] Vangay P, Ward T, Gerber JS, Knights D. Antibiotics, pediatric dysbiosis, and disease. Cell Host Microbe. 2015;17(5):553-64.

[281] Muegge BD, Kuczynski J, Knights D, Clemente JC, Gonzalez A, Fontana L, et al. Diet drives convergence in gut microbiome functions across mammalian phylogeny and within humans. Science. 2011;332(6032):970-4.

[282] Delzenne NM, Neyrinck AM, Cani PD. Modulation of the gut microbiota by nutrients with prebiotic properties: consequences for host health in the context of obesity and metabolic syndrome. Microb Cell Fact. 2011;10 Suppl 1:S10.

[283] Tilg H, Moschen AR. Microbiota and diabetes: an evolving relationship. Gut. 2014;63(9):1513-21.

[284] Rosenfeld CS. Microbiome Disturbances and Autism Spectrum Disorders. Drug Metab Dispos. 2015;43(10):1557-71.

[285] Galloway S, Jian L, Johnsen R, Chew S, Mamo JC. beta-amyloid or its precursor protein is found in epithelial cells of the small intestine and is stimulated by high-fat feeding. J Nutr Biochem. 2007;18(4):279-84.

[286] Galloway S, Takechi R, Pallebage-Gamarallage MM, Dhaliwal SS, Mamo JC. Amyloid-beta colocalizes with apolipoprotein B in absorptive cells of the small intestine. Lipids Health Dis. 2009;8:46.

[287] Nam KN, Mounier A, Wolfe CM, Fitz NF, Carter AY, Castranio EL, et al. Effect of high fat diet on phenotype, brain transcriptome and lipidome in Alzheimer's model mice. Sci Rep. 2017;7(1):4307.

[288] Lin B, Hasegawa Y, Takane K, Koibuchi N, Cao C, Kim-Mitsuyama S. High-Fat-Diet Intake Enhances Cerebral Amyloid Angiopathy and Cognitive Impairment in a Mouse Model of Alzheimer's Disease, Independently of Metabolic Disorders. J Am Heart Assoc. 2016;5(6).

[289] Goedert M. NEURODEGENERATION. Alzheimer's and Parkinson's diseases: The prion concept in relation to assembled Abeta, tau, and alpha-synuclein. Science. 2015;349(6248):1255555.

[290] Ano Y, Sakudo A, Nakayama H, Onodera T. Uptake and dynamics of infectious prion protein in the intestine. Protein Pept Lett. 2009;16(3):247-55.

[291] Yoshioka H, Takeda T, Higuchi K, Ohshio G, Miyake T, Sugiyama T, et al. Immunohistochemical examination of Peyer's patches in senescence-accelerated mice. Autoimmunity. 1990;8(1):25-35.

[292] Kimura I, Inoue D, Maeda T, Hara T, Ichimura A, Miyauchi S, et al. Short-chain fatty acids and ketones directly regulate sympathetic nervous system via G protein-coupled receptor 41 (GPR41). Proc Natl Acad Sci U S A. 2011;108(19):8030-5.

[293] Tan FHP, Liu G, Lau SA, Jaafar MH, Park YH, Azzam G, et al. Lactobacillus probiotics improved the gut microbiota profile of a *Drosophila melanogaster* Alzheimer's disease model and alleviated neurodegeneration in the eye. Benef Microbes. 2020;11(1):79-89.

[294] Feltzin V, Wan KH, Celniker SE, Bonini NM. Role and impact of the gut microbiota in a *Drosophila* model for parkinsonism. 2019:718825.

[295] Scheperjans F, Aho V, Pereira PA, Koskinen K, Paulin L, Pekkonen E, et al. Gut microbiota are related to Parkinson's disease and clinical phenotype. Mov Disord. 2015;30(3):350-8.

[296] Chen K, Luan X, Liu Q, Wang J, Chang X, Snijders AM, et al. *Drosophila* Histone Demethylase KDM5 Regulates Social Behavior through Immune Control and Gut Microbiota Maintenance. Cell Host Microbe. 2019;25(4):537-52 e8.

[297] Ryu JH, Kim SH, Lee HY, Bai JY, Nam YD, Bae JW, et al. Innate immune homeostasis by the homeobox gene caudal and commensal-gut mutualism in *Drosophila*. Science. 2008;319(5864):777-82.

[298] Ha EM, Oh CT, Bae YS, Lee WJ. A direct role for dual oxidase in *Drosophila* gut immunity. Science. 2005;310(5749):847-50.

[299] Ha EM, Oh CT, Ryu JH, Bae YS, Kang SW, Jang IH, et al. An antioxidant system required for host protection against gut infection in *Drosophila*. Dev Cell. 2005;8(1):125-32.

[300] Yu X, Waltzer L, Bienz M. A new *Drosophila* APC homologue associated with adhesive zones of epithelial cells. Nat Cell Biol. 1999;1(3):144-51.

[301] Tian A, Benchabane H, Ahmed Y. Wingless/Wnt Signaling in Intestinal Development, Homeostasis, Regeneration and Tumorigenesis: A *Drosophila* Perspective. J Dev Biol. 2018;6(2).

[302] Cordero JB, Stefanatos RK, Myant K, Vidal M, Sansom OJ. Non-autonomous crosstalk between the Jak/Stat and Egfr pathways mediates Apc1-driven intestinal stem cell hyperplasia in the *Drosophila* adult midgut. Development. 2012;139(24):4524-35.

[303] Cordero JB, Ridgway RA, Valeri N, Nixon C, Frame MC, Muller WJ, et al. c-Src drives intestinal regeneration

DOI: http://dx.doi.org/10.5772/intechopen.96503

and transformation. EMBO J. 2014;33(13):1474-91.

[304] Christofi T, Apidianakis Y. Ras-oncogenic *Drosophila* hindgut but not midgut cells use an inflammation-like program to disseminate to distant sites. Gut Microbes. 2013;4(1):54-9.

[305] Ghosh S, Tibbit C, Liu JL. Effective knockdown of *Drosophila* long non-coding RNAs by CRISPR interference. Nucleic Acids Res. 2016;44(9):e84.

[306] Miguel-Aliaga I, Jasper H, Lemaitre B. Anatomy and Physiology of the Digestive Tract of *Drosophila melanogaster*. Genetics. 2018;210(2):357-96.

Section 2

Animal Models of Skeletal and Cardiac Muscle Diseases

Chapter 4

Duchenne Muscular Dystrophy Animal Models

Tatiana V. Egorova, Ivan I. Galkin, Yulia V. Ivanova and Anna V. Polikarpova

Abstract

Duchenne muscular dystrophy is a complex and severe orphan disease. It develops when the organism lacks the expression of dystrophin - a large structural protein. Dystrophin is transcribed from the largest gene in the human genome. At the moment, there is no cure available. Dozens of groups all over the world search for cure. Animal models are an important component of both the fundamental research and therapy development. Many animal models reproducing the features of disease were created and actively used since the late 80's until present. The species diversity spans from invertebrates to primates and the genetic diversity of these models spans from single mutations to full gene deletions. The models are often non-interchangeable; while one model may be used for particular drug design it may be useless for another. Here we describe existing models, discuss their advantages and disadvantages and potential applications for research and therapy development.

Keywords: Duchenne muscular dystrophy, DMD, dystrophin, animal models, *mdx*, genome editing, exon-skipping, gene therapy

1. Introduction

Duchenne muscular dystrophy (DMD) was primarily described in 1834–1836 by Neapolitan physicians Giovanni Semmola and Gaetano Conte. Dr. Guillaume Duchenne de Boulogne made a significant contribution to the description of the disease in 1860s [1]. DMD is considered a rare, or orphan, disease but it is definitely one of the most frequent among muscular dystrophies. About one male in 3500 is diagnosed with DMD. DMD is an X-linked recessive disease so women are affected with a frequency of 1 case per 50 million [2–4]. Many attempts of various groups and organizations are set towards the search for the cure. Different strategies such as genome editing, replacement therapy, anti-inflammatory and antioxidative drug treatment are developed [5]. These therapies target different components of an extremely complex scheme of DMD pathogenesis. So animal models are important for study of the disease, research and development of the therapies. Many animal models were created or, in some cases, adapted from natural sources.

It is important to understand the mechanism of DMD pathogenesis and progression in order to discuss origins, purposes and potential uses of animal disease models. DMD develops when the organism lacks dystrophin expression. Dystrophin is encoded by the largest gene in the genome (*DMD*) that consists of more than 2.3

megabases (Mb). The gene contains 7 promoters and two polyadenylation signal sequences which orchestrate expression of 17 known isoforms. Three large isoforms are produced by three distant promoters. These isoforms are brain isoform Dp427c, muscle isoform Dp427m and Purkinje isoform Dp427p [6]. Each of them consists of 79 exons which include the first unique exon and 78 common exons. Several smaller isoforms are operated by 4 internal promoters and some of them have alternatively spliced variants. These isoforms are retinal Dp260, Dp140 which is prevalent in central nervous system (CNS) and kidney, Dp116 which is expressed in Schwann cells and ubiquitously expressed Dp71 and Dp40 [6, 7]. Muscle isoform Dp427m is the most characterized and widely studied due to its crucial role in DMD manifestation. Most of the mutations that lead to DMD progression are large insertions, exon deletions or duplications which lead to the shift of the reading frame in the Dp427m [8]. Usually these mutations produce preliminary stop codon leading to the complete absence of the protein [8]. Point mutations (deletions, insertions or substitutions) are responsible for a small portion of all DMD cases [8]. Other isoforms are studied less. The deficiency of most of them is usually linked to CNS and behavioral disorders while Dp260 deficiency is linked to retinal impairment [6, 7].

Muscle dystrophin is a very complicated molecular machine. The function of muscle dystrophin is formation of dystrophin-associated protein complex (DAPC) and absorption of mechanical tensions which occur due to muscle constriction [9]. Muscle dystrophin is 427 kDa protein that consists of 3685 amino acids [10]. The protein is usually divided in four functional and structural superdomains. The N-terminal superdomain consists of two calpain-homology domains and provides binding of the protein to actin. The second superdomain is called rod domain. It is the largest domain that includes 24 spectrin-like repeats and 4 unstructured hinge domains. It acts as a spring that adsorbs mechanical tensions. The third superdomain (referred to as cysteine-rich domain, or CR) includes WW-motif, two EF motifs and ZZ-motif. This domain binds dystrophin to the sarcolemmal proteins being the central driver of DAPC formation. C-terminal domain binds to several proteins performing mostly signal functions [10].

DAPC is located in sarcolemma and provides the linkage between dystrophin and external proteins such as laminin and collagen. The complex includes α- and β-dystroglycans, α-,β-, γ-,δ-,ε-sarcoglycans which interact with CR domain of dystrophin; and dystrobrevin, α1, β1, and β2-syntrophins, neuronal nitric oxide synthase (nNOS) and several other proteins which interact with C-terminal domain. The deficiency of these proteins also induces several pathologies such as limb-girdle muscular dystrophy, myotonia and some others [9].

The loss of dystrophin leads to several consequences. The initial one is the loss of membrane integrity and toughness. This causes membrane damage during muscle contractions and consequent membrane leakage. The homeostasis of extra- and intracellular components (calcium ions being the most important of all) is disrupted. This leads to calcium signaling imbalance, mitochondrial dysfunction (as mitochondria acts as calcium depo), proinflammatory and apoptotic signaling activation and other damaging consequences [11]. Finally, this results in muscle cell death and its replacement by new muscle cells originating from satellite predecessor cells that finally leads to depletion of the pool of satellite cells. Damaged and regenerating muscle tissue is characterized by central nuclei. The fraction of central nucleated myofibers is a quantitative marker of DMD progression and therapeutic treatment [12]. Normal muscular tissue is also replaced by connective tissue (fibrosis) and adipose tissue in addition to regeneration. Neutrophil and macrophage infiltration also accompanies the disease progression [13].

The first symptoms of DMD usually arise at the age of 16–18 months. The children may experience issues with walking, running or rising, toe walking or Gower's sign. At the age of 2–3 years old the muscles of lower limbs begin to degrade. The children suffer from extensive weakness and obtain specific gait patterns. Scoliosis and flexion contractures of the limbs also develop in DMD patients. At the age of 10–12 years old children begin to use a wheelchair. Later, at 14 y.o., some patients develop dilated cardiomyopathy and arrhythmia. Patients usually die at 20 years due to heart failure or respiratory distress in absence of proper treatment. Female carriers do not suffer from severe symptoms; they usually have cardiomyopathy, mild respiratory issues, creatine kinase (CK) level enhancement and pseudo hypertrophy of the backside of the shin [14].

If any suspicious symptoms are observed CK level estimation is the first diagnostic procedure. This is a cheap and fast but not selective test as CK growth is a symptom of various muscle and nonmuscle (i.e. liver) diseases. So further diagnostics is required. If the CK is elevated the screening for exon deletion or duplication should be performed. About 30% of mutations may not be identified by these techniques (multiplex ligation-dependent probe amplification or comparative genomic hybridisation array) and full sequencing of the gene is required. The mutation location and character may help to predict the type and severity of the disease. If the mutation is still unidentified the muscle biopsy sample should be tested for dystrophin protein presence by immunohistochemistry or western blot [14].

In some cases, mutations in *DMD* gene do not lead to reading frame shift or do not cause severe instability or protein dysfunction. If the function of the protein is slightly affected the milder form of muscular dystrophy develops. This disease is referred to as Becker muscular dystrophy (BMD). BMD is characterized by a very wide spectrum of symptoms. In some cases disease may be almost as severe as DMD while in other cases it may develop comparatively mild phenotype [15]. In 1990 a patient with a large part (>50%) of the *DMD* gene deletion was discovered [16]. The patient was active at 61-year-old and demonstrated mild myodystrophy phenotype further described as BMD. The analysis of the mutant gene and its product revealed extremely valuable data on the mechanism of dystrophin molecular action. The deletion of the part of the gene did not lead to reading frame shift and functional protein was expressed. This protein lacked most of the rod domain while N-terminal, cysteine rich and C-terminal domains remained intact. Obviously the rod domain which is the largest part of the protein may be truncated without complete function loss. The second important outcome is the frameshift rule formulation. The restoration of the reading frame may lead to the synthesis of truncated but still partly functional protein and shift the DMD type to BMD type. These findings set the initial point for development of several antiDMD therapies [5].

Currently no ultimate cure for DMD exists. Several treatment strategies are currently applied and many approaches are waiting for approval or being developed [5]. Most of the approved treatments target the farther consequences of dystrophin loss [5, 11]. Glucocorticosteroids suppress fibrosis and inflammation and mechanical ventilation helps patients with respiratory deficits. Anti-inflammatory and antioxidant drugs are also used or being tested [11]. But these approaches do not target the primary issue and are capable of lengthening the lifespan for about a decade. Several more complex approaches are now being developed. One of the most promising candidate therapies is the gene replacement therapy [17]. The idea is the delivery of a shortened but still functional gene copy to the muscles lacking its natural variant. The delivery may be provided via various types of vectors such as viral vectors, nanoparticles or even plasmids [18]. Several difficulties complicate the path to success. These are extremely high research and production costs, immune response and comparatively large size of the protein and corresponding genetic construct. Another class of therapies being developed is restoration of the reading frame [19]. This may be achieved by introduction of antisense oligonucleotide, genome editing or some other techniques. The next class of therapies is utrophin modulation. Utrophin is an autosomal paralog of dystrophin which shares almost similar domain organization and high sequence correlation with dystrophin. In embryonic muscles utrophin localizes similarly to dystrophin and performs the same functions. In muscles utrophin is replaced by dystrophin in early childhood and in adults it is present in such non-muscle tissues as renal epithelia. In the adult organism utrophin expression is extremely low. In the case of dystrophin deficiency the expression of utrophin starts to increase but its level is still insufficient for dystrophin replacement in humans. Several approaches such as transcription modulators may potentially increase utrophin expression and slow down the disease progression [20]. Interestingly, several species such as mice are able to increase utrophin expression to sufficient level without any modulators [21]. This may provide fundamental data about dystrophy compensation mechanisms. However, it questions the adequacy of the DMD model based on these species. Other strategies include cell-based therapies which are being developed for a long time and interesting exosome-based approach which originated from cell-based one [22].

As can be seen from the above, the existing and potent strategies for DMD therapy include genome editing, pre-mRNA splicing and cell modification, gene or cell delivery, and others [5]. All of them require animal models to be tested. In most cases these models are not interchangeable. For example, if one develops an exon-skipping strategy for a rare mutation, they will need an animal model with a corresponding mutation. So ideally a unique model is essential for every single mutation (at least for most common of them). The type and location of mutation is also important as, despite almost all mutations lead to absence of three major isoforms, the presence or absence of short isoforms depends on mutation location and type. So different mutations on similar backgrounds may have different phenotypes and may be valuable both for research and drug development. Many animal (mostly mouse) models with different specific mutations were developed both for fundamental studies of the gene and protein function and role of short isoforms and for proof-of-concept and preclinical studies of potential therapies.

Despite mouse models of DMD being the most common due to their relative cheapness they possess a significant disadvantage. All dystrophin-deficient animals have dystrophic symptoms but the severity of them does not often correlate with the disease severity in DMD patients. For example the lifespan of classic mouse model *mdx* is about 80% of normal [23, 24] while the lifetime of a human with DMD is not more than one third of healthy. To circumvent these demerits, several other species were used to reproduce the phenotype of DMD in animals. These are large animal models (dogs, pigs, primates) or mouse models with mutations in additional genes, or crossbreed models. In some cases the genetic structure of these models does not correspond to any known DMD mutation in humans but similar phenotype makes them useful for studies of the disease and several symptomatic therapies.

Here we describe animal models starting from classic *mdx* identified in 80's to the newest ones introduced in 2020. The list of model species includes species from such invertebrates as *D. melanogaster* and *C. elegans* to monkeys. The origin, genotype, phenotype and purpose of these models are very diverse. We basically divide the models into two large groups. Chapter 1 will focus mostly on phenotypic properties of the most common models, the comparison of their advantages and disadvantages and their use in research and drug development. Chapter 2 will focus on the models created for development of unique and precision therapies. These are mostly murine models with various spectrum of mutations suitable for targeted drug design such as exon skipping.

2. Animal models to study the pathogenesis of DMD

The most widely used and well described animal model for Duchenne muscular dystrophy (DMD) research is the *mdx* mouse. Spontaneous X chromosome-linked mutation arose in inbred C57BL/10 colony of mice and produced viable and fertile homozygous animals. Mutant mice exhibited specific features similar to human DMD such as elevated plasma pyruvate kinase and CK levels and histological lesions of skeletal muscles. Later, the nature of the mutation was established. Nonsense point mutation caused by a single base substitution of C for T within an exon 23 leads to a premature termination of the dystrophin translation [24]. In addition to the absence of dystrophin all proteins of the DAPC such as sarcoglycans, syntrophin, nNOS, dystrobrevin, α-dystroglycan are significantly reduced at the sarcolemma in *mdx* skeletal muscle [9]. The absence of dystrophin and destabilization of the DAPC complex are believed to make muscle cells susceptible to stretch-induced damage and increased intracellular calcium influx. These pathological processes lead to skeletal and cardiac muscle degeneration [9]. Despite the absence of full-length dystrophin, *mdx* mice have mild symptoms of muscular dystrophy compared to DMD patients or the golden retriever muscular dystrophy (GRMD) dog model [24]. The pathogenesis of muscular dystrophy, physiological, biochemical and histological characteristics have been well studied in *mdx* mice of various ages. Birth body weight and neonatal death rates do not differ from their wild type counterparts. Significant histopathological abnormalities begin to be observed in *mdx* muscles at 3–4 weeks. The occurrence of extensive necrosis followed by regeneration and involving skeletal muscles was documented in *mdx* mice as young as 16–17 days [25]. In humans DMD is characterized by muscle hypertrophy in the early ages and atrophy in the late stages of disease. Contrary, in *mdx* mice myofibers pass through progressive hypertrophy from week 24 till the end of life without atrophy signs. Myofiber branching increased with the age and contributed to the hypertrophy. Aged *mdx* myofibers are also hypernucleated. The "extra" nuclei are central nuclei which highlight that the muscle undergoes continuous cycles of degeneration-regeneration. The estimation of synapse number indicated significant myofiber loss in *mdx* mice with the age [26]. The damaged skeletal muscle fibers with impaired function lead to a 20–30% loss in maximum specific force depending on mice age. The weakness is more severe in muscles of old *mdx* than in younger mice and healthy control mice [27]. *Mdx* muscle also demonstrates high susceptibility to contraction-induced injury [28]. Except skeletal muscles the diaphragm is severely damaged in *mdx* mice showing progressive deterioration, as is also typical for affected humans [24]. Compared to the voluntarily moving limb muscles, diaphragm fibers in *mdx* mice are subjected to early contraction-induced membrane rupture due to continuous action in the absence of dystrophin [24]. Histopathological changes of *mdx* diaphragm start to be observed at 4 weeks and include myofiber degeneration, necrosis, mineralization and large areas of fibrosis. But in contrast to the limb skeletal muscles, which are constantly affected to cycles of degeneration and regeneration, diaphragm undergoes progressive degeneration. By 16 months of age the *mdx* diaphragm looks pale due to extensive myofiber necrosis and replacement fibrosis. Changes in the physiological properties of *mdx* diaphragm correlate to histopathological lesions. Another muscular organ that is affected in *mdx* mice as in DMD patients is the heart. Echocardiographic signs of cardiomyopathy arise after ~8 months of age, while histological evidence of interstitial cardiac fibrosis does not appear until about 17 months [29].

Similar to DMD patients, *mdx* mice have increased levels of CK, marker of muscle damage, wherein CK levels were shown to increase with age, exercise, and male gender [30].

Since the pathogenesis of DMD in the *mdx* mice is genetically, biochemically and histologically similar to DMD patients, they have been extensively used as a preclinical model for DMD over the last 20 years. These mice are used to study the mechanisms of disease occurrence and dystrophin function, to test pharmaceutical drugs and to establish proof-of-concept for gene and cell therapy focusing on restoration of dystrophin expression [24, 30, 31]. The efficacy of a large number of pharmacological agents such as prednisone, deflazacort and other immunosuppressive and anti-inflammatory drugs currently used in therapy of DMD patients was tested in *mdx* mice in preclinical trials [30]. Also *mdx* mice were used in preclinical trials of replacement gene therapy on adeno-associated viruses carrying the dystrophin microgene/minigene. This therapy is currently in clinical trials [17].

Although *mdx* mice are the most commonly used animal model for DMD, its main disadvantage is the mild phenotype compared to DMD patients. To enhance muscular dystrophy pathology a lot of animal models with a more severe phenotype were created. Several approaches were used to create new murine models with DMD symptoms: N-ethylnitrosourea (ENU) mutagenesis (mdx^{2Cv}, mdx^{3Cv}, mdx^{4Cv}, mdx^{5Cv} mice models), generation of humanized transgenic mice with yeast artificial chromosomes (YAC) (hDMD mice), CRISPR/Cas9 (Clustered Regularly Interspaced Palindromic Repeats/CRISPR associated protein 9) and homologous recombination in embryonic stem cells (different murine models with exons deletion/duplication), Cre-loxP (Cre is from gene name *cre* that means "causes recombination"; loxP is for Locus of Crossover in P1) recombination system (*Dmd*-null mice), breeding *mdx* mice with other backgrounds (DBA/2-*mdx* mice, albino-*mdx* mice, BALB/c-*mdx* mice, immune deficient *mdx* mice) or other knockout (KO) murine models (*hDMD/mdx* mice, *hDMD/Dmd* null mice, *mdx*/Cmah−/−, *hDMD/mdx/Utrn*−/−, *mdx/Utrn*−/−, *mdx*/a7−/−, *mdx/MyoD*−/−).

Four new mdx murine models (mdx^{2Cv}, mdx^{3Cv}, mdx^{4Cv}, mdx^{5Cv}) were generated with ENU chemical mutagenesis [32]. Nature of these mutations was characterized. It was established that mdx^{2Cv} allele results from mutation affecting mRNA splicing, and is located in the splice acceptor of intron 42 [33]. The mdx^{3Cv} allele arises from a mutant splice acceptor site in intron 65 [32]. Similar to the mdx^{2Cv} allele, the mdx^{3Cv} splice acceptor mutation generates a complex pattern of aberrant splicing that generates multiple transcripts. But, in contrast to the mdx^{3cv} mutation, alternative transcripts generated from mdx^{2Cv} allele do not preserve the normal open reading frame [33]. In the case of the mdx^{4Cv} allele, mutation is a C to T transition in exon 53, creating a stop codon (CAA to TAA). In the mdx^{5Cv} allele, the dystrophin mRNA contains a 53 base pairs deletion and a single A to T transversion in exon 10 which does not alter the encoded amino acid. But a new splice donor was created (GTGAG) that generates a frameshifting deletion in the processed mRNA [33]. Despite all four new mutants show elevated serum CK level and muscle pathology similar to original *mdx* mice [32], each strain of mutant mice has unique features. Although each strain of mutant mice has unique features. The mdx^{3Cv} mice exhibit abnormal breeding behavior and cognitive defects in addition to dystrophic muscle pathology. The levels of DAPC proteins and full-length dystrophin were decreased. So mdx^{3Cv} mice may act as a useful model for studying the effect of subtherapeutic level of dystrophin on DMD phenotype recovery. Surprisingly, skeletal muscle strength was only slightly reduced compared to wild type mice and muscles were partially protected from eccentric contraction-induced injury [34]. Histopathological analysis of skeletal muscles, heart and diaphragm of the mdx^{4Cv} and mdx^{5Cv} mutants indicates 10-fold fewer revertants than in the muscles of *mdx* mice [24]. Also *mdx*^{5Cv} mice have a more severe skeletal muscle phenotype than *mdx* mice. These mice showed pronounced functional deficits and lower interindividual variability in motor activity tests compared with *mdx* mice which is a great advantage in studies with small numbers of animals [24, 30, 31]. Both of these murine models *mdx*^{4Cv} and *mdx*^{5Cv} are currently used in preclinical trials of gene therapy [35].

There are several models of mice obtained by crossing *mdx* mice with other genetic backgrounds such as albino mice [36], BALB/c mice, DBA2 mice [37], C57BL/6 mice, C3H mice [38], FVB mice and immune deficient mice [24]. In some cases background does not dramatically alter dystrophic phenotype of *mdx* mice (BALB/c-*mdx* mice, C57BL/6-*mdx* mice, FVB-*mdx* mice). But some murine models obtained during the crossing showed new phenotypic features and more severe phenotypes than *mdx* mice (albino *mdx* mice, DBA2/*mdx* mice). For example, albino-*mdx* mice combined signs of muscular dystrophy (histopathology of skeletal muscles, increased serum CK level, body and muscle weights) with signs of oculocutaneous albinism (skin, fur and eye depigmentation) [36]. In contrast to original black *mdx* mice, albino-*mdx* mice showed slow geotaxis, which can indicate a deterioration of neurological state of DMD [39], and increased circulating cytokines levels [40].

The most phenotypically relevant to the human DMD murine model was created on the DBA2 background. The DBA2 inbred mouse strain carries a naturally occuring in-frame deletion within the latent TGFβ-Binding Protein 4 (LTBP4) gene. This promotes enhanced inflammation and loss of ambulation in DMD patients [41]. The DBA2-*mdx* (D2-*mdx*) mice showed progressive development of muscular dystrophy. These mice had severe histopathological features, including the rapid progression of fibrosis in diaphragm and skeletal muscles. In addition, all muscles of these mice had zones of extensive calcification. In contrast to original *mdx* mice D2-*mdx* mice developed cardiomyopathy at an earlier age, moreover, more fibrous tissue was observed in the hearts of D2-*mdx* mice [37]. The more pronounced dystrophic phenotype and faster progression of the disease in D2-*mdx* mice compared to *mdx* mice on C57BL/10 background makes D2-*mdx* mouse strain more suitable for evaluation of treatment efficacy in preclinical trials [42]. Immune-deficient *mdx* mice are used to test cell therapies as one of the approaches to treating muscular dystrophy. These strains were created by crossing of *mdx* mice with different strains of mice with mutations in different genes (c-kit receptor gene, IL-2 receptor gene, DNA-dependent protein kinase catalytic subunit deficient and others) and deficiency of B cells, T cells and NK cells [43], cytokine signaling deficiency [43], hematopoietic cells deficiency [44] or with severe combined immunodeficiency [45]. Severity of phenotypical features in immune-deficient dystrophic mice are usually similar to *mdx* mice. But these murine strains are a good model for preclinical trials of cell transplantation therapies.

Mdx murine model lacking dystrophin expression demonstrates less pronounced degenerative changes in comparison with DMD in humans. This may be attributed to various species-specific compensatory mechanisms in mice, increased expression of other membrane proteins in murine muscles, or the characteristics of the skeletal and cardiac muscles themselves. To study the effect of compensatory mechanisms in mice, double-knockout (DKO) murine models and humanized murine models were created. Compensation for the lack of dystrophin with structurally related proteins possibly leads to a milder DMD phenotype in *mdx* mice than in DMD patients. In *mdx* mice, unlike humans, the expression of utrophin, in skeletal muscles, diaphragm, heart and non-muscular tissues persists throughout life [46]. The amino acid sequence of utrophin repeats largely dystrophin and can hypothetically substitute it on the sarcolemma and participate in muscle contraction [9].

Therefore, upregulation of utrophin may be one of the treatment options for DMD. To test such drugs as well as to study DMD pathogenesis, mice deficient in both dystrophin and utrophin were created. This double-knockout (*mdx/utrn*$^{-/-}$, u-dko) murine model was derived from breeding dystrophin deficient *mdx* mice with utrophin deficient mice [47]. In contrast to *mdx* mice u-dko mice were smaller and weaker and developed severe muscular dystrophy phenotype similar to phenotype in DMD patients. All clinical signs of the disease (pathohistology of skeletal and cardiac muscles, muscle functions) were more pronounced in u-dko mice than in *mdx* mice. These mice also started to show DMD symptoms at an earlier age [47]. This murine model is currently used in preclinical trials of gene therapy drugs based on adeno-associated or adenoviruses carrying shortened utrophin genes. Several studies have shown that utrophin-delivering therapy is equally effective as micro/minidystrophin-delivering therapies [48]. Another protein that can replace the absent dystrophin and perform complementary function in *mdx* muscles is the membrane protein integrin α7. Dystrophin and integrin α7 double knockout mice (*mdx*/α7$^{-/-}$), as well as u-dko mice, showed a more apparent dystrophic phenotype compared to original *mdx* mice [49]. Dystrophin- and integrin α7-deficient mice had reduced body mass compared to *mdx* mice and demonstrated early lethality (4 weeks after birth). Skeletal and cardiac muscles of double-knockout *mdx*/α7$^{-/-}$ mice were more severely affected and exhibited loss of membrane integrity, more prominent histopathological and functional characteristics [49].

Another explanation for the less pronounced dystrophic phenotype in *mdx* mice may be the increased regeneration of muscle fibers after necrosis which presents in formation of fibers with centrally located nuclei and muscle pseudohypertrophy [23]. To test this hypothesis, several murine models with reduced muscle regeneration were created. Since activated satellite cells are involved in the regeneration of skeletal muscle fibers, murine models with knockout of genes involved in the activation of satellite cells, were created to limit regenerative capacity. The first approach is a knockout of myogenic basic-helix–loop–helix transcription factors MyoD which plays an important role in myogenesis [50]. Mice lacking both MyoD and dystrophin (*mdx*/MyoD/$^{-/-}$) created by breeding of *mdx* mice with MyoD mutant mice developed a severe cardiomyopathy and muscle hypertrophy leading to premature death [51]. Phenotypically these mice are much closer to DMD patients. The second approach to enhance DMD phenotype in mice is a modeling of the telomerase RNA absence. It was established that telomere length in human dystrophic cardiomyocytes and skeletal muscles is shorter than in normal muscles [52]. To create such a murine model, *mdx* mice were crossed with mice lacking telomerase RNA (*mdx*/mTR KO) [52]. *Mdx*/mTR KO showed a severe dystrophic phenotype and significantly reduced lifespan compared to *mdx* or mTR KO controls. Also aged mice showed explicit skeletal deformity (kyphosis) [52]. Double knockout mice make a significant contribution to the study of DMD pathogenesis and the assessment of DMD drug therapy effectiveness, however, these murine models do not directly explain the differences in phenotype between mice and humans. Therefore, so-called humanized murine models were created.

Humanization makes phenotype of *mdx* mice closer to the phenotype of DMD patients. Mice have reduced inflammatory and immunologic reactivity compared to humans. For example, mice, unlike humans, evolutionally retained the cytidine monophosphate-sialic acid hydroxylase (*Cmah*) gene. Introduction of human-like inactivating deletion of Cmah gene into *mdx* mice prevented synthesis of the sialic acid N-glycolylneuraminic acid [53]. The *mdx*/Cmah/$^{-/-}$ mice had genotypic and phenotypic similarities to human DMD, enhanced DMD severity and shortened lifespan compared to *mdx* mice. Cardiac muscle of mutant mice shows large areas of fibrosis and mononuclear infiltration. These features make

DOI: http://dx.doi.org/10.5772/intechopen.96738

mdx/Cmah/$^{-/-}$ murine model suitable for evaluating effects of new DMD therapy on dystrophic cardiac muscle.

Dystrophin function, as well as pathogenesis and treatment strategies for DMD have been well studied in different murine models (*mdx*, *mdx/Utrn*$^{-/-}$ dko and many others). All these murine strains lack full-length dystrophin expression and show specific dystrophic features. However, the expression of small isoforms of dystrophin may remain in some models. To study the contribution of small isoforms to the DMD pathogenesis, a model with a completely deleted dystrophin gene was created. Using the Cre-loxP recombination system Dmd gene was completely removed in mice. The resulting mutants (*Dmd*-null mice) were viable, but the males were sterile. The mice showed an evident dystrophic phenotype and behavioral abnormalities [54].

Murine models are the most convenient and widely used for studying protein function, pathogenesis and treatment options for the disease. Many preclinical trials of drugs that are currently used or tested in clinical trials have been performed on DMD murine models. However, many laboratories use not only mice for their studies, but also other species of animals, including non-mammalian models, other rodents or large mammals. Non-mammalian DMD models were generated in zebrafish *Danio rerio*, *Drosophila melanogaster* and *Caenorhabditis elegans* [24, 30, 31, 55]. Non-mammalian DMD models have some advantages over mammals. Fishes, worms and insects are eukaryotic models and have some valuable features: small size, high reproduction rate, fast growth and development, a large number of offsprings and fully sequenced genomes. Dystrophin amino acid sequence and subcellular localization are highly conserved between humans and zebrafish. The zebrafish *dmdta222a* mutants (*sapje*) with dystrophin deficiency showed muscle degeneration which was more severe than in *mdx* mice and died at an early larval stage [56]. Zebrafish DMD model is a good model to test exon-skipping therapeutic strategy. For example, FDA approved drug Ataluren (Translarna) was tested on zebrafish and led to restoration of muscle contractile functions [57]. One more non-mammalian DMD model is dystrophin deficient *Drosophila melanogaster*. Muscle-specific RNAi-mediated knockdown of all dystrophin isoforms in flies led to severe muscle degeneration, cardiomyopathy phenotype and climbing deficits [58, 59]. Nematode worm *Caenorhabditis elegans* is also used for DMD model creation. These worms have dystrophin homolog gene dys-1. Loss-of-function in dys-1 resulted in worm hyperactivity and hypercontraction [55].

In addition to mice, larger animal models are now available. All DMD canine and feline models have been identified in natural populations. Porcine, rat, monkey and rabbit models were created with CRISPR/Cas9 technology [24, 31]. The most popular DMD models in large animals are canine models. Spontaneous mutations in the dystrophin gene causing the development of dystrophic phenotype have been identified in 14 dog breeds [60]. Some of them are currently bred in nurseries as a DMD canine model, others were discovered in natural populations as individual cases and described in the literature. The first group includes the well known golden retriever muscular dystrophy dog model (GRMD), Cavalier King Charles spaniel model [61], Welsh corgi model Australian Labradoodle model, German short-haired pointer and new labrador retriever model with inversion in dystrophin gene [60]. The most widely used and well described canine model of DMD is the GRMD model. The GRMD mutation was first reported in four animals in the early 1980s [62]. It was established that GRMD dogs had a splice site mutation (transition A > G) in intron 6 causing abnormal mRNA splicing and loss of exon 7 of dystrophin gene. GRMD dogs had severe dystrophic phenotype including elevated CK level, skeletal muscle atrophy with contractures, dyspnoea, dysphagia, dilated cardiomyopathy, large fibrosis and fat tissue areas. The GRMD dog population also showed heterogeneity of dystrophic features between different individuals, what also makes this model similar to DMD in humans [60]. A clinical course of GRMD dogs is more similar to DMD patients in contrast to *mdx* mice. Large body size, severe muscular dystrophic phenotype, humoral and cellular immune response to viral vector and transgene, as well as transplanted cells similar to human, make GRMD dogs a more suitable model for preclinical trials to test pharmaceutical drugs, gene replacement therapies and cell therapies [31]. The GRMD dogs model was used in different preclinical trials of gene and cell therapies. The advantage of using GRMD dogs in these studies is the experiment design similar to clinical trials. For example, in clinical trials, the inclusion criterion is the intake of immunosuppressive drugs. In dogs, in contrast to mice, the immune reactivity is similar to that of humans, which makes it possible to reproduce this design as well as to study the obvious adverse reactions associated with the activation of host immunity [63]. The mutation of Cavalier King Charles spaniel (CKCS) model is a splice site mutation (transition G > T) in intron 50 causing the deletion of exon 50 [61]. CKCS dogs show elevated levels of serum CK and typical areas of necrosis and regeneration in skeletal muscles and heart. Dogs of this breed seem to be suitable for testing due to their small body mass and amiable temperament. CKCS canine model can be used to test exon 51 skipping, the therapy that may be suitable for many patients, as DMD mutation hotspot is located between exons 45 and 55 [61]. The mutation of Welsh corgi model, Australian Labradoodle model and German short-haired pointer model (GSHPMD) are LINE-1 insertion in intron 13, point mutation in exon 21 and whole *DMD* gene deletion respectively [60]. These dogs show severe dystrophic phenotype including muscle degeneration, mineralization and inflammatory infiltration. It is important to note that GSHPMD dog model with completely absent dystrophin is the most suitable preclinical model for the prediction of immune responses to gene therapy due to the lack of immunological tolerance to dystrophin [64]. One more interesting canine DMD model is the recently identified labrador retriever (LRMD) model with an inversion in dystrophin gene. 2.2-Mb spontaneous inversion disrupting the *DMD* gene within intron 20 was found in two young labrador retriever dogs. The clinical signs of disease included elevated CK level in serum, specific histopathological lesions of skeletal and cardiac muscles, myopathic electrodiagnostic profile, high neonatal lethality. The LRMD dogs had detected expression of Dp71 isoforms of dystrophin. But unlike the GRMD dogs with absent Dp71 isoform, the LRMD dogs have more severe dystrophic phenotype. This may indicate that the presence of the Dp71 isoform in muscles does not provide a functional advantage [60].

In addition to dystrophic dog colonies maintained in nurseries several cases of spontaneous mutations in dogs of different breeds have also been described. The interesting case is 7 base pair deletion in exon 42 in Cavalier King Charles spaniel, the second CKCS model with mutation in the *DMD* gene hotspot area. These dogs had generalized skeletal muscle atrophy of the temporal region, limbs and thoracolumbar spine [65]. One more case of spontaneous mutation in dystrophin gene was revealed in Miniature Poodle dog. Dogs had whole *DMD* gene deletion and showed all dystrophic clinical signs including muscle degeneration, lumbar kyphosis, stiff gait and abnormal posture. Neurological examination also revealed reluctance to exercise in these dogs [66]. One case of disease development was also recently detected in the Jack Russell Terrier population. The dog had deletion of exons 3–21 causing severe dystrophic phenotype and death at the young age [67]. Progressive muscle weakness was also detected in a male border collie dog. Its mutation was a single nucleotide deletion in canine DMD exon 20, minor DMD mutation hotspot, resulting in generalized muscle atrophy, muscle fatigue and dysphagia [68].

Unequivocally, canine models have a significant advantage over murine models due to their more pronounced dystrophic phenotype and possible immune response to treatment. However, as well as *mdx* mice, GRMD and other dogs have some disadvantages associated with the high cost of keeping dog colonies and training of personnel caring for sick animals. In addition, due to a greater body weight than in mice, large amounts of drugs are required for dogs, which is essential for gene therapy based on viral delivery. Nevertheless, studies in dogs are considered more informative than studies in mice. The results of the dog trials provide a better indication of future clinical trials. In this regard, it is important to use not only widespread mice but also dogs in the design of preclinical trials.

The first case of hypertrophic feline muscular dystrophy (HFMD) in domestic cats was described in 1989 [69]. Spontaneous mutation causing dystrophic phenotype was established as a deletion of the dystrophin promoter and first exons corresponding to dystrophin from muscle and Purkinje cells. Dystrophic cats showed pronounced appendicular and axial muscle hypertrophy, involving of tongue and diaphragm, histopathological lesions in skeletal muscles, diaphragm and heart, including different fiber diameter and acute necrosis and cardiomyopathy [70]. The HFMD model is rarely used in DMD preclinical research because tongue hypertrophy and diaphragm defects lead to difficulties in feeding, animal welfare and early death.

The CRISPR/Cas9 technology has made it possible to create several more models of DMD in such animals as pigs, rats, rabbits and monkeys. Rats are the most convenient animals for biomedical research, therefore several rat models have been created. The first rat model was created using CRISPR/Cas9 gene editing [71] and had exon 3–6 deleted in dystrophin gene. Dystrophin deficient rats showed reduced muscle strength and specific dystrophic phenotype of skeletal muscles, diaphragm and heart. Also these rats showed age-dependent decline of cardiac functions similar to DMD patients [72]. Later, based on this model, another rat model with an in-frame mutation in the dystrophin gene was generated [73]. New mutant rats had reduced expression of truncated dystrophin and mild phenotype similar to BMD patients. These rats can be useful to study BMD pathogenesis and efficiency of dystrophin recovery. The third rat model was created using TALEN (Transcription activator-like effector nucleases) technology. Its mutation was a frame shifting 11 base pairs deletion in exon 23 generating premature stop codon [74]. Animals exhibited reduced muscle strength, cardiomyopathy, large muscle necrosis and fibrosis. This model can be used for preclinical research as a small DMD animal model.

Several mice models were created that may be suitable mostly for scientific use. One of them is the $\text{Dmd}^{\text{mdx-bgeo}}$ model [75]. It contains the beta-Geo marker inserted after exon 63. The protein product translated from the resulting allele lacks cysteine-rich and C-terminal domains and is not functional. The $\text{Dmd}^{\text{mdx-bgeo}}$ model mostly resembles the $\textit{mdx}^{3cv}$ model as both of them lack all dystrophin isoforms including Dp71 and Dp40. Hemizygous $\text{Dmd}^{\text{mdx-bgeo}}$ animals demonstrate phenotypic properties similar to other *mdx* models. LacZ (β-galactosidase-mediated) staining helps to visualize the expression of dystrophin in various tissues on different stages of development including embryonic. Nevertheless, the dysfunctionality of dystrophin-lacZ chimeric protein should always be taken into account.

Dmd^{EGFP} reporter mouse [76] lacks the disadvantage of $\text{Dmd}^{\text{mdx-bgeo}}$ model. The eGFP (enhanced green fluorescent protein) coding sequence was introduced behind the exon 79 and the chimeric protein remains functional. The transgenic mice did not show any signs of pathology. This approach allows us to observe almost all major dystrophin isoforms except for those having alternative C-terminal domain. The studies with this model may provide valuable data on dystrophin expression and localization in muscle and non-muscle tissues and shed the light on its functions.

In 1999 the Dp71-null mouse model was described [77]. The first and unique exon of Dp71 is located between exons 62 and 63 of the *Dmd* gene. It is replaced by promotorless b-geo gene in Dp71-null mice leaving all other dystrophin isoforms intact (except for Dp40). The resulting construction provided the expression of β-Galactosidase regulated by Dp71 promoter while the native product, Dp71, was absent. This model acts as a valuable tool for examination of the role and functions of Dp71 isoform both by Dp71 promoter activity estimation by LacZ staining and Dp71-null phenotype examination. The further experiments demonstrated that Dp71 deficiency causes retinal vascular inflammation, increases retinal vascular permeability. AAV-mediated delivery of Dp71 restored retinal homeostasis and prevented retinal oedema [78] and restored defective electroretinographic responses [79]. Dp71 expression in neurons plays a regulatory role in synapse organization, formation and function and inactivation of Dp71 may lead to increased severity of mental retardation and intellectual disability [80].

3. Animal models to test precision medicine approaches

Genetic testing revealed the incredible diversity of mutations in *DMD* gene. However, mutations are not equally presented throughout the gene. As much as 80% of all mutations are concentrated in exons 2–20 and 45–55 representing two hotspots. Mutations can be divided into two groups: frequent (one or more exons deletions and duplications) and rare (point substitutions in exons and introns, small deletions and duplications) [81]. Mutation-specific precision medicine approaches are mostly based on the reading frame rule and convert mutations from Duchenne to Becker type. In the presence of frameshift generating mutations additional removal of one or several exons can restore the reading frame and cause expression of shortened yet functional dystrophin protein. For exons removal during splicing process antisense oligonucleotides (ASO, AON) are used. AON binds specifically to the splice sites of selected exons hiding them from cellular splicing machinery and leading to their exclusion from mRNA. Different chemical structures are used for reduced AON cleavage, prolonged circulation, better cellular and nuclear penetration. The most popular backbones are presented by PMO (phosphorodiamidate morpholino oligomers), 2-OMePS (2'O-methylated phosphorothioate), vivo-morpholino (morpholino oligo covalently linked to octaguanidine dendrimer), LNA (locked nucleic acids), tcDNA (tricyclo-DNA). Indeed, AON can be delivered naked or in the lipid complex, fused with targeting peptides or other molecules enhancing biodistribution. In addition to AON, vectorized drug candidates are tested for exon skipping. Their design is based on U7 snRNA, naturally participating in histone pre-mRNA processing. Deletion of additional exons directly from genomic DNA (gDNA) is also proposed as a mutation-specific therapeutic strategy for DMD. For this purpose viral delivery of one or two single guide RNA (sgRNA) and Cas9 encoding sequences is tested. Targeted Cas9-induced double strand cleavage is also applied for indel generation in affected or neighborhood exons. Indels lead to +1 or – 1 frameshifts with a certain probability. This approach is known as reframing. Exon can be excluded from mRNA due to another DNA modification - base editing in conservative splice site sequence. For this approach Cas9 fused with base editing enzymes is utilized. Both for U7 snRNA (U7 small nuclear RNA) and Cas9 delivery viral vectors such as lentiviruses and AAV are used. Majority of experiments for mutation-specific approach examinations are conducted on patients-derived cell cultures and modified human embryonic stem (ES) cells. However, complexity of the disease and limitations of functional tests applicable *in vitro* force to generate and use genetically modified animal models.

Mice with various mutations in the dystrophin gene, replicating mutations found in individual patients or groups of patients are the most common among the genome-edited models. The timeline of disease progression and traits of new models are usually not well studied. Main DMD symptoms are similar to those found in *mdx* mice. The purpose of these "genetic" models is to test mutation-specific therapies and show not only restoration of dystrophin expression but also improvement in locomotor activity, illustrating the functionality of the shortened protein. The ease of maintenance and reproduction, extensive experience in obtaining and speed of reproduction, together with the high conservativeness of the dystrophin gene, make mice the optimal objects for such work, nevertheless, there are other, larger animal models with mutations often found in patients with DMD.

Deletions of one or more exons are the most common mutations in the DMD gene. They account for 68% of all mutations. Among them, deletions of single exon 44 (3%), 45 (4%), 50 (2%), 51 (3%), 52 (3%) are represented with approximately the same frequency [81]. Directed mutations in the dystrophin gene in laboratory animals were obtained for the purpose of selecting drugs for exon-skipping. Exon structures of popular models with deletions in mutation hotspot are shown on **Figure 1**. The first models were obtained by homologous recombination using embryonic stem cells. In 1997 a mouse model *mdx52* with a deletion of exon 52 was created [82], where this exon was replaced with a neomycin resistance cassette. This mouse model was used to test various drug candidates: PS-modified tcDNA (phosphorothioate-modified Tricyclo-DNA) based ASO for skipping of the exon 51 [83], PMO for exon 51 skipping [84, 85], AAV9-U7snRNA for exon 51 skipping [86],

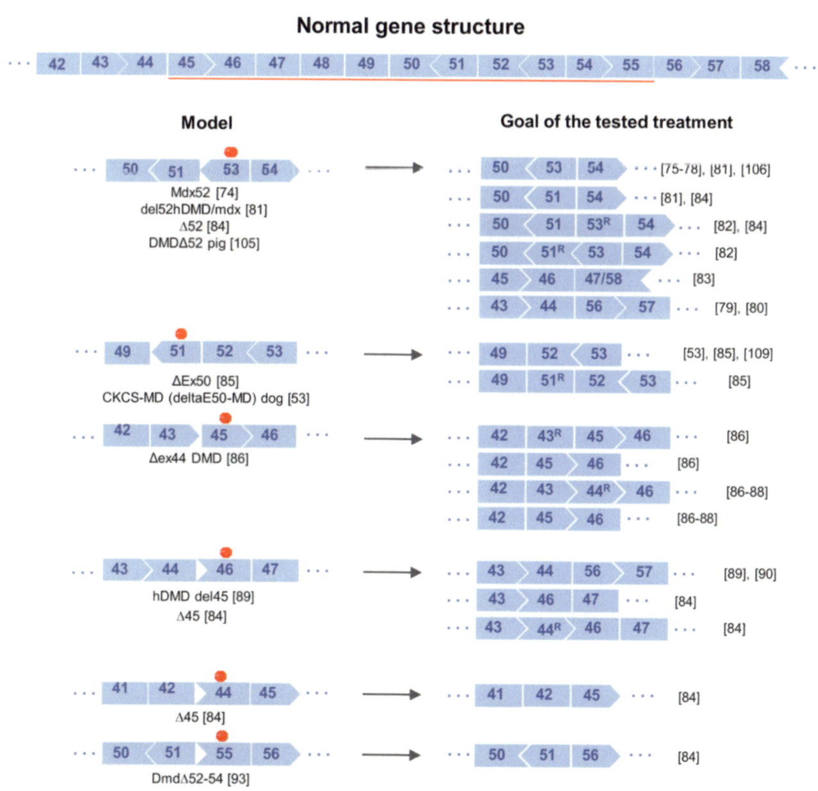

Figure 1.
Animal models representing DMD exon deletions in mutation hotspot. Gene fragment structures around exon with frameshift mutation are shown on the left. Currently tested therapeutic approaches and resulting exon structures are shown on the right.

mix of vivo-morpholinos for simultaneous skipping of the exons 45–55 [87, 88]. With the advent of effective genome editing techniques, frequent mutations were the first to be reproduced in animals. TALEN were used to create mice with exon 52 deletion resulting in **del52hdmd/***mdx* model [89]. This model is notable for the fact that the mutation was introduced into the sequence of the human gene. Thus, **del52hdmd/***mdx* model can be used to test drugs that are designed to target unique human sequences. The authors showed the effectiveness of AON for skipping exons 51 and 53 to the human sequence during intramuscular delivery [89]. This line was used to test CRISPR/Cas9 genome editing complexes for reframing in exons 51 and 53 during lentiviral delivery [90]. AAV9 double SaCas9 (*Staphylococcus aureus* Cas9 ortholog) and guide mix was tested for deletion with borders within exons 47 and 58 for himeric exon formation [91]. Later, another mouse model with a deletion of exon 52, **Δ52**, was obtained using CRISPR/Cas9 genome editing system [92]. This model was used to test CRISPR/Cas9-based drugs for exon 53 removal or reframing [92].

Reframing in exon 51 was also tested in mouse models with deletion of exon 50 **ΔEx50** and **ΔEx50-Dmd-Luc** [93]. In the *Dmd* gene of **ΔEx50-Dmd-Luc** mice, in addition to the deletion of exon 50, the luciferase gene sequence is also introduced at the C-terminus, connected to the protein sequence via an autocatalytic 2A peptide. Thus, luminescence was observed during the restoration of the reading frame, which allowed to assess the effectiveness of drugs *in vivo* without resorting to invasive methods [93]. Bioluminescence was detected both after intramuscular and systemic delivery of Cas9 and sgRNA-51 by AAV9. The presence of bioluminescence was shown to correlate with dystrophin expression as verified by western blotting and immunohistochemistry (IHC) [93].

One of the most frequent deletions, the deletion of exon 44, was reproduced in mice **Δex44 DMD** [94]. Correction of exon 44 deletions by gene editing of surrounding exons could potentially restore the reading frame of dystrophin in ~12% of patients with DMD. Authors created AAV9-Cas9 and AAV9-sgRNA mix targeting 5′-end of exon 45 and tested them *in vivo* during intramuscular injections on this model. The most perspective guide sequence 6 (G6) was used for systemic delivery and selection of a better Cas9 to sgRNA AAV particles ratio. Selected conditions lead to force increase from 59% to 107% in the extensor digitorum longus (EDL) muscle of **ΔEx44 DMD** mice [94]. 20-fold lower dose of self-complementary adeno-associated virus (scAAV) bearing Cas9 + sgRNA was used for exon 45 skipping and reframing on the same model [95]. Weekly injection of (1,2-dioleoyl-3-trimethyl-ammonium-propane) LNPs (lipid nanoparticles) encapsulating Cas9/sgDMD RNPs (ribonucleoproteins) into Tibialis Anterior (TA) muscles was tested on **ΔEx44 DMD** mice. The expression of dystrophin in TA muscles was successfully restored after skipping or reframing of exon 45 induced by treatment, as demonstrated by immunofluorescence and western blot analysis. Quantitative analysis of the western blot result showed that 4.2% of dystrophin protein was restored [96].

CRISPR/Cas9 genome edited **hDMD del45** model represents deletion of exon 45 in human dystrophin gene in the presence of wild type *Dmd* gene while **hDMD del45** *mdx* **D2** has dystrophic phenotype due to *Dmd* gene knock-out [97]. In the same paper exons 45–55 deletion strategy (Cas9 + gRNAs to introns 44 and 55) aiming to help 60–65% of patients was tested [97, 98]. A more realistic approach from the clinical application point of view is multiple exon 45–55 skipping using U7 snRNAs [99]. It was tested on **hDMD/***mdx* model [100]. Similar multiple exon-skipping strategy using PMOs cocktail [98] was tested on **hDMD/Dmd Null** mice [85]. The **hDMD/Dmd Null** model compares favorably with the previous models, since it does not have a mouse dystrophin sequence and allows us to quantify the level of exon skipping and compare the effectiveness of different sequences and drugs with each other, which is demonstrated by the example of exon 51 skipping [85]. Moreover, the presence of normal dystrophin in some models leads to the absence of the necessary symptoms for the delivery of oligonucleotides and viruses, such as inflammation in the muscles and intact cellular membranes. It's necessary to point out the crucial role of **hDMD** mouse model with full-length *DMD* gene integrated into chromosome 5 [100]. It is not very useful for any drug substances by itself due to simultaneous expression of wild type human and murine dystrophin proteins. But when crossing to *mdx* or other *Dmd* knockout mice (**hDMD/*mdx*, hDMD/Dmd Null**) it becomes an extremely important background for creation of new models. Any antisense or guide molecules designed and tested on subsequent animals can be transferred to human cells without sequence adaptation.

Models with single exon deletions **Δ43** (exon 43 deletion), **Δ45** (exon 45 deletion) were reported together with **Δ52** (exon 52 deletion) **DMD** mice [92]. These mouse models were used to test single guide genome editing procedures aiming at exon skipping or reframing. AAV9 and scAAV9 viruses with a guide and Cas9 sequences were used. Intramuscular delivery of guide RNA to exon 44 and Cas9 encoding viruses to TA muscle restored dystrophin expression in both **Δ43** and **Δ45 DMD** models. Interestingly, the selected guide generated both exon reframed and exon skipped transcripts in **Δ45 DMD** muscle, but only exon skipped transcripts in **Δ43 DMD** muscle. Restoration of dystrophin in **Δ45 DMD** muscle was more efficient than in **Δ43 DMD** muscle when using the same sgRNA for gene editing [92].

Deletions of several exons are quite common in patients, but to date only one mouse model with an extended mutation in the hotspot is known. Deletion of exons 52–54 was simulated in **Dmd Δ52–54** in which authors declare severe cardiac dysfunction in addition to common skeletal muscle symptoms. CRISPR-mediated single sgRNA exon skipping of exon 55 was tested on this model. Also another model with deletion of exons 52–55 was created to check potential benefit of the treatment [101]. CRISPR/Cas9 system popularity, easy to use and high efficiency allow to generate such 100% skipping (editing) models to check generated shortened dystrophin protein functionality.

Duplications of one or several exons are also highly widespread mutations, affecting 5–10% of all DMD patients [102]. The most common duplication in the patient population **Dup2** (duplication of exon 2) was recreated in the mouse model created in 2015 [103]. Correction of the mutation was shown on this model after intramuscular injections of AAV1.U7-ACCA [104]. Main attribute of this mutation and corresponding model is that precision skipping of a duplicated exon results in full-length dystrophin expression. Thus, it is the rare case when exon-skipping converts Duchenne type mutation to wild type rather than Becker type. At the same time it is a challenge to accurately skip only copy of exon 2 not affecting the main sequence.

Nonsense mutations are also very common in the human population affecting approximately 25% of the patients [102]. The most popular *mdx* mouse model representing nonsense mutation was found in the natural population [105]. A lot of treatment strategies targeting downstream disease mechanisms were tested on this model. Precision medicine approach on *mdx* model includes stop codon readthrough [106]. Targeted single nucleotide mutation was created in **DMD-KO** (D108) mouse [107] representing C-to-T conversion generating stop codon in exon 20 (Q871Stop). This mouse model was used for adenine base editing using guided SpCas9 (*Streptococcus pyogenes* Cas9 ortholog) nickase [108]. Created by ENU mutagenesis, *mdx*^{4cv} model also has C-to-T conversion in exon 53 generating TAA stop codon [33]. Adenine base editor was also tested on this mouse model with modified Cas9 recognizing relaxed minimal PAM (protospacer adjacent motif) sequence - NG [109]. Both *mdx* and *mdx*^{4cv} models were used for trans-splicing method efficiency demonstration [110]. Intramuscular delivery of AAV vectors expressing trans-splicing template (PTM) allowed detectable levels of dystrophin in *mdx* and *mdx*^{4cv}, illustrating that a given PTM can be suitable for a variety of mutations.

Rare mutations found in patients were repeated in models to test precision gene editing methods. Those contain big deletion of exons 8–34 in **DmdDel8–34** mouse model (Egorova et al., 2019). Reading frame in this model can be restored by simultaneous skipping of exons 6 and 7. The fact that the N-terminal actin binding domain is partly encoded by these exons, gives the opportunity to better understand structure-functional interplay in dystrophin protein and its shortened forms. Several approaches including vivo-morpholino induced exon-skipping and CRISPR/Cas9 gene editing are tested on this model ([111]; unpublished data). Other variants of rare mutations generated by Koo and colleagues, represent small frameshift mutations [112]. In vivo treatment with AAV vectors encoding CjCas9 (*Campylobacter jejuni* Cas9 ortholog) and single guide to the affected exon restored the reading frame and enhanced muscle strength.

Large mammalian models have more pronounced DMD symptoms in comparison to murine models. But limited availability and less extensive experience in their genome modification led to reduced use in precision medicine approaches testing. Pig model with deletion of exon 52 **DMDΔ52** was created using somatic nuclear transfer from bacterial artificial chromosome (BAC)-edited cells [113]. AAV9 vector with intein splitted Cas9 and two guides around exon 51 was tested on these animals reaching widespread dystrophin expression, prolonged survival and reduced arrhythmogenic vulnerability [114]. Another example of CRISPR/Cas9 Dmd gene targeting in pigs resulted in indels in exon 27 which lead to premature piglet death at day 52 [115]. So this model was not tested yet for any treatment approach.

DMD KO rabbits represent different mutations in exon 51 which is within the mutation hotspot in human *DMD* gene [116]. Many of these mutations are small deletions or insertions, disrupting the reading frame of the *DMD* gene, resulting in frameshift and complete absence of dystrophin expression followed by main phenotypic features in skeletal muscles and cardiomyopathy. Animals could benefit from 50–51, 51–52 or 45–55 exons skipping, however this model animals were not used for any precision medicines testing.

Identified in natural population **CKCS-MD** (deltaE50-MD) dogs have a splice site missense mutation in intron 50 of the *DMD* gene, causing out-of-frame skipping of exon 50 and resulting in a lack of dystrophin and a severe dystrophic phenotype resembling DMD [61]. In the same paper authors show that additional skipping of exon 51 could restore dystrophin expression on cultured myoblasts [61]. Single guide genome editing aiming at exon 51 skipping or reframing shows big potential after intramuscular and intravenous delivery [117].

Naturally occurring intron splice site mutation that leads to the loss of exon 7 was identified in Golden retriever dogs leading to generation of **GRMD (CXMDJ)** canine model [62]. It is the most widespread canine model which is used in numerous studies including exons 6 and 8 skipping driven by PMO and 2'OMePS [118, 119], AAV1-U7snRNA [120], rAAV6-U7snRNA [121], AAV8-U7snRNA [122].

The next model stands out and its value is more in demonstrating the possibility of creating new models than in itself. The new mice obtained by transgenesis carry randomly embedded copies of the EGFP under the CAG promoter (strong synthetic promoter that consists of regulatory elements from **C**MV, chicken beta-**a**ctin gene and rabbit beta-**g**lobin gene), which are separated by exon 23 with the murine *mdx* mutation. EGFP expression is possible only in case of exon 23 skipping, which was demonstrated using PMO and LNA/2'-OMe based AONs [123]. Thus, the resulting mouse model allows noninvasive assessment of the effectiveness of exon skipping, as well as studying the bio-distribution of drugs. The creation of similar mouse models for testing exon skipping, more applicable to patients, will allow more intensive studies of future drugs.

4. Conclusions

Here we described several dozens of Duchenne muscular dystrophy models. The list of species used to create these models includes worms, fruit flies, fishes, dogs, cats, mice, pigs, rats and monkeys. Some of them were found in natural populations, while the others were artificially created. The spectrum of genetic interventions spans from point mutations to complete deletion of the largest gene - *Dmd* gene, double knockouts and humanized constructions. The genetic and phenotypic diversity provides great opportunities for fundamental studies and drug development.

The correspondence of the model phenotype to human DMD phenotype is extremely important for drug testing. Some of the models, especially based on small animal species, could not represent DMD features correctly. The same goes for many mice models. The mouse model which has mutation identical to a certain DMD case may not correctly represent the DMD phenotype. Vice versa, several double knockout mice models reproduce the DMD phenotype much closer while being an inadequate genetic model. The models based on larger species are more useful as their phenotype is usually closer to DMD. But the creation, maintenance and cost of these animals complicates their use and restricts diversity. Indeed, no ideal DMD model is still created. However, the development of novel promising DMD treatment strategies requires both genetically similar models for precision drugs testing and phenotypically appropriate models for disease study and design of therapies. We should expect the expansion of the DMD-related animal models list in the nearest future.

Author details

Tatiana V. Egorova[1,2]*, Ivan I. Galkin[1,2], Yulia V. Ivanova[1,2] and Anna V. Polikarpova[1,2]

1 Institute of Gene Biology RAS, Moscow, Russia

2 Marlin Biotech LLC, Moscow, Russia

*Address all correspondence to: egorovatv@genebiology.ru

References

[1] Emery AEH, Emery MLH. The History of a Genetic Disease: Duchenne Muscular Dystrophy Or Meryon's Disease. OUP Oxford; 2011. 231 p.

[2] Moat SJ, Bradley DM, Salmon R, Clarke A, Hartley L. Newborn bloodspot screening for Duchenne muscular dystrophy: 21 years experience in Wales (UK). Eur J Hum Genet. 2013 Oct;21(10):1049-1053.

[3] Ryder S, Leadley RM, Armstrong N, Westwood M, de Kock S, Butt T, et al. The burden, epidemiology, costs and treatment for Duchenne muscular dystrophy: an evidence review. Orphanet J Rare Dis. 2017 Apr 26;12(1):79.

[4] Ishizaki M, Kobayashi M, Adachi K, Matsumura T, Kimura E. Female dystrophinopathy: Review of current literature. Neuromuscul Disord. 2018 Jul;28(7):572-581.

[5] Shieh PB. Emerging Strategies in the Treatment of Duchenne Muscular Dystrophy. Neurotherapeutics. 2018 Oct;15(4):840-848.

[6] Culligan KG, Mackey AJ, Finn DM, Maguire PB, Ohlendieck K. Role of dystrophin isoforms and associated proteins in muscular dystrophy (review). Int J Mol Med. 1998 Dec;2(6):639-648.

[7] Doorenweerd N, Mahfouz A, van Putten M, Kaliyaperumal R, T' Hoen PAC, Hendriksen JGM, et al. Timing and localization of human dystrophin isoform expression provide insights into the cognitive phenotype of Duchenne muscular dystrophy. Sci Rep. 2017 Oct 3;7(1):12575.

[8] Aartsma-Rus A, Ginjaar IB, Bushby K. The importance of genetic diagnosis for Duchenne muscular dystrophy. J Med Genet. 2016 Mar;53(3):145-151.

[9] Lapidos Karen A., Kakkar Rahul, McNally Elizabeth M. The Dystrophin Glycoprotein Complex. Circ Res. 2004 Apr 30;94(8):1023-1031.

[10] Le Rumeur E, Winder SJ, Hubert J-F. Dystrophin: more than just the sum of its parts. Biochim Biophys Acta. 2010 Sep;1804(9):1713-1722.

[11] Guiraud S, Davies KE. Pharmacological advances for treatment in Duchenne muscular dystrophy. Curr Opin Pharmacol. 2017 Jun;34:36-48.

[12] Folker ES, Baylies MK. Nuclear positioning in muscle development and disease. Front Physiol. 2013 Dec 12;4:363.

[13] Rosenberg AS, Puig M, Nagaraju K, Hoffman EP, Villalta SA, Rao VA, et al. Immune-mediated pathology in Duchenne muscular dystrophy. Sci Transl Med. 2015 Aug 5;7(299):299rv4.

[14] Birnkrant DJ, Bushby K, Bann CM, Apkon SD, Blackwell A, Brumbaugh D, et al. Diagnosis and management of Duchenne muscular dystrophy, part 1: diagnosis, and neuromuscular, rehabilitation, endocrine, and gastrointestinal and nutritional management. Lancet Neurol. 2018 Mar;17(3):251-267.

[15] Bushby KM, Gardner-Medwin D, Nicholson LV, Johnson MA, Haggerty ID, Cleghorn NJ, et al. The clinical, genetic and dystrophin characteristics of Becker muscular dystrophy. II. Correlation of phenotype with genetic and protein abnormalities. J Neurol. 1993 Feb;240(2):105-112.

[16] England SB, Nicholson LV, Johnson MA, Forrest SM, Love DR, Zubrzycka-Gaarn EE, et al. Very mild muscular dystrophy associated with the deletion of 46% of dystrophin. Nature. 1990 Jan 11;343(6254):180-182.

[17] Duan D. Systemic AAV Micro-dystrophin Gene Therapy for Duchenne Muscular Dystrophy. Mol Ther. 2018 Oct 3;26(10):2337-2356.

[18] Nance ME, Hakim CH, Yang NN, Duan D. Nanotherapy for Duchenne muscular dystrophy. Wiley Interdiscip Rev Nanomed Nanobiotechnol [Internet]. 2018 Mar;10(2). Available from: http://dx.doi.org/10.1002/wnan.1472

[19] Schneider A-FE, Aartsma-Rus A. Developments in reading frame restoring therapy approaches for Duchenne muscular dystrophy. Expert Opin Biol Ther. 2020 Oct 19;1-17.

[20] Guiraud S, Roblin D, Kay DE. The potential of utrophin modulators for the treatment of Duchenne muscular dystrophy. Expert Opinion on Orphan Drugs. 2018 Mar 4;6(3):179-192.

[21] Weir AP, Burton EA, Harrod G, Davies KE. A- and B-utrophin Have Different Expression Patterns and Are Differentially Up-regulated in mdx Muscle *. J Biol Chem. 2002 Nov 22;277(47):45285-45290.

[22] Sienkiewicz D, Kulak W, Okurowska-Zawada B, Paszko-Patej G, Kawnik K. Duchenne muscular dystrophy: current cell therapies. Ther Adv Neurol Disord. 2015 Jul;8(4):166-177.

[23] Chamberlain JS, Metzger J, Reyes M, Townsend D, Faulkner JA. Dystrophin-deficient mdx mice display a reduced life span and are susceptible to spontaneous rhabdomyosarcoma. FASEB J. 2007 Jul;21(9):2195-2204.

[24] McGreevy JW, Hakim CH, McIntosh MA, Duan D. Animal models of Duchenne muscular dystrophy: from basic mechanisms to gene therapy. Dis Model Mech. 2015 Mar;8(3):195-213.

[25] Muntoni F, Mateddu A, Marchei F, Clerk A, Serra G. Muscular weakness in the mdx mouse. J Neurol Sci. 1993 Dec 1;120(1):71-77.

[26] Massopust RT, Lee YI, Pritchard AL, Nguyen V-KM, McCreedy DA, Thompson WJ. Lifetime analysis of mdx skeletal muscle reveals a progressive pathology that leads to myofiber loss. Sci Rep. 2020 Oct 14;10(1):17248.

[27] Lynch GS, Hinkle RT, Chamberlain JS, Brooks SV, Faulkner JA. Force and power output of fast and slow skeletal muscles from mdx mice 6-28 months old. J Physiol. 2001 Sep 1;535(Pt 2):591-600.

[28] Dellorusso C, Crawford RW, Chamberlain JS, Brooks SV. Tibialis anterior muscles in mdx mice are highly susceptible to contraction-induced injury. J Muscle Res Cell Motil. 2001;22(5):467-475.

[29] Quinlan JG, Hahn HS, Wong BL, Lorenz JN, Wenisch AS, Levin LS. Evolution of the mdx mouse cardiomyopathy: physiological and morphological findings. Neuromuscul Disord. 2004 Sep;14(8-9):491-496.

[30] Spurney CF, Gordish-Dressman H, Guerron AD, Sali A, Pandey GS, Rawat R, et al. Preclinical drug trials in the mdx mouse: assessment of reliable and sensitive outcome measures. Muscle Nerve. 2009 May;39(5):591-602.

[31] Wasala NB, Chen S-J, Duan D. Duchenne muscular dystrophy animal models for high-throughput drug discovery and precision medicine. Expert Opin Drug Discov. 2020 Apr;15(4):443-456.

[32] Chapman VM, Miller DR, Armstrong D, Caskey CT. Recovery of induced mutations for X chromosome-linked muscular dystrophy in mice. Proc Natl Acad Sci U S A. 1989 Feb;86(4):1292-1296.

[33] Im WB, Phelps SF, Copen EH, Adams EG, Slightom JL, Chamberlain JS. Differential expression of dystrophin isoforms in strains of mdx mice with different mutations. Hum Mol Genet. 1996 Aug;5(8):1149-1153.

[34] Li D, Yue Y, Duan D. Preservation of muscle force in Mdx3cv mice correlates with low-level expression of a near full-length dystrophin protein. Am J Pathol. 2008 May;172(5):1332-1341.

[35] Ramos JN, Hollinger K, Bengtsson NE, Allen JM, Hauschka SD, Chamberlain JS. Development of Novel Micro-dystrophins with Enhanced Functionality. Mol Ther. 2019 Mar 6;27(3):623-635.

[36] Krivov LI, Stenina MA, Yarygin VN, Polyakov AV, Savchuk VI, Obrubov SA, et al. A new genetic variant of mdx mice: study of the phenotype. Bull Exp Biol Med. 2009 May;147(5):625-629.

[37] van Putten M, Putker K, Overzier M, Adamzek WA, Pasteuning-Vuhman S, Plomp JJ, et al. Natural disease history of the D2-mdx mouse model for Duchenne muscular dystrophy. FASEB J. 2019 Jul;33(7):8110-8124.

[38] Schmidt WM, Uddin MH, Dysek S, Moser-Thier K, Pirker C, Höger H, et al. DNA damage, somatic aneuploidy, and malignant sarcoma susceptibility in muscular dystrophies. PLoS Genet. 2011 Apr;7(4):e1002042.

[39] Thiessen DD, Lindzey G. Negative geotaxis in mice: effect of balancing practice on incline behaviour in C57BL-6J male mice. Anim Behav. 1967 Jan;15(1):113-116.

[40] Stenina MA, Krivov LI, Voevodin DA, Yarygin VN. Phenotypic differences between mdx black mice and mdx albino mice. Comparison of cytokine levels in the blood. Bull Exp Biol Med. 2013 Jul;155(3):376-379.

[41] Flanigan KM, Ceco E, Lamar K-M, Kaminoh Y, Dunn DM, Mendell JR, et al. LTBP4 genotype predicts age of ambulatory loss in Duchenne muscular dystrophy. Ann Neurol. 2013 Apr;73(4):481-488.

[42] Hammers DW, Hart CC, Matheny MK, Wright LA, Armellini M, Barton ER, et al. The D2.mdx mouse as a preclinical model of the skeletal muscle pathology associated with Duchenne muscular dystrophy. Sci Rep. 2020 Aug 21;10(1):14070.

[43] Vallese D, Negroni E, Duguez S, Ferry A, Trollet C, Aamiri A, et al. The Rag2^{-}Il2rb^{-}Dmd^{-} mouse: a novel dystrophic and immunodeficient model to assess innovating therapeutic strategies for muscular dystrophies. Mol Ther. 2013 Oct;21(10):1950-1957.

[44] Walsh S, Nygren J, Pontén A, Jovinge S. Myogenic reprogramming of bone marrow derived cells in a W^{41}Dmd(mdx) deficient mouse model. PLoS One. 2011 Nov 28;6(11):e27500.

[45] Farini A, Meregalli M, Belicchi M, Battistelli M, Parolini D, D'Antona G, et al. T and B lymphocyte depletion has a marked effect on the fibrosis of dystrophic skeletal muscles in the scid/mdx mouse. J Pathol. 2007 Oct;213(2):229-238.

[46] Pons F, Robert A, Marini JF, Léger JJ. Does utrophin expression in muscles of mdx mice during postnatal development functionally compensate for dystrophin deficiency? J Neurol Sci. 1994 Apr;122(2):162-170.

[47] Deconinck AE, Rafael JA, Skinner JA, Brown SC, Potter AC, Metzinger L, et al. Utrophin-dystrophin-deficient mice as a model for Duchenne muscular dystrophy. Cell. 1997 Aug 22;90(4):717-727.

[48] Odom GL, Gregorevic P, Allen JM, Finn E, Chamberlain JS. Microutrophin

delivery through rAAV6 increases lifespan and improves muscle function in dystrophic dystrophin/utrophin-deficient mice. Mol Ther. 2008 Sep;16(9):1539-1545.

[49] Rooney JE, Welser JV, Dechert MA, Flintoff-Dye NL, Kaufman SJ, Burkin DJ. Severe muscular dystrophy in mice that lack dystrophin and alpha7 integrin. J Cell Sci. 2006 Jun 1;119 (Pt 11):2185-2195.

[50] Rudnicki MA, Braun T, Hinuma S, Jaenisch R. Inactivation of MyoD in mice leads to up-regulation of the myogenic HLH gene Myf-5 and results in apparently normal muscle development. Cell. 1992 Oct 30;71(3):383-390.

[51] Megeney LA, Kablar B, Perry RL, Ying C, May L, Rudnicki MA. Severe cardiomyopathy in mice lacking dystrophin and MyoD. Proc Natl Acad Sci U S A. 1999 Jan 5;96(1):220-225.

[52] Mourkioti F, Kustan J, Kraft P, Day JW, Zhao M-M, Kost-Alimova M, et al. Role of telomere dysfunction in cardiac failure in Duchenne muscular dystrophy. Nat Cell Biol. 2013 Aug;15(8):895-904.

[53] Wood CL, Suchacki KJ, van 't Hof R, Cawthorn WP, Dillon S, Straub V, et al. A comparison of the bone and growth phenotype of mdx, mdx:Cmah−/− and mdx:Utrn +/− murine models with the C57BL/10 wild-type mouse. Dis Model Mech [Internet]. 2020 Jan 10;13(2). Available from: http://dx.doi.org/10.1242/dmm.040659

[54] Kudoh H, Ikeda H, Kakitani M, Ueda A, Hayasaka M, Tomizuka K, et al. A new model mouse for Duchenne muscular dystrophy produced by 2.4 Mb deletion of dystrophin gene using Cre-loxP recombination system. Biochem Biophys Res Commun. 2005 Mar 11;328(2):507-516.

[55] Chamberlain JS, Benian GM. Muscular dystrophy: the worm turns to genetic disease. Curr Biol. 2000 Nov 2;10(21):R795–R797.

[56] Bassett DI, Bryson-Richardson RJ, Daggett DF, Gautier P, Keenan DG, Currie PD. Dystrophin is required for the formation of stable muscle attachments in the zebrafish embryo. Development. 2003 Dec;130(23):5851-5860.

[57] Li M, Andersson-Lendahl M, Sejersen T, Arner A. Muscle dysfunction and structural defects of dystrophin-null sapje mutant zebrafish larvae are rescued by ataluren treatment. FASEB J. 2014 Apr;28(4):1593-1599.

[58] Taghli-Lamallem O, Akasaka T, Hogg G, Nudel U, Yaffe D, Chamberlain JS, et al. Dystrophin deficiency in Drosophila reduces lifespan and causes a dilated cardiomyopathy phenotype. Aging Cell. 2008 Mar;7(2):237-249.

[59] Shcherbata HR, Yatsenko AS, Patterson L, Sood VD, Nudel U, Yaffe D, et al. Dissecting muscle and neuronal disorders in a Drosophila model of muscular dystrophy. EMBO J. 2007 Jan 24;26(2):481-493.

[60] Barthélémy I, Calmels N, Weiss RB, Tiret L, Vulin A, Wein N, et al. X-linked muscular dystrophy in a Labrador Retriever strain: phenotypic and molecular characterisation. Skelet Muscle. 2020 Aug 7;10(1):23.

[61] Walmsley GL, Arechavala-Gomeza V, Fernandez-Fuente M, Burke MM, Nagel N, Holder A, et al. A duchenne muscular dystrophy gene hot spot mutation in dystrophin-deficient cavalier king charles spaniels is amenable to exon 51 skipping. PLoS One. 2010 Jan 13;5(1):e8647.

[62] Kornegay JN. The golden retriever model of Duchenne muscular dystrophy. Skelet Muscle. 2017 May 19;7(1):9.

[63] Lorant J, Larcher T, Jaulin N, Hedan B, Lardenois A, Leroux I, et al. Vascular Delivery of Allogeneic MuStem Cells in Dystrophic Dogs Requires Only Short-Term Immunosuppression to Avoid Host Immunity and Generate Clinical/Tissue Benefits. Cell Transplant. 2018 Jul;27(7):1096-1110.

[64] VanBelzen DJ, Malik AS, Henthorn PS, Kornegay JN, Stedman HH. Mechanism of Deletion Removing All Dystrophin Exons in a Canine Model for DMD Implicates Concerted Evolution of X Chromosome Pseudogenes. Mol Ther Methods Clin Dev. 2017 Mar 17;4:62-71.

[65] Nghiem PP, Bello L, Balog-Alvarez C, López SM, Bettis A, Barnett H, et al. Whole genome sequencing reveals a 7 base-pair deletion in DMD exon 42 in a dog with muscular dystrophy. Mamm Genome. 2017 Apr;28(3-4):106-113.

[66] Sánchez L, Beltrán E, de Stefani A, Guo LT, Shea A, Shelton GD, et al. Clinical and genetic characterisation of dystrophin-deficient muscular dystrophy in a family of Miniature Poodle dogs. PLoS One. 2018 Feb 23;13(2):e0193372.

[67] Brunetti B, Muscatello LV, Letko A, Papa V, Cenacchi G, Grillini M, et al. X-Linked Duchenne-Type Muscular Dystrophy in Jack Russell Terrier Associated with a Partial Deletion of the Canine DMD Gene. Genes [Internet]. 2020 Oct 8;11(10). Available from: http://dx.doi.org/10.3390/genes11101175

[68] Mata López S, Hammond JJ, Rigsby MB, Balog-Alvarez CJ, Kornegay JN, Nghiem PP. A novel canine model for Duchenne muscular dystrophy (DMD): single nucleotide deletion in DMD gene exon 20. Skelet Muscle. 2018 May 29;8(1):16.

[69] Carpenter JL, Hoffman EP, Romanul FC, Kunkel LM, Rosales RK, Ma NS, et al. Feline muscular dystrophy with dystrophin deficiency. Am J Pathol. 1989 Nov;135(5):909-919.

[70] Blunden AS, Gower S. Hypertrophic feline muscular dystrophy: diagnostic overview and a novel immunohistochemical diagnostic method using formalin-fixed tissue. Vet Rec. 2011 May 14;168(19):510.

[71] Nakamura K, Fujii W, Tsuboi M, Tanihata J, Teramoto N, Takeuchi S, et al. Generation of muscular dystrophy model rats with a CRISPR/Cas system. Sci Rep. 2014 Jul 9;4:5635.

[72] Sugihara H, Kimura K, Yamanouchi K, Teramoto N, Okano T, Daimon M, et al. Age-Dependent Echocardiographic and Pathologic Findings in a Rat Model with Duchenne Muscular Dystrophy Generated by CRISPR/Cas9 Genome Editing. Int Heart J. 2020 Nov 28;61(6):1279-1284.

[73] Teramoto N, Sugihara H, Yamanouchi K, Nakamura K, Kimura K, Okano T, et al. Pathological evaluation of rats carrying in-frame mutations in the dystrophin gene: a new model of Becker muscular dystrophy. Dis Model Mech [Internet]. 2020 Sep 28;13(9). Available from: http://dx.doi.org/10.1242/dmm.044701

[74] Larcher T, Lafoux A, Tesson L, Remy S, Thepenier V, François V, et al. Characterization of dystrophin deficient rats: a new model for Duchenne muscular dystrophy. PLoS One. 2014 Oct 13;9(10):e110371.

[75] Wertz K, Füchtbauer EM. Dmd(mdx-beta geo): a new allele for the mouse dystrophin gene. Dev Dyn. 1998 Jun;212(2):229-241.

[76] Petkova MV, Morales-Gonzales S, Relizani K, Gill E, Seifert F, Radke J, et al. Characterization of a Dmd (EGFP) reporter mouse as a tool to investigate dystrophin expression. Skelet Muscle. 2016 Jul 5;6:25.

[77] Sarig R, Mezger-Lallemand V, Gitelman I, Davis C, Fuchs O, Yaffe D, et al. Targeted inactivation of Dp71, the major non-muscle product of the DMD gene: differential activity of the Dp71 promoter during development. Hum Mol Genet. 1999 Jan;8(1):1-10.

[78] Vacca O, Charles-Messance H, El Mathari B, Sene A, Barbe P, Fouquet S, et al. AAV-mediated gene therapy in Dystrophin-Dp71 deficient mouse leads to blood-retinal barrier restoration and oedema reabsorption. Hum Mol Genet. 2016 Jul 15;25(14):3070-3079.

[79] Barboni MTS, Vaillend C, Joachimsthaler A, Liber AMP, Khabou H, Roux MJ, et al. Rescue of Defective Electroretinographic Responses in Dp71-Null Mice With AAV-Mediated Reexpression of Dp71. Invest Ophthalmol Vis Sci. 2020 Feb 7;61(2):11.

[80] Miranda R, Nudel U, Laroche S, Vaillend C. Altered presynaptic ultrastructure in excitatory hippocampal synapses of mice lacking dystrophins Dp427 or Dp71. Neurobiol Dis. 2011 Jul;43(1):134-141.

[81] Bladen CL, Salgado D, Monges S, Foncuberta ME, Kekou K, Kosma K, et al. The TREAT-NMD DMD Global Database: analysis of more than 7,000 Duchenne muscular dystrophy mutations. Hum Mutat. 2015 Apr;36(4):395-402.

[82] Araki E, Nakamura K, Nakao K, Kameya S, Kobayashi O, Nonaka I, et al. Targeted disruption of exon 52 in the mouse dystrophin gene induced muscle degeneration similar to that observed in Duchenne muscular dystrophy. Biochem Biophys Res Commun. 1997 Sep 18;238(2):492-497.

[83] Aupy P, Echevarría L, Relizani K, Zarrouki F, Haeberli A, Komisarski M, et al. Identifying and Avoiding tcDNA-ASO Sequence-Specific Toxicity for the Development of DMD Exon 51 Skipping Therapy. Mol Ther Nucleic Acids. 2020 Mar 6;19:371-383.

[84] Aoki Y, Nakamura A, Yokota T, Saito T, Okazawa H, Nagata T, et al. In-frame dystrophin following exon 51-skipping improves muscle pathology and function in the exon 52-deficient mdx mouse. Mol Ther. 2010 Nov;18(11):1995-2005.

[85] Echigoya Y, Lim KRQ, Trieu N, Bao B, Miskew Nichols B, Vila MC, et al. Quantitative Antisense Screening and Optimization for Exon 51 Skipping in Duchenne Muscular Dystrophy. Mol Ther. 2017 Nov 1;25(11):2561-2572.

[86] Aupy P, Zarrouki F, Sandro Q, Gastaldi C, Buclez P-O, Mamchaoui K, et al. Long-Term Efficacy of AAV9-U7snRNA-Mediated Exon 51 Skipping in mdx52 Mice. Mol Ther Methods Clin Dev. 2020 Jun 12;17:1037-1047.

[87] Aoki Y, Yokota T, Wood MJA. Development of multiexon skipping antisense oligonucleotide therapy for Duchenne muscular dystrophy. Biomed Res Int. 2013 Jul 31;2013:402369.

[88] Echigoya Y, Aoki Y, Miskew B, Panesar D, Touznik A, Nagata T, et al. Long-term efficacy of systemic multiexon skipping targeting dystrophin exons 45-55 with a cocktail of vivo-morpholinos in mdx52 mice. Mol Ther Nucleic Acids. 2015 Feb 3;4:e225.

[89] Veltrop M, van Vliet L, Hulsker M, Claassens J, Brouwers C, Breukel C, et al. A dystrophic Duchenne mouse model for testing human antisense oligonucleotides. PLoS One. 2018 Feb 21;13(2):e0193289.

[90] Lyu P, Yoo KW, Yadav MK, Atala A, Aartsma-Rus A, van Putten M, et al. Sensitive and reliable evaluation of single-cut sgRNAs to restore dystrophin by a GFP-reporter assay. PLoS One. 2020 Sep 24;15(9):e0239468.

[91] Duchêne BL, Cherif K, Iyombe-Engembe J-P, Guyon A, Rousseau J, Ouellet DL, et al. CRISPR-Induced Deletion with SaCas9 Restores Dystrophin Expression in Dystrophic Models In Vitro and In Vivo. Mol Ther. 2018 Nov 7;26(11):2604-2616.

[92] Min Y-L, Chemello F, Li H, Rodriguez-Caycedo C, Sanchez-Ortiz E, Mireault AA, et al. Correction of Three Prominent Mutations in Mouse and Human Models of Duchenne Muscular Dystrophy by Single-Cut Genome Editing. Mol Ther. 2020 Sep 2;28(9):2044-2055.

[93] Amoasii L, Li H, Zhang Y, Min Y-L, Sanchez-Ortiz E, Shelton JM, et al. In vivo non-invasive monitoring of dystrophin correction in a new Duchenne muscular dystrophy reporter mouse. Nat Commun. 2019 Oct 4;10(1):4537.

[94] Min Y-L, Li H, Rodriguez-Caycedo C, Mireault AA, Huang J, Shelton JM, et al. CRISPR-Cas9 corrects Duchenne muscular dystrophy exon 44 deletion mutations in mice and human cells. Sci Adv. 2019 Mar;5(3):eaav4324.

[95] Zhang Y, Li H, Min Y-L, Sanchez-Ortiz E, Huang J, Mireault AA, et al. Enhanced CRISPR-Cas9 correction of Duchenne muscular dystrophy in mice by a self-complementary AAV delivery system. Sci Adv. 2020 Feb;6(8):eaay6812.

[96] Wei T, Cheng Q, Min Y-L, Olson EN, Siegwart DJ. Systemic nanoparticle delivery of CRISPR-Cas9 ribonucleoproteins for effective tissue specific genome editing. Nat Commun. 2020 Jun 26;11(1):3232.

[97] Young CS, Mokhonova E, Quinonez M, Pyle AD, Spencer MJ. Creation of a Novel Humanized Dystrophic Mouse Model of Duchenne Muscular Dystrophy and Application of a CRISPR/Cas9 Gene Editing Therapy. J Neuromuscul Dis. 2017;4(2):139-145.

[98] Echigoya Y, Lim KRQ, Melo D, Bao B, Trieu N, Mizobe Y, et al. Exons 45-55 Skipping Using Mutation-Tailored Cocktails of Antisense Morpholinos in the DMD Gene. Mol Ther. 2019 Nov 6;27(11):2005-2017.

[99] Goyenvalle A, Wright J, Babbs A, Wilkins V, Garcia L, Davies KE. Engineering multiple U7snRNA constructs to induce single and multiexon-skipping for Duchenne muscular dystrophy. Mol Ther. 2012 Jun;20(6):1212-1221.

[100] 't Hoen PAC, de Meijer EJ, Boer JM, Vossen RHAM, Turk R, Maatman RGHJ, et al. Generation and characterization of transgenic mice with the full-length human DMD gene. J Biol Chem. 2008 Feb 29;283(9):5899-907.

[101] Wong TWY. Utilization of CRISPR/Cas9-mediated gene editing for correction of deletion mutations in DMD [Internet]. 2020 [cited 2021 Jan 21]. Available from: https://tspace.library.utoronto.ca/handle/1807/103696

[102] Flanigan KM, Dunn DM, von Niederhausern A, Soltanzadeh P, Gappmaier E, Howard MT, et al. Mutational spectrum of DMD mutations in dystrophinopathy patients: application of modern diagnostic techniques to a large cohort. Hum Mutat. 2009 Dec;30(12):1657-1666.

[103] Vulin A, Wein N, Simmons TR, Rutherford AM, Findlay AR, Yurkoski JA, et al. The first exon duplication mouse model of Duchenne muscular dystrophy: A tool for therapeutic development. Neuromuscul Disord. 2015 Nov;25(11):827-834.

[104] Wein N, Simmons T, Gumienny F, Huang N, Heller K, Yurkoski J, et al. A single neonatal injection of an AAV9.

U7snRNA virus mediating skipping of dmd exon 2 allows dystrophin expression preventing apparition of pathologic features in the Dup2 mouse one year post injection. Neuromuscul Disord. 2017 Oct 1;27:S187.

[105] Bulfield G, Siller WG, Wight PA, Moore KJ. X chromosome-linked muscular dystrophy (mdx) in the mouse. Proc Natl Acad Sci U S A. 1984 Feb;81(4):1189-1192.

[106] Malik V, Rodino-Klapac LR, Viollet L, Mendell JR. Aminoglycoside-induced mutation suppression (stop codon readthrough) as a therapeutic strategy for Duchenne muscular dystrophy. Ther Adv Neurol Disord. 2010 Nov;3(6):379-389.

[107] Kim K, Ryu S-M, Kim S-T, Baek G, Kim D, Lim K, et al. Highly efficient RNA-guided base editing in mouse embryos. Nat Biotechnol. 2017 May;35(5):435-437.

[108] Ryu S-M, Koo T, Kim K, Lim K, Baek G, Kim S-T, et al. Adenine base editing in mouse embryos and an adult mouse model of Duchenne muscular dystrophy. Nat Biotechnol. 2018 Jul;36(6):536-539.

[109] Xu L, Zhang C, Li H, Wang P, Gao Y, Mohler PJ, et al. Efficient precise in vivo base editing in adult dystrophic mice [Internet]. Cold Spring Harbor Laboratory. 2020 [cited 2021 Jan 21]. p. 2020.06.24.169292. Available from: https://www.biorxiv.org/content/10.1101/2020.06.24.169292v1

[110] Lorain S, Peccate C, Le Hir M, Griffith G, Philippi S, Précigout G, et al. Dystrophin rescue by trans-splicing: a strategy for DMD genotypes not eligible for exon skipping approaches. Nucleic Acids Res. 2013 Sep;41(17):8391-8402.

[111] Egorova T, Reshetov D, Polikarpova A, Vassilieva S, Vlodavets D, Deikin A. DMD TREATMENT: ANIMAL MODELS: P.203Exons 6 and 7 skipping test on new murine model of Duchenne muscular dystrophy. Neuromuscul Disord. 2018 Oct 1;28:S94.

[112] Koo T, Lu-Nguyen NB, Malerba A, Kim E, Kim D, Cappellari O, et al. Functional Rescue of Dystrophin Deficiency in Mice Caused by Frameshift Mutations Using Campylobacter jejuni Cas9. Mol Ther. 2018 Jun 6;26(6):1529-1538.

[113] Klymiuk N, Blutke A, Graf A, Krause S, Burkhardt K, Wuensch A, et al. Dystrophin-deficient pigs provide new insights into the hierarchy of physiological derangements of dystrophic muscle. Hum Mol Genet. 2013 Nov 1;22(21):4368-4382.

[114] Moretti A, Fonteyne L, Giesert F, Hoppmann P, Meier AB, Bozoglu T, et al. Somatic gene editing ameliorates skeletal and cardiac muscle failure in pig and human models of Duchenne muscular dystrophy. Nat Med. 2020 Feb;26(2):207-214.

[115] Yu H-H, Zhao H, Qing Y B, Pan W-R, Jia B-Y, Zhao H-Y, et al. Porcine Zygote Injection with Cas9/sgRNA Results in DMD-Modified Pig with Muscle Dystrophy. Int J Mol Sci [Internet]. 2016 Oct 9;17(10). Available from: http://dx.doi.org/10.3390/ijms17101668

[116] Sui T, Lau YS, Liu D, Liu T, Xu L, Gao Y, et al. A novel rabbit model of Duchenne muscular dystrophy generated by CRISPR/Cas9. Dis Model Mech [Internet]. 2018 Jun 4;11(6). Available from: http://dx.doi.org/10.1242/dmm.032201

[117] Amoasii L, Hildyard JCW, Li H, Sanchez-Ortiz E, Mireault A, Caballero D, et al. Gene editing restores dystrophin expression in a canine model of Duchenne muscular dystrophy. Science. 2018 Oct 5;362(6410):86-91.

[118] Yokota T, Hoffman E, Takeda S 'ichi. Antisense oligo-mediated multiple exon skipping in a dog model of duchenne muscular dystrophy. Methods Mol Biol. 2011;709:299-312.

[119] Nakamura A, Aoki Y, Tsoumpra M, Yokota T, Takeda S 'ichi. In Vitro Multiexon Skipping by Antisense PMOs in Dystrophic Dog and Exon 7-Deleted DMD Patient. Methods Mol Biol. 2018;1828:151-63.

[120] Vulin A, Barthélémy I, Goyenvalle A, Thibaud J-L, Beley C, Griffith G, et al. Muscle function recovery in golden retriever muscular dystrophy after AAV1-U7 exon skipping. Mol Ther. 2012 Nov;20(11):2120-2133.

[121] Bish LT, Sleeper MM, Forbes SC, Wang B, Reynolds C, Singletary GE, et al. Long-term restoration of cardiac dystrophin expression in golden retriever muscular dystrophy following rAAV6-mediated exon skipping. Mol Ther. 2012 Mar;20(3):580-589.

[122] Le Guiner C, Montus M, Servais L, Cherel Y, Francois V, Thibaud J-L, et al. Forelimb treatment in a large cohort of dystrophic dogs supports delivery of a recombinant AAV for exon skipping in Duchenne patients. Mol Ther. 2014 Nov;22(11):1923-1935.

[123] Hara Y, Mizobe Y, Inoue YU, Hashimoto Y, Motohashi N, Masaki Y, et al. Novel EGFP reporter cell and mouse models for sensitive imaging and quantification of exon skipping. Sci Rep. 2020 Jun 22;10(1):10110.

Chapter 5

Left Ventricular Noncompaction Cardiomyopathy: From Clinical Features to Animal Modeling

Enkhsaikhan Purevjav, Michelle Chintanaphol, Buyan-Ochir Orgil, Nelly R. Alberson and Jeffrey A. Towbin

Abstract

Cardiomyopathy or disease of the heart muscle involves abnormal enlargement and a thickened, stiff, or spongy-like appearance of the myocardium. As a result, the function of the myocardium is weakened and does not sufficiently pump blood throughout the body nor maintain a normal pumping rhythm, leading to heart failure. The main types of cardiomyopathies include dilated hypertrophic, restrictive, arrhythmogenic, and noncompaction cardiomyopathy. Abnormal trabeculations of the myocardium in the left ventricle are classified as left ventricular noncompaction cardiomyopathy (LVNC). Myocardial noncompaction most frequently is observed at the apex of the left ventricle and can be associated with chamber dilation or muscle hypertrophy, systolic or diastolic dysfunction, or both, or various forms of congenital heart disease. Animal models are incredibly important for uncovering the etiology and pathogenesis involved in this disease. This chapter will describe the clinical and pathological features of LVNC in humans and present the animal models that have been used for the study of the genetic basis and pathogenesis of this disease.

Keywords: animal models, noncompaction, cardiomyopathy, mutation, cardiac development

1. Introduction

Left ventricular noncompaction (LVNC) is a unique form of cardiomyopathy that is distinguished by a distinctive ("spongy") morphological appearance of the left ventricle (LV) myocardium [1]. This "spongy" appearance encompasses hypertrabeculation, deep intertrabecular recesses or sinusoids, and a bilayered ventricular myocardium with a noncompacted endocardium and compacted epicardium [2]. Although LVNC is rare, the prevalence of LVNC is reported to be <0.3% in adults and < 0.0001% in children. It is the third most common form of inherited cardiomyopathies and accounts for 9% of all pediatric cardiomyopathy cases [3]. Prevalence was reported as 0.014–1.3% in adult patients who underwent echocardiography. In heart failure patients, the prevalence of LVNC is estimated at 3–4% [4]. LVNC is characterized as genetic, primary cardiomyopathy by the 2006 American Heart Association classification model, whereas the European Society of Cardiology has not classified LVNC as distinct cardiomyopathy due to its phenotypic heterogeneity [5, 6].

Clinical presentation of LVNC is variable, and Towbin et al. have described nine distinct subtypes: 1) benign, 2) arrhythmogenic, 3) dilated, 4) hypertrophic, 5) mixed hypertrophic and dilated, 6) restrictive, 7) right ventricular with the normal left ventricle, 8) biventricular, and 9) associated with congenital heart disease [7]. Some of the LVNC phenotypes are shown in **Figure 1**. Complications of LVNC include chronic heart failure, arrhythmias, cardioembolism, chest pain, dyspnea, syncope, myocardial infarction, and sudden cardiac death (SCD) [8]. Patients with LVNC associated with neuromuscular disease may present with exercise intolerance, fatigue, muscle pain, muscle stiffness, and muscle weakness. Heart failure associated with LVNC is often due to either systolic or diastolic ventricular dysfunction. Electrocardiogram (ECG) abnormalities are very common (88–94% and 88%, respectively) in both adult and pediatric cases. Common arrhythmias are atrial fibrillation, atrial flutter, paroxysmal supraventricular tachycardia, and atrioventricular block. Heart failure and arrhythmias are the greatest cause of concern for mortality in LVNC patients [9].

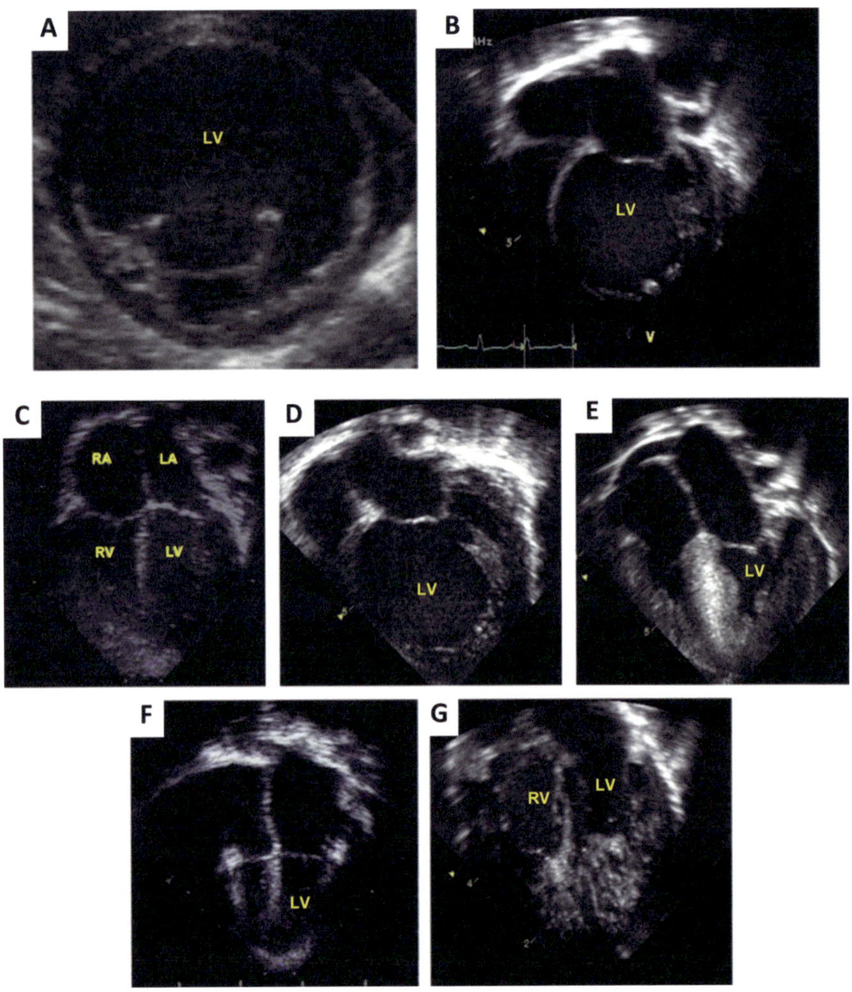

Figure 1.
Echocardiographic images of heterogeneous forms of left ventricular noncompaction phenotype. A. Parasternal short-axis view of a dilated form of LVNC with trabeculations noted at the apex. B. An apical 4-chamber view with trabeculations noted at the right side of the image. C-G, Heterogeneous phenotypes associated with LVNC. LVNC with normal LV size, thickness, and function (C), dilated form of LVNC (D), hypertrophic form of LVNC (E), restrictive form of LVNC (F), biventricular LVNC (G). LV, left ventricle; RV, right ventricle; LA, left atrium, RA, right atrium.

The etiology, pathogenesis, and natural history of LVNC are not clearly understood. The genetic causes of LVNC are heterogeneous [10, 11], involving final common pathways initiated by primary (the sarcomere) and developmental (NOTCH pathway) genetic abnormalities, often *via* a disturbance of protein–protein binding caused by the primary genetic mutation [12]. Doppler echocardiography, cardiac magnetic resonance imaging, or LV angiography are used for the diagnosis. Due to heritable nature, patients with LVNC and at-risk first-degree relatives are recommended to undergo genetic screening and counseling [13, 14]. Clinical symptoms associated with myocardial dysfunction, significant arrhythmias, congenital heart disease, or neuromuscular disease combined with the results of genetic testing dictate the outcome and therapeutic management of LVNC [15]. Family studies and animal models are incredibly important for uncovering the genetic basis and pathways involved in this disease. In this chapter, we describe trabeculation and compaction events during cardiogenesis, morphopathological features of LVNC, and possible genetic mechanisms of LVNC. We will also describe the animal models that have been used for the study of LVNC.

2. Embryonic development of compacted myocardium

The underlying mechanisms for LVNC remain largely unknown, but many studies associate it with the failure of compaction of trabecular myocardium during embryogenesis [16]. The development of the functionally competent, compacted, and multilayered myocardial wall is a two-part process consisting of trabeculation followed by a compaction process set at the midgestational period of cardiogenesis [17]. When the myocardial spiral system enfolds, myocyte recruitment and proliferation lead to myocardial maturation with the development of protrusions into the lumen. Endocardial cells invaginate, and cardiomyocytes in specific regions along the inner wall of the heart form sheet-like protrusions into the lumen to give rise to the trabecular myocardium [16]. The intertrabecular recesses communicate with the blood-filled cavity of the heart tube to increase the surface area for gas exchange and blood. This mechanism favors the concomitant increase in myocardial mass despite the absence of a distinct epicardial coronary circulation [18].

The trabecular myocardium starts undergoing compaction between weeks 5 and 8 of human embryonic development and coincides with the invasion of the developing coronary vasculature from the epicardium. Compaction is gradual, from the epicardial to the endocardial surface and from the basal segments of the ventricle moving toward the apex [19]. Vascular endothelial growth factor (VEGF) and angiopoietin-1 may be involved with triggering compaction [2]. As a result of the compaction process, the intertrabecular recesses disappear almost entirely leaving a smooth endocardial ventricular surface. Compaction is more pronounced in the LV than in the right ventricle (RV), therefore the RV endomyocardial surface is more heavily trabeculated (**Figure 2**) [19]. On the other hand, noncompaction indicates failure of compact myocardium formation, leaving spongy myocardium and deep intertrabecular recesses [20].

2.1 Etiopathophysiology of LVNC and genotype: phenotype correlation

While the etiology of LVNC is not clearly understood, it is largely considered that hypertrabeculation or noncompaction in LVNC has a genetic origin with typically autosomal dominant inheritance if the implicated genes encode components of the sarcomere, Z-disc, or cytoskeleton [21]. Autosomal recessive, X-linked, and mitochondrial inheritance patterns have also been found [3, 22]. One large retrospective multicenter study showed that nearly one-third of the LVNC patients had genetic variants in at least one cardiomyopathy-causative gene [14]. LVNC

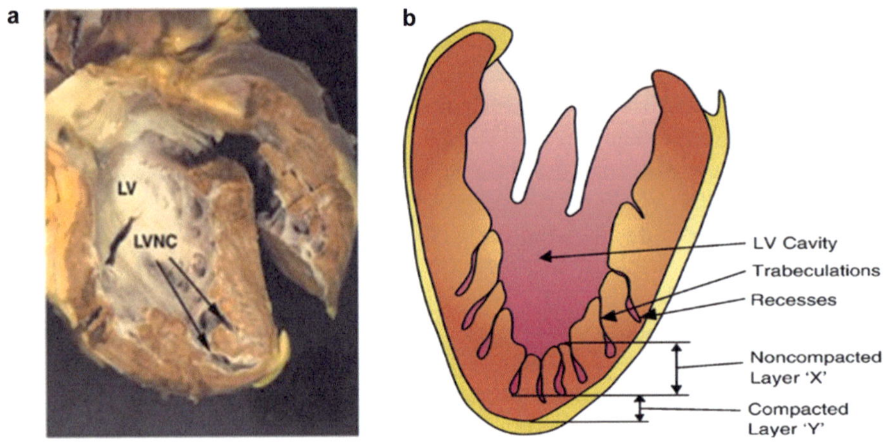

Figure 2.
Gross morphopathologic appearance of LVNC. a. Heart from a individual with left ventricular noncompaction. Note the spongy appearance of the ventricular wall, caused by 'holes' in the myocardium, which represent deep trabeculations. The heart is thick and has a dilated chamber (that is, hypertrophic and dilated). In life this ventricle functioned poorly. LV, left ventricle; LVNC, trabeculations of left ventricular noncompaction. b. Numerous excessive prominent trabeculations and deep intertrabecular recesses is noted by arrows. The trabecular zone (noncompacted layer, X) in the LV is at least twice thick as the compact layer (Y) of the ventricular wall. (Adopted from Towbin and Bowles, Nature 415, 227–233. 2002).

has also been reported in many complex syndromes [23, 24] and neuromuscular disorders [25–27]. LVNC can also be considered congenital or acquired, and several hypotheses have been proposed for the development of LVNC [28]. The primary hypothesis for congenital LVNC is the embryonic hypothesis, which attributes the hypertrabeculation of LVNC to the arrest in normal ventricular compaction during myocardial embryogenesis [29]. The etiology of LVNC can be described as having two components, congenital and modifier factors.

Genetically, LVNC is heterogeneous and has been associated with chromosomal defects and genetic mutations in myosin heavy chain 7 (*MYH7*) [21, 30], LIM domain-binding protein 3 (*ZASP*), α-dystrobrevin (*DTNA*), tafazzin (*TAZ/G4.5*), ion channels, and proteins found in the sarcomere, cytoskeleton, and mitochondria. Alterations in the NOTCH signaling pathway, associated with morphological development, and WNT pathway signaling, embryonically involved in body axis patterning and cell polarity, are also linked to LVNC [20, 31]. In some categories of LVNC, the genotype–phenotype correlation is identifiable. Tafazzin mutations, one of the first mutations linked to LVNC, are characteristic of Barth syndrome, an X-linked genetic disorder that commonly presents with LVNC. Tafazzin, an inner mitochondrial membrane protein, catalyzes phospholipid cardiolipin synthesis, which is essential for mitochondrial integrity and energy production in cardiomyocytes [29, 32]. Family studies have identified mutations in hyperpolarization-activated cyclic nucleotide-gated channel 4 (*HCN4*), sodium voltage-gated channel alpha subunit 5 (*SCN5A*), and ankyrin 2 (*ANK2*) as genetic abnormalities underlying sinus bradycardia-associated LVNC [33]. Lamin A/C (*LMNA*) mutations, which are also found in dilated cardiomyopathies, are associated with the early onset of advanced atrioventricular block [34]. A 6.8-megabase locus on chromosome 11p15, containing muscle LIM protein (*MLP/CSRP3*) and SOX6, was implicated in an autosomal dominant pedigree of LVNC [35]. The V470I variant in bone morphogenetic protein 10 (*BMP10*) and W143X variant in neuregulin (*NRG1*) were identified in two unrelated LVNC probands and their affected family members [36]. Impaired BMP receptor binding ability, perturbed proliferation and differentiation processes, and intolerance to stretch in mutant cardiomyoblasts may underlie myocardial noncompaction in these families.

The causal nature of genetic defects is further complicated by the overlap of genetic mutations in distinct cardiomyopathies. LVNC can be categorized based on its association with dilated cardiomyopathy (DCM), hypertrophic cardiomyopathy (HCM), and other forms of heart muscle disease. Using next-generation sequencing, several groups revealed a wide range of pathogenic variants in LVNC patients and an association between pathogenic variants and poor prognoses, especially in those patients harboring multiple pathogenic variants [10, 11, 37, 38]. Variants in *MYH7* were associated with HCM, DCM, and restrictive cardiomyopathy (RCM). Patients with sarcomeric genes variants had more frequent findings of trabeculations and likelihood fibrosis in the interventricular septum of the myocardium [11]. Variants in mindbomb homolog 1 (*MIB1*), *LMNA*, and *MLP* were linked to LVNC associated with DCM. Myosin-binding protein C (*MYBPC3*) mutations are associated with LVNC-hypertrophic cardiomyopathy, while *SCN5A* and *DSP* variants are reported causative for arrhythmogenic cardiomyopathy (ACM), DCM, and cardiac conduction system dysfunction disorders including Brugada syndrome and long QT syndrome. Interestingly, truncating variants in the *LAMP2* gene that is causative for Danon disease were identified in LVNC patients by Li et.al [37]. In addition, mitochondrial genome mutations [39], chromosomal abnormalities such as 1p36 deletion, 7p14·3p14·1 deletion, 18p subtelomeric deletion, 22q11·2 deletion, distal 22q11·2, 8p23·1 deletion trisomies 18 and 13, and tetrasomy 5q35·2–5q35 have been associated with syndromic LVNC [40–44]. Patients with Coffin–Lowry syndrome (*RPS6KA3* mutation), Sotos syndrome (*NSD1* mutation), and Charcot–Marie–Tooth disease type 1A (*PMP22* duplication) have also been reported to manifest clinical signs of LVNC [23, 45–47]. Titin encoded by the *TTN* gene with 364 exons is the largest protein, expressed in striated muscles [48]. A missense variant *TTN* A178D identified by high throughput next-generation whole-genome sequencing techniques that have been implicated in clinical genetics practice over the last decade has recently been associated with autosomal dominant LVNC and DCM [49]. Nonetheless, a genotype–phenotype correlation may not be identifiable for all mutations and variants. Genetic defects may have incomplete penetrance and variable expressivity or have no causal relationship between genotype and phenotype [2].

The embryonic hypothesis does not explain acquired LVNC that presents after birth, some forms of which are potentially reversible. Acquired LVNC, has been identified in athletes, pregnant women, and patients with sickle cell anemia, myopathies, and chronic renal failure [50]. The etiology of acquired LVNC is merely speculative. One such hypothesis argues that mild LVNC can remain undetected until transient LV dilation allows LVNC to become visible under precise and accurate imaging [51]. It is also speculated that acquired LVNC may be due to cardiac remodeling from increased preload and altered hemodynamics [29]. Ventricular trabeculation in athletes, particularly in the LV apex, allows for increased compliance which reduces wall stress and strain [52]. Given the high risk of possible cardiac embolic events from thrombus formation in the intertrabecular recesses, clinical trials for thromboembolic events in isolated LVNC have been suggested [53–55].

2.2 Diagnosis and therapeutic strategy

The clinical manifestations of LVNC vary widely, including no symptoms, thromboembolic events (ventricular or systemic arterial), LV dilation, impaired contractility with heart failure leading to pulmonary edema, arrhythmia including ventricular tachycardia and atrial fibrillation, and sudden cardiac death. Patients with neuromuscular disorder and LVNC may present with elevation in muscle form of creatine kinase, CK-MM (creatine kinase, muscle isoform) consistent with skeletal myopathy [7].

Echocardiography is the first-line diagnostic routine and an accessible technique to detect abnormal trabeculations or a "spongy" appearance of the myocardium. Several diagnostic criteria have been developed to define LVNC through echocardiographic analysis. A ratio of >2:1 in thickness of noncompacted to compacted layers during diastole is deemed diagnostic for LVNC [56, 57]. Compared with echocardiography, cardiac magnetic resonance (CMR) imaging offers more in-depth anatomic and functional features of the noncompacted myocardium. Late gadolinium enhancement specifically provides detection of cardiac fibrosis. CMR criteria developed by Petersen et al. to accurately diagnose pathologic noncompaction is based on a noncompaction to compaction ratio at end-diastole of >2.3 [58]. Quantitative CMR criteria by Jacquier *et al*. define LV noncompacted mass > 20% of the total mass for accurate LVNC diagnosis [59], while Grothoff et al. propose LV mass > 25% of the total mass as well as a noncompacted mass > 15 g/m^2 [60]. Despite all these proposed criteria, there are wide inconsistencies and poor specificity, and it remains difficult to accurately differentiate normal variants in trabeculations from pathological LVNC [61]. Therefore, data matrices 0f echocardiography and CMR imaging measurements, electrocardiogram features, and clinical genetics of the patient and relatives are helpful for confirming the clinical diagnosis [7].

Genetic testing in patients with LVNC and family members has been important in identifying genetic causes of cardiac dysfunction. Testing can be done on genes known to be associated with LVNC and other forms of cardiomyopathy as well as genes involved in syndromic diseases such as metabolic abnormalities, mitochondrial dysfunction, Barth syndrome, and storage diseases. Identification of pathogenic variants in probands and family members can be followed by segregation studies in the family [15].

Treatment strategy in LVNC depends on clinical presentations and complications, and clinical needs are managed according to corresponding guidelines [62]. The key targets of clinical management are the treatment of heart failure (including beta-blockers, angiotensin-converting enzyme inhibitors, angiotensin-II receptor blockers, aldosterone antagonists, diuretics, and heart transplantation), arrhythmias (including ablation and implantation of an implantable cardioverter-defibrillator in patients with life-threatening events), and oral anticoagulation. In patients with congenital heart disease and LVNC, surgery for the congenital abnormalities takes precedence when feasible. In many cases, palliative surgery ultimately fails because of the myocardial abnormality, and cardiac transplantation is required [63].

3. Animal models of LVNC

LVNC is an overlap disorder and it appears that any of these "final common pathways" can be involved depending on the specific form of LVNC [64]. Combining information about disease-causing genes with murine models is crucial in identifying pathways involved in ventricular noncompaction. For instance, Barth syndrome is caused by tafazzin mutations, and tafazzin knockdown mice were engineered using a short-hairpin RNA-inducible transgenic approach. These mice demonstrated hypertrabeculation and noncompaction, and the knockdown mice died prenatally at E12.5–14.5 [65]. New powerful cutting-edge gene-editing technologies using transcription activator-like effector nucleases (TALENs) and clustered regularly interspaced short palindromic repeats-CRISPR-associated protein 9 (CRISPR-Cas9) have been used for modeling LVNC [66–69]. Patient-specific induced pluripotent stem cells (iPSCs) derived cardiomyocytes have emerged as a useful tool for investigating pathological mechanisms of many cardiovascular diseases including LVNC [70, 71].

Gene	Animal model	Signaling	Ref #
FKBP12	KO mouse	Decrease in Notch1 activity, increase in BMP10	[79]
BMP10	KO E9.0–13.5 mouse	TGF-b	[80]
BMP10	Overexpression adult mouse	TGF-b	[81]
NUMB/NUMBL	Double KO mouse	Inhibition of Notch1, Smad6 and Smad7, WNT	[82]
SMAD7	Mutant mouse	BMP10, TGF-b	[86]
TBX20	Overexpression mouse	T-box family, TBX1	[87]
MIB1	Mutant zebrafish	Reduces Notch1	[89]
MIB1	Decifient zebrafish	Reduces Notch1	[89]
VEGF	Overexpression mouse	Notch1, Flk-1	[90]
Daam1	Decifient mouse	PCP and WNT	[92]
NKX2–5	KO mouse	MEF2, HAND1, HAND2, GATA, BMP10	[96]
NFATC1	Mutant mouse	NFAT	[99]
TAZ	Inducible knockdown	Cardiolipin remodeling	[102]
TAZ	KO mouse	Cardiolipin remodeling	[65]
TTN	Mutant mouse	Telethonin loss	[104]

Table 1.
Animal models of LVNC.

Several signaling pathways such as the Dll4-NOTCH [72], MIB1 [73], BMP [74], and TGF-β [71] have been demonstrated to regulate myocardial trabecular compaction as well as to be involved in the development of LVNC. While zebrafish and *Drosophila* have been used to study LVNC in addition to patient-specific iPSCs derived cardiomyocytes, mice are more commonly used to genetically engineer LVNC phenotypes as shown in **Table 1** [75, 76].

3.1 Animal models related to the Notch signaling pathway

The Notch signaling pathway is a highly conserved intercellular pathway involved with multisystem differentiation. Particularly in the cardiovascular system, Notch1 mediates ventricular morphogenesis, coronary vessel development, and communication between the endocardium and myocardium for cardiomyocyte proliferation and differentiation. Mutations in the Notch signaling pathway cause congenital heart disease [77]. Mammals have Notch 1–4, a group of transmembrane receptors with an extracellular domain and an intracellular domain. The Notch extracellular domain (NECD) interacts with ligands of the Delta and Jagged family, and these receptor-ligand interactions are modulated by manic fringe (Mfng) glycosyltransferase. Delta and Jagged ligands are ubiquitinated by Mib1, an E3 ubiquitin ligase, and trigger endocytosis of the ligand. Mib1 activity exposes the receptor to ADAM metalloproteases for Notch cleavage. In response, the Notch intracellular domain (NICD) translocates to the nucleus and acts as a transcription factor. The NICD is comprised of the RBPJ domain and ANK repeats [77].

The first murine model for LVNC was the Fkbp1a (or FKBP12)-deficient mouse. Deficiency in FKBP1a, a binding protein of the immunophilin family, causes ventricular noncompaction, thin ventricular walls, hypertrabeculation, and ventricular septal defects [20, 78]. Fkbp1a is a negative modulator of activated Notch 1. In Fkbp1a-deficient mice, activated Notch1 is upregulated. In Fkb1a-deficient mice, Fkbp1a overexpression significantly reduced activated

Notch1 [79]. Fkbp1a deficiency upregulates BMP10, a peptide growth factor in the TGF-β family involved in the cardiac compaction process. BMP10 upregulation in Fkbp1a-deficient mice indicates the importance of this gene in the trabeculation and compaction process.

In mouse embryogenesis, Bmp10 is transiently expressed in ventricular myocardium at E9.0–13.5 during myocardial maturation and in the atria E16.5–18.5 [74]. BMP10-deficient mice embryos appear unaffected at E8.5–9.0, arrest at E9.0–9.5, and die at E10.5. Immunostaining of mutant embryos exhibited thin ventricular walls and primitive trabecular ridges. The localization of BMP10 to the ventricular myocardium for the brief period at E9.0–13.5 suggests that BMP10 is crucial for continued myocardial development. Postnatal cardiac-specific BMP10 overexpression compromised cardiac growth, caused subaortic narrowing and concentric myocardial thickening [80]. Human atrial natriuretic factor (hANF) promoter can be used to overexpress BMP10 in mice. Overexpression of BMP10 demonstrated hypertrabeculation and severe heart failure [81]. Like in Fkbp1a-deficient mice and cardiac overexpression models, BMP10 is also upregulated in NUMB/NUMBL-deficient mice (myocardial double-knockout mice) [82]. NUMB and NUMBL proteins of the NUMB family are cell fate determinants for hemopoietic stem cells, muscle satellite cells, cancer stem cells, and hemangioblast progenitor cell types and maintain the fate of neural stem cells as well as regulate their differentiation [83]. Both NUMB and NUMBL inhibit Notch1 signaling and are crucial for trabeculation, cardiomyocyte proliferation and differentiation, and trabecular thickness [84]. On the other hand, inhibitory intracellular transducers such as Smad6 and Smad7 negatively regulate the BMP/ TGF-β signaling pathway [85]. Smad7 is expressed by endothelial cells in the major arteries in mice, and Smad7 deficiency causes increased Smad 1, 5, and 8 in the endocardial endothelium [81, 86]. Unsurprisingly, Smad7 mutant mice demonstrate ventricular noncompaction, thin ventricular walls, and ventricular septal defect. One of the key mediators of BMP10 signaling in ventricular myocardial development and maturation is TBX20, a member of the TBX1 subfamily of the T-box family transcription factors [87]. In murine embryos, Tbx20 can be detected in the cardiac precursor cells at E7·5 and the developing myocardium and endocardium at E8·0 [88]. Cardiac-specific overexpression of TBX20 results in severe DCM, ventricular hypertrabeculation, and abnormal muscular septum, consistent with the DCM type of LVNC [87].

Another Notch pathway element, Mib1, is associated with the LVNC phenotype of biventricular noncompaction with dilation and heart failure [20]. Genetic sequencing of 100 European patients revealed two autosomal dominant mutations—V943F and R530X. Injection of Mib1-mutated mRNA, corresponding to the V943F and R530X mutations, into zebrafish embryos disrupts Notch signaling [89]. Inactivation of Mib1 reduces Notch1 signaling and myocardial arrest. Mutant Mib1 mice produce an LVNC phenotype of immature trabeculae and noncompaction [89].

Vascular endothelial growth factor (VEGF) is produced by the myocardium and plays a role in endocardium-myocardium communication by binding to endocardial receptor Flk-1 [20]. Overexpression of VEGF-A in mice causes hypertrabeculation, abnormalities in cardiac morphology and coronary vessels, and embryonic lethality at E12.5–14.0 [90].

3.2 Animal models related to the WNT signaling pathway

The planar cell polarity (PCP) pathway is a β-catenin-independent Wnt pathway that was first studied in *Drosophila*. The PCP pathway plays a role in the epithelial orientation of hair and sensory bristles, apical-basolateral polarity, gastrulation, and neurulation [31, 91]. Disheveled-associated activator of morphogenesis I

(Daam1) is a mediator of the PCP pathway and a formin protein found in the plasma membrane and cytoplasmic vesicles. Daam1 is involved with cardiac morphogenesis and is highly expressed in murine cardiac tissue. Daam1-deficient mice have been shown to cause an LVNC phenotype with ventricular noncompaction and the thin ventricular wall. It is likely that the abnormalities seen in Daam1-deficient mice are due to cytoskeletal dysfunction since Daam1 is involved with F-actin assembly and sarcomere organization. Interestingly, the absence of Daam1 does not alter BMP10 expression nor cardiomyocyte proliferation, which offers another pathogenic model of LVNC through disruption in myofibrillogenesis, cytoskeleton organization, and cardiomyocyte polarization [31, 92].

NUMB is also a component of the adherens junction by forming complexes with β-catenin to regulate cellular adhesion *via* Wnt signaling [82]. It also interacts with integrin-β subunits to regulate cell migration and promote their endocytosis for directional cell migration. Deletion of NUMB and NUMBL from mouse hearts results in LVNC with congenital heart disease with atrioventricular septal defects, truncus arteriosus, and double outlet right ventricle *in vivo* [82]. This model shows that NUMB family proteins regulate trabecular thickness by inhibiting Notch1 signaling and control cardiac morphogenesis in a Notch1-independent manner.

3.3 Animal models related to other signaling pathways

NKX2–5, a cardiac homeobox gene, is a transcription factor that regulates heart development, working along with MEF2, HAND1, and HAND2 transcription factors to direct heart looping during early heart development [93]. Genetic variants in *NKX2–5* are associated with progressive cardiomyopathy and conduction defects in humans [94, 95]. Ventricular-muscle-cell-restricted knockout of *NKX2–5* in mice leads to progressive atrioventricular block with conduction system cell dropout and fibrosis [96]. LVNC is a prominent feature in neonatal mice, with progressive biventricular dilation and heart failure developing early. It directly activates *MEF2* to control cardiomyocyte differentiation and operates in a positive feedback loop with GATA transcription factors to regulate cardiomyocyte formation. A high-level BMP10 expression in the adult ventricular myocardium has been also observed.

The expression of early response genes in lymphocytes is regulated by NFAT transcription factors [97]. *NFATC1* mutant mouse embryos have cardiac abnormalities including myocardial developmental abnormalities, narrowing or occlusion of the ventricular outflow tract, defective septum morphogenesis, and underdevelopment of valves [98, 99]. Ventricular hypertrophy and noncompaction with hypertrabeculation were seen in 40% of mutant mice, suggesting that NFAT signaling pathways are important for hypertrabeculation and noncompaction as well as the development of valves and the septum.

Barth syndrome is caused by mutations in the X-linked *TAZ* and is associated with LVNC and abnormal cardiolipin remodeling [12, 100]. Tafazzin catalyzes cardiolipin maturation reactions at the final stage of cardiolipin biosynthesis [101]. Inducible knockdown of *TAZ* (TAZKD) in murine models using short-hairpin RNA (shRNA) exhibited an adult-onset LVNC associated with abnormal cardiolipin profiles and mitochondrial structural abnormalities [102]. Knockout of *TAZ* at the embryonic stage leads to unique developmental cardiomyopathy characterized by ventricular myocardial hypertrabeculation and noncompaction and early lethality, suggesting that mitochondrial function is important for proper myocardial development [65].

Cytoskeletal and sarcomeric proteins encoding gene mutations have been shown to account for 20% or more of LVNC [7]. Truncating variants in *TTN* are well-documented to cause skeletal myopathies and cardiomyopathies including LVNC

[48, 49, 103]. Homozygous mouse model carrying titin A178D mutation created by using CRISPR-Cas9 gene-editing displayed features of mild DCM, but not LVNC phenotype [104]. These mice showed complete loss of telethonin from the Z-disc and induction of a proteo-toxic response in the heart upon aging and adrenergic stress.

4. Conclusions

The pathogenesis of LVNC, a recently classified cardiomyopathy, remains largely unclear. With over 40 genes linked to LVNC, both genotype variation and phenotype variation are vast. Genetic testing in families and individuals with LVNC shas proved useful in identifying disease-causing variants. While the Notch signaling pathway is implicated in the pathogenesis of LVNC, there may be other pathways leading to congenital and acquired forms of LVNC. Identifying specific pathway elements is crucial for diagnosis and treatment. Modeling LVNC variants can help us to determine the genetic basis and pathogenesis of the disease.

Conflict of interest

The authors have no conflicts of interest.

Author details

Enkhsaikhan Purevjav[1,2]*, Michelle Chintanaphol[1], Buyan-Ochir Orgil[1,2], Nelly R. Alberson[1,2] and Jeffrey A. Towbin[1,2,3]

1 Department of Pediatrics, Heart Institute, University of Tennessee Health Science Center, Memphis, TN, United States

2 Children's Foundation Research Institute, Le Bonheur Children's Hospital Memphis, Memphis, TN, United States

3 Pediatric Cardiology, St. Jude Children's Research Hospital, Memphis, TN, United States

*Address all correspondence to: epurevja@uthsc.edu

References

[1] Maron BJ et al. Contemporary definitions and classification of the cardiomyopathies: An American Heart Association Scientific Statement from the Council on Clinical Cardiology, Heart Failure and Transplantation Committee; Quality of Care and Outcomes Research and Functional Genomics and Translational Biology Interdisciplinary Working Groups; and Council on Epidemiology and Prevention. Circulation. 2006;**113**(14):1807-1816

[2] Finsterer J, Stöllberger C, Towbin JA. Left ventricular noncompaction cardiomyopathy: Cardiac, neuromuscular, and genetic factors. Nature Reviews Cardiology. 2017;**14**(4):224-237

[3] Towbin JA, Jefferies JL. Cardiomyopathies due to left ventricular noncompaction, mitochondrial and storage diseases, and inborn errors of metabolism. Circulation Research. 2017;**121**(7):838-854

[4] Goud A, Padmanabhan S. A rare form of cardiomyopathy: Left ventricular non-compaction cardiomyopathy. Journal of Community Hospital Internal Medicine Perspectives. 2016;**6**(1):29888

[5] Maron BJ. The 2006 American Heart Association classification of cardiomyopathies is the gold standard. Circulation: Heart Failure. 2008;**1**(1):72-76

[6] Elliott P et al. Classification of the cardiomyopathies: A position statement from the european society of cardiology working group on myocardial and pericardial diseases. European Heart Journal. 2007;**29**(2):270-276

[7] Towbin JA, Lorts A, Jefferies JL. Left ventricular non-compaction cardiomyopathy. Lancet. 2015;**386**(9995):813-825

[8] Brescia ST et al. Mortality and sudden death in pediatric left ventricular noncompaction in a tertiary referral center. Circulation. 2013;**127**(22):2202-2208

[9] Finsterer J. Cardiogenetics, neurogenetics, and pathogenetics of left ventricular hypertrabeculation/noncompaction. Pediatric Cardiology. 2009;**30**(5):659-681

[10] Wang C et al. A wide and specific spectrum of genetic variants and genotype-phenotype correlations revealed by next-generation sequencing in patients with left ventricular noncompaction. Journal of the American Heart Association. 2017;**6**(9):e006210

[11] Miszalski-Jamka K et al. Novel genetic triggers and genotype-phenotype correlations in patients with left ventricular noncompaction. Circulation Cardiovascular Genetics, 2017;**10**(4):e001763

[12] Towbin JA. Left ventricular noncompaction: A new form of heart failure. Heart Failure Clinics, 2010;**6**(4):453-469

[13] Hoedemaekers YM et al. The importance of genetic counseling, DNA diagnostics, and cardiologic family screening in left ventricular noncompaction cardiomyopathy. Circulation Cardiovascular Genetics. 2010;**3**(3):232-239

[14] van Waning JI et al. Cardiac phenotypes, genetics, and risks in familial noncompaction cardiomyopathy. Journal of the American College of Cardiology. 2019;**73**(13):1601-1611

[15] Towbin JA, Jefferies JL. Cardiomyopathies due to left ventricular noncompaction, mitochondrial and

storage diseases, and inborn errors of metabolism. Circulation Research. 2017;**121**(7):838-854

[16] Zhang W et al. Molecular mechanism of ventricular trabeculation/compaction and the pathogenesis of the left ventricular noncompaction cardiomyopathy (LVNC). American Journal of Medical Genetics. Part C, Seminars in Medical Genetics. 2013;**163C**(3):144-156

[17] Sedmera D et al. Developmental patterning of the myocardium. The Anatomical Record. 2000;**258**(4): 319-337

[18] Sedmera D et al. Developmental patterning of the myocardium. The Anatomical Record. 2000;**258**(4): 319-337

[19] Engberding R, Yelbuz TM, Breithardt G. Isolated noncompaction of the left ventricular myocardium - a review of the literature two decades after the initial case description. Clinical Research in Cardiology. 2007;**96**(7): 481-488

[20] Ichida F. Left ventricular noncompaction – risk stratification and genetic consideration . Journal of Cardiology. 2020;**75**(1):1-9

[21] Sasse-Klaassen S et al. Isolated noncompaction of the left ventricular myocardium in the adult is an autosomal dominant disorder in the majority of patients. American Journal of Medical Genetics. Part A. 2003;**119A**(2):162-167

[22] Xing Y et al. Genetic analysis in patients with left ventricular noncompaction and evidence for genetic heterogeneity. Molecular Genetics and Metabolism. 2006;**88**(1):71-77

[23] Martinez HR et al. Left ventricular noncompaction in Sotos syndrome. American Journal of Medical Genetics. Part A. 2011;**155A**(5):1115-1118

[24] Saccucci P et al. Isolated left ventricular noncompaction in a case of sotos syndrome: A casual or causal link? Cardiology Research and Practice. 2011;**2011**:824095

[25] Finsterer J et al. Acquired noncompaction in Duchenne muscular dystrophy. International Journal of Cardiology. 2006;**106**(3):420-421

[26] Hofer M, Stollberger C, Finsterer J. Acquired noncompaction associated with myopathy. International Journal of Cardiology. 2007;**121**(3):296-297

[27] Stollberger C et al. Neuromuscular and cardiac comorbidity determines survival in 140 patients with left ventricular hypertrabeculation/noncompaction. International Journal of Cardiology. 2011;**150**(1):71-74

[28] Okumura T, Murohara T. Unsolved issue in left ventricular noncompaction: is the strange form of myocardium congenital or acquired? Cardiology. 2019;**143**(3-4):105-106

[29] Wengrofsky P et al. Left ventricular trabeculation and noncompaction cardiomyopathy: A review. EC Clinical and Experimental Anatomy. 2019;**2**(6):267-283

[30] Villard E et al. Mutation screening in dilated cardiomyopathy: Prominent role of the beta myosin heavy chain gene. European Heart Journal. 2005;**26**(8):794-803

[31] Liu Y, Chen H, Shou W. Potential common pathogenic pathways for the left ventricular noncompaction cardiomyopathy (LVNC). Pediatric Cardiology. 2018;**39**(6):1099-1106

[32] Phoon CKL et al. Tafazzin knockdown in mice leads to a developmental cardiomyopathy with early diastolic dysfunction preceding myocardial noncompaction. Journal of the American Heart Association. 2012;**1**(2):jah3-e000455

[33] Milano A et al. HCN4 mutations in multiple families with bradycardia and left ventricular noncompaction cardiomyopathy. Journal of the American College of Cardiology. 2014; **64**(8):745-756

[34] Saga A et al. Lamin A/C gene mutations in familial cardiomyopathy with advanced atrioventricular block and arrhythmia. The Tohoku Journal of Experimental Medicine. 2009;**218**(4): 309-316

[35] Sasse-Klaassen S et al. Novel gene locus for autosomal dominant left ventricular noncompaction maps to chromosome 11p15. Circulation. 2004;**109**(22):2720-2723

[36] Hirono K et al. Familial left ventricular non-compaction is associated with a rare p.V407I variant in bone morphogenetic protein 10. Circulation Journal. 2019;**83**(8):1737-1746

[37] Li S et al. Genotype-positive status is associated with poor prognoses in patients with left ventricular noncompaction cardiomyopathy. Journal of the American Heart Association. 2018;**7**(20):e009910

[38] van Waning JI et al. Genetics, clinical features, and long-term outcome of noncompaction cardiomyopathy. Journal of the American College of Cardiology. 2018;**71**(7):711-722

[39] Tang S et al. Left ventricular noncompaction is associated with mutations in the mitochondrial genome. Mitochondrion. 2010;**10**(4):350-357

[40] Digilio MC et al. Syndromic non-compaction of the left ventricle: Associated chromosomal anomalies. Clinical Genetics. 2013;**84**(4):362-367

[41] Beken S et al. A neonatal case of left ventricular noncompaction associated with trisomy 18. Genetic Counseling. 2011;**22**(2):161-164

[42] Blinder JJ et al. Noncompaction of the left ventricular myocardium in a boy with a novel chromosome 8p23.1 deletion. American Journal of Medical Genetics. Part A. 2011;**155A**(9):2215-2220

[43] Yukifumi M et al. Trisomy 13 in a 9-year-old girl with left ventricular noncompaction. Pediatric Cardiology. 2011;**32**(2):206-207

[44] Sellars EA et al. Ventricular noncompaction and absent thumbs in a newborn with tetrasomy 5q35.2-5q35.3: An association with Hunter-McAlpine syndrome? American Journal of Medical Genetics. Part A. 2011;**155A**(6): 1409-1413

[45] Martinez HR et al. Coffin-Lowry syndrome and left ventricular noncompaction cardiomyopathy with a restrictive pattern. American Journal of Medical Genetics. Part A. 2011; **155A**(12):3030-3034

[46] Zechner U et al. Familial Sotos syndrome caused by a novel missense mutation, C2175S, in NSD1 and associated with normal intelligence, insulin dependent diabetes, bronchial asthma, and lipedema. European Journal of Medical Genetics. 2009;**52**(5):306-310

[47] Corrado G et al. Left ventricular hypertrabeculation/noncompaction with PMP22 duplication-based Charcot-Marie-Tooth disease type 1A. Cardiology. 2006;**105**(3):142-145

[48] Labeit S, Kolmerer B, Linke WA. The giant protein titin. Emerging roles in physiology and pathophysiology. Circulation Research. 1997;**80**(2): 290-294

[49] Hastings R et al. Combination of whole genome sequencing, linkage, and functional studies implicates a missense mutation in titin as a cause of autosomal dominant cardiomyopathy with features of left ventricular noncompaction.

Circulation. Cardiovascular Genetics. 2016;**9**(5):426-435

[50] Arbustini E et al. Left ventricular noncompaction. Journal of the American College of Cardiology. 2016;**68**(9):949-966

[51] Angelini P. Can left ventricular noncompaction be acquired, and can it disappear? Texas Heart Institute Journal. 2017;**44**(4):264-265

[52] Abela M, D'Silva A. Left ventricular trabeculations in athletes: Epiphenomenon or phenotype of disease? Current Treatment Options in Cardiovascular Medicine. 2018;**20**(12):100-100

[53] Lestienne F et al. Ischemic stroke in a young patient heralding a left ventricular noncompaction cardiomyopathy. Case Reports in Neurology. 2017;**9**(2):204-209

[54] Kulhari A, Kalra N, Sila C. Noncompaction cardiomyopathy and stroke: Case report and literature review. Journal of Stroke and Cerebrovascular Diseases. 2015;**24**(8):e213-e217

[55] Finsterer J, Stollberger C. Stroke due to Chagas' cardiomyopathy or noncompaction. Arquivos Brasileiros de Cardiologia. 2011;**96**(5):427 author reply 428

[56] Ichida F. Left ventricular noncompaction—Risk stratification and genetic consideration. Journal of Cardiology. 2020;**75**(1):1-9

[57] Jenni R et al. Echocardiographic and pathoanatomical characteristics of isolated left ventricular non-compaction: A step towards classification as a distinct cardiomyopathy. Heart. 2001;**86**(6):666-671

[58] Petersen SE et al. Left ventricular non-compaction: Insights from cardiovascular magnetic resonance imaging. Journal of the American College of Cardiology. 2005;**46**(1):101-105

[59] Jacquier A et al. Measurement of trabeculated left ventricular mass using cardiac magnetic resonance imaging in the diagnosis of left ventricular non-compaction. European Heart Journal. 2010;**31**(9):1098-1104

[60] Grothoff M et al. Value of cardiovascular MR in diagnosing left ventricular non-compaction cardiomyopathy and in discriminating between other cardiomyopathies. European Radiology. 2012;**22**(12): 2699-2709

[61] Rhee JW, Grove ME, Ashley EA. Navigating genetic and phenotypic uncertainty in left ventricular noncompaction. Circulation. Cardiovascular Genetics, 2017;**10**(4): e001857

[62] Yancy CW et al. 2013 ACCF/AHA guideline for the management of heart failure: A report of the American College of Cardiology Foundation/ American Heart Association Task Force on Practice Guidelines. Journal of the American College of Cardiology. 2013;**62**(16):e147-e239

[63] Yu WZ et al. Congenital heart surgery in patients with ventricular noncompaction. Journal of Cardiac Surgery. 2015;**30**(2):179-184

[64] Towbin JA. Inherited cardiomyopathies. Circulation Journal. 2014;**78**(10):2347-2356

[65] Phoon CK et al. Tafazzin knockdown in mice leads to a developmental cardiomyopathy with early diastolic dysfunction preceding myocardial noncompaction. Journal of the American Heart Association, 2012;**1**(2):jah3-e000455

[66] Doudna JA, Charpentier E. Genome editing. The new frontier of genome

engineering with CRISPR-Cas9. Science. 2014;**346**(6213):1258096

[67] Gaj T et al. Genome-editing technologies: Principles and applications. Cold Spring Harbor Perspectives in Biology. 2016;**8**(12):a023754

[68] German DM et al. Therapeutic genome editing in cardiovascular diseases. JACC Basic Translational Science. 2019;**4**(1):122-131

[69] Nishiga M, Qi LS, Wu JC. Therapeutic genome editing in cardiovascular diseases. Advanced Drug Delivery Reviews. 2021;**168**:147-157

[70] Kim C et al. Studying arrhythmogenic right ventricular dysplasia with patient-specific iPSCs. Nature. 2013;**494**(7435):105-110

[71] Kodo K et al. iPSC-derived cardiomyocytes reveal abnormal TGF-beta signalling in left ventricular non-compaction cardiomyopathy. Nature Cell Biology. 2016;**18**(10):1031-1042

[72] D'Amato G, Luxan G, de la Pompa JL. Notch signalling in ventricular chamber development and cardiomyopathy. The FEBS Journal. 2016;**283**(23):4223-4237

[73] Luxan G et al. Mutations in the NOTCH pathway regulator MIB1 cause left ventricular noncompaction cardiomyopathy. Nature Medicine. 2013;**19**(2):193-201

[74] Chen H et al. BMP10 is essential for maintaining cardiac growth during murine cardiogenesis. Development. 2004;**131**(9):2219-2231

[75] Arbustini E, Weidemann F, Hall JL. Left ventricular noncompaction: A distinct cardiomyopathy or a trait shared by different cardiac diseases? Journal of the American College of Cardiology. 2014;**64**(17):1840-1850

[76] Purevjav E. Animal Models of Cardiomyopathies. Eva T, Sarat Chandra Y, (Eds). Animal Models in Medicine and Biology. IntechOpen; 15th October 2019. Available from: https://www.intechopen.com/chapters/68936 2020. DOI: 10.5772/intechopen.89033

[77] D'Amato G, Luxán G, De La Pompa JL. Notch signalling in ventricular chamber development and cardiomyopathy. The FEBS Journal. 2016;**283**(23):4223-4237

[78] Towbin JA, Lorts A, Jefferies JL. Left ventricular non-compaction cardiomyopathy. The Lancet. 2015;**386**(9995):813-825

[79] Chen H et al. Fkbp1a controls ventricular myocardium trabeculation and compaction by regulating endocardial Notch1 activity. Development. 2013;**140**(9):1946-1957

[80] Chen H et al. Overexpression of bone morphogenetic protein 10 in myocardium disrupts cardiac postnatal hypertrophic growth. The Journal of Biological Chemistry. 2006;**281**(37):27481-27491

[81] Chen H et al. Analysis of ventricular hypertrabeculation and noncompaction using genetically engineered mouse models. Pediatric Cardiology. 2009;**30**(5):626-634

[82] Yang J et al. Inhibition of Notch2 by Numb/Numblike controls myocardial compaction in the heart. Cardiovascular Research. 2012;**96**(2):276-285

[83] Dho SE et al. Characterization of four mammalian numb protein isoforms. Identification of cytoplasmic and membrane-associated variants of the phosphotyrosine binding domain. The Journal of Biological Chemistry. 1999;**274**(46):33097-33104

[84] Zhao C et al. Numb family proteins are essential for cardiac morphogenesis

and progenitor differentiation. Development. 2014;**141**(2):281-295

[85] Lin SJ et al. The structural basis of TGF-beta, bone morphogenetic protein, and activin ligand binding. Reproduction. 2006;**132**(2):179-190

[86] Chen Q et al. Smad7 is required for the development and function of the heart. The Journal of Biological Chemistry. 2009;**284**(1):292-300

[87] Zhang W et al. Tbx20 transcription factor is a downstream mediator for bone morphogenetic protein-10 in regulating cardiac ventricular wall development and function. The Journal of Biological Chemistry. 2011;**286**(42): 36820-36829

[88] Shelton EL, Yutzey KE. Tbx20 regulation of endocardial cushion cell proliferation and extracellular matrix gene expression. Developmental Biology. 2007;**302**(2):376-388

[89] Luxán G et al. Mutations in the NOTCH pathway regulator MIB1 cause left ventricular noncompaction cardiomyopathy. Nature Medicine. 2013;**19**(2):193-201

[90] Miquerol L, Langille BL, Nagy A. Embryonic development is disrupted by modest increases in vascular endothelial growth factor gene expression. Development. 2000;**127**(18):3941-3946

[91] Komiya Y, Habas R. Wnt signal transduction pathways. Organogenesis. 2008;**4**(2):68-75

[92] Li D et al. Dishevelled-associated activator of morphogenesis 1 (Daam1) is required for heart morphogenesis. Development. 2011;**138**(2):303-315

[93] Lints TJ et al. Nkx-2.5: A novel murine homeobox gene expressed in early heart progenitor cells and their myogenic descendants. Development. 1993;**119**(3):969

[94] Jhaveri S, Aziz PF, Saarel E. Expanding the electrical phenotype of NKX2-5 mutations: Ventricular tachycardia, atrial fibrillation, and complete heart block within one family. HeartRhythm Case Report. 2018;**4**(11):530-533

[95] Benson DW et al. Mutations in the cardiac transcription factor NKX2.5 affect diverse cardiac developmental pathways. The Journal of Clinical Investigation. 1999;**104**(11):1567-1573

[96] Pashmforoush M et al. Nkx2-5 pathways and congenital heart disease; loss of ventricular myocyte lineage specification leads to progressive cardiomyopathy and complete heart block. Cell. 2004;**117**(3):373-386

[97] Aramburu J et al. Selective inhibition of NFAT activation by a peptide spanning the calcineurin targeting site of NFAT. Molecular Cell. 1998;**1**(5):627-637

[98] Liu J et al. Calcineurin is a common target of cyclophilin-cyclosporin A and FKBP-FK506 complexes. Cell. 1991;**66**(4):807-815

[99] de la Pompa JL et al. Role of the NF-ATc transcription factor in morphogenesis of cardiac valves and septum. Nature. 1998;**392**(6672): 182-186

[100] Ichida F et al. Novel gene mutations in patients with left ventricular noncompaction or Barth syndrome. Circulation. 2001;**103**(9):1256-1263

[101] Xu Y et al. The enzymatic function of tafazzin. The Journal of Biological Chemistry. 2006;**281**(51):39217-39224

[102] Acehan D et al. Cardiac and skeletal muscle defects in a mouse model of human Barth syndrome. The Journal of Biological Chemistry. 2011;**286**(2):899-908

[103] Peled Y et al. Titin mutation in familial restrictive cardiomyopathy. International Journal of Cardiology. 2014;**171**(1):24-30

[104] Jiang H et al. Functional analysis of a gene-edited mouse model to gain insights into the disease mechanisms of a titin missense variant. Basic Research in Cardiology. 2021;**116**(1):14

Section 3

Animal Models of Acute Injury and Pain

Chapter 6

Experimental Animal Models of Cerebral Ischemic Reperfusion Injury

Prabhakar Orsu and Y. Srihari

Abstract

Restitution of blood flow in the ischemic region helps liberate cells from mortification in any tissue or organ. Reperfusion post cerebral ischemia worsen the condition and lead to "cerebral reperfusion injury". In cerebral reperfusion injury, significant changes observed are infarct size, behavioural deficits, hematoma formation, inflammatory mediators, and oxidative stress markers representing the extent of brain injury. Experimental *In vivo* models mimicking pathological and neurological processes are key tools in researching cerebral reperfusion injury and potential therapeutic agents' development. This review explains currently used *In vivo* models like middle cerebral artery occlusion model, emboli stroke model, two-vessel occlusion model of forebrain ischemia, four-vessel occlusion model of forebrain ischemia, photochemical stroke model, collagenase induced brain haemorrhage model, autologous whole blood induced haemorrhage model. This review provides contemplative facts to setup authentic and relevant animal models to study cerebral reperfusion injury.

Keywords: Ischemia, Reperfusion injury, In vivo models, Stroke

1. Introduction

The cerebrovascular system refers to the transport of blood to and from the brain. Ischemia is a condition initiated with reduced blood flow to the brain regions affecting its normal function. Reperfusion injury, also called Ischemic reperfusion injury, is defined as illogical damage to cells post-restoration of blood flow to ischemic cells.

Cerebrovascular disorders (CVD) comprise a group of signs, symptoms, and damage mechanisms in the brain tissue cells. The damage is associated with various blood supply abnormalities that include haemorrhage, blockage or malformation that prevent brain cells from receiving enough blood supply leading to cerebrovascular disorder. CVD has a transient ischemic attack, aneurysm, stroke and vascular malformation [1]. CVD manifests as acute accidents (commonly known as stroke), which may be either ischemic or haemorrhagic, where the outcome ranges from complete recovery to immediate death.

Cerebral reperfusion injury is a condition where ischemia is worsened but protects the brain tissue after reperfusion. Thrombolysis and embolectomy are considered important contributors to reperfusion injury. Thus, understanding reperfusion injury is essential to know possible diagnosis and treatment of stroke [2].

Cerebrovascular disease (CVD) or stroke are leading causes of morbidity and mortality in humans. In 2001 it was estimated that approximately around 5.5 million deaths were due to stroke [3]. In Europe, about 1 million deaths were due to stroke in the year 2015 [4]. Studies suggest that stroke is the fifth major cause of death in the USA [5]. Certain studies reveal that 15 million people are affected by stroke every year; about 6 million have died. Throughout the western world, stroke is a cause of death of 10 to 12% of its population [6]. Reports conclude that CVD people are about 13–33 people per one lac population in India [7]. Stroke is associated with risk factors such as sex, age, lifestyle, smoking, alcohol, diet and physiological characteristics such as fibrinogen, serum cholesterol and high blood pressure [8]. Research has revealed that high blood pressure is the most critical risk factor contributing to 50% of ischemic stroke [9]. The use of tobacco increases the risk of hemorrhagic stroke by two-fold [10].

Treatment of stroke is mainly focused on improving blood supply, decreasing the severity of brain tissue injuries. Few clinical studies have revealed that reperfusion after thrombolysis has improved clinical outcome in few patients with stroke. Still, in a few patients, reperfusion has worsened the condition by causing fatal edema and intracranial haemorrhage following thrombolysis [2]. Cerebrovascular disease is an age-linked disease with severe vascular complications and comorbidities. Therefore there is an urgency to develop different therapeutic approaches to treat the disease. Thus, researchers could focus on Animal models which reproduce similar pathophysiological condition of human stroke. These animal models support emerging new strategies for stroke treatment in humans. This chapter explains in detail different rodents models for cerebral ischemia along with their advantages and disadvantages.

2. Rodent models of cerebral ischemia

MCAO [intra-arterial suture occlusion of the middle cerebral artery (MCA)]: This model is the most widely accepted and has several advantages in mimicking the human stroke. MCAO was first used by Kozuimi et al. [11] and was further revised using a silicone-coated suture technique to control the premature reperfusion subarachnoid haemorrhage [12, 13]. MCAO technique starts with transecting the external carotid artery and temporarily closing the common carotid artery using the thread knot. The suture is passed into an internal carotid artery to the middle and anterior cerebral arteries' junction through the external carotid artery trunk. The suture is left at the junction for a stipulated time and then removed to produce reperfusion. The typical duration of suture occlusion of the MCA in the rat would be 60 min, 90 min, 120 min and permanent occlusion. In this technique, craniotomy is not required, and it produces occlusion of the cerebral artery similar to that seen in the human stroke. MCAO technique will reduce the cerebral blood flow bilaterally and produce around 12% subarachnoid haemorrhage even after using coated suture [14, 15]. Transection of the external carotid artery affects the function of muscles of mastication that produces difficulty in swallowing. This technique is also associated with inadequate behavioural performance outcome measures [16].

MCAO produces ischemic cell death in the frontal, parietal, temporal, occipital cortex and variable damage in the substantia nigra, cervicomedullary junction, hypothalamus and thalamus [17–19]. Damage to diverse brain region will produce complex sensory, motor, autonomic and cognitive deficits. In suture occlusion of 60 min or more, it will impact the hypothalamus significantly [17, 20].

Hypothalamic ischemia produces a hypothermic response in rats that exist for at least 24 hrs after the animal's recovery. Hypothermia worsens cell death, which confirms that temperature fluctuations have to be considered the primary reason for ischemic cell death in MCAO [19–21]. In MCAO, the cell death pattern follows with the formation of early infarct in the striatum and the formation of delayed infarct in the dorsolateral cortex in the striatum. Striatum infarcts are necrotic and are highly resistant to neuroprotective agents [22–27]. Cortical infarct formation takes a longer duration to show a high level of programmed cell death when compared to striatal infarction [16, 22, 28, 29].

In MCAO, with reperfusion, the striatum will be remained as the core of the ischemic, whereas the cortex region returns to normal blood flow levels [30]. In MCAO, the striatal infarction is the core region of ischemia and cortical infarction where delayed and progressive cell death occurs. The progressive cell death in the region cortex is due to the delayed release of inflammatory mediator TNF-α (Tumor necrosis factor-α), interleukins-1, neutrophil invasion, cytokines release, COX-2 (Cyclooxygenase) activation and oxidative cell injury [31].

Merits of MCAO:

- The delayed process of cell death in the region of the cortex is very close to human stroke.
- This model helps in finding targets such as oxidative injury and inflammatory mediators for studying neuroprotective activities [32, 33].
- Highly reproducible [34].
- Assessing the lesions formed by observing histopathological changes [34].
- To know the Cerebral blood flow pattern during ischemia by comparing histopathological modifications [35].
- The mortality rate of animals is low as animals survive a few weeks after surgery [36].
- As the mortality rate of animals is sufficient low, data would be available to conduct statistical analysis and investigate the changes after focal cerebral ischemia [36].

Demerits of MCAO: [37].

- Visual confirmation of MCAO cannot be achieved in this model.
- Filament dimensions majorly affect reproducibility.
- The use of a specific type of filaments increases the risk of bleeding.
- Few cases of mortality may be observed with large strokes of more than 24 h.
- Thrombolytic agents cannot be investigated.

3. Research envisaged using the MCAO model in rats

Michael Chopp et al., in their study, found that administration of anti-Mac-1(Macrophage-1) antibody after one hour of focal cerebral ischemia induced by MCAO inhibits lesion volume, post-ischemic weight loss and hinders the movement of leukocyte adhesion molecules into the cortical ischemic region. These studies support the hypothesis that leukocyte adhesion molecules' involvement in ischemic brain damage, and these molecules' blockings would be a new therapeutic approach in treating ischemic brain cell damage [38].

James.W. Simpkins et al., found that administration of oestrogens in ovariectomized female rats before or after MCAO has significantly altered the mortality rate, which was accompanied by a decrease in the ischemic region of the brain. Thus, these results confirm the use of oestrogens as a neuroprotective agent in stroke [39].

Meenakshi ST and SS. Sharma, in their study, found that administration of Curcumin significantly produced neuroprotection in MCAO induced cerebral ischemia. Administration of curcumin inhibited lipid peroxidation, decrease in peroxynitrite production and activation of the antioxidant defence system. The antioxidant potential of curcumin may be attributed to its neuroprotection in MCAO induced focal cerebral ischemia [40].

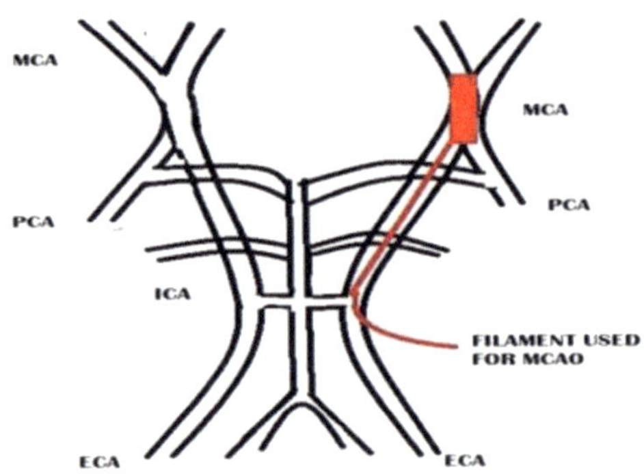

Figure 1.
MCAO method.

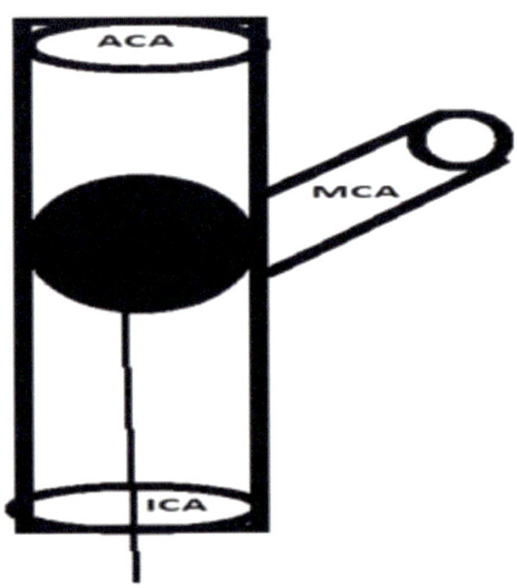

Figure 2.
MCAO.

Kurozumi K et al., in their studies, reported that the use of mesenchymal stem cells improved functional deficits in MCAO induced stroke model. This activity was due to the secretion of cytokines by mesenchymal stem cells. These studies confirmed the role of mesenchymal stem cells transfected along with brain-derived neurotrophic factor (BDNF) gene or glial cell line-derived neurotrophic factor (GDNF) gene resulted in improving functional abnormalities and decreasing ischemic brain cell damage. Studies reveal that gene-modified cell therapy is a new therapeutic approach to treating ischemic stroke [41] (**Figures 1–5**).

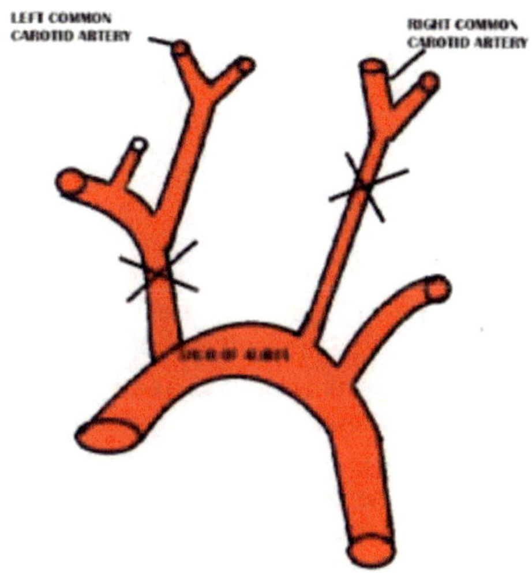

Figure 3.
Two vessel occlusion model.

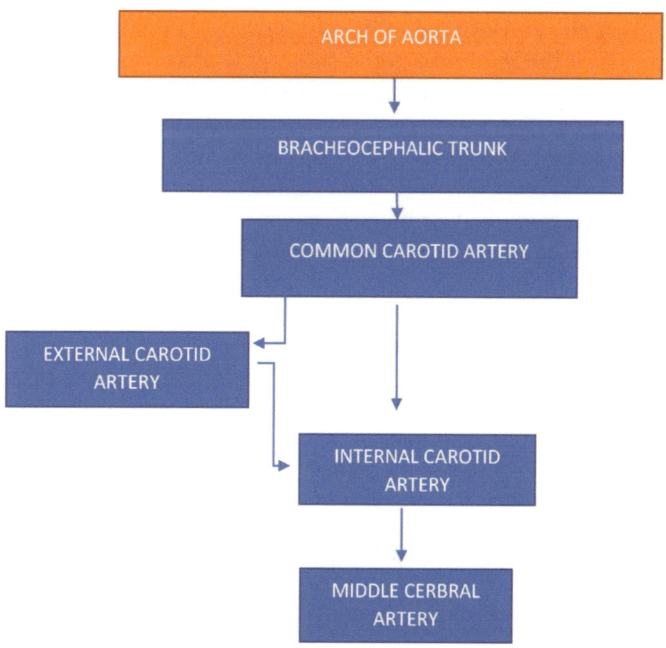

Figure 4.
Schematic diagram of blood vessels.

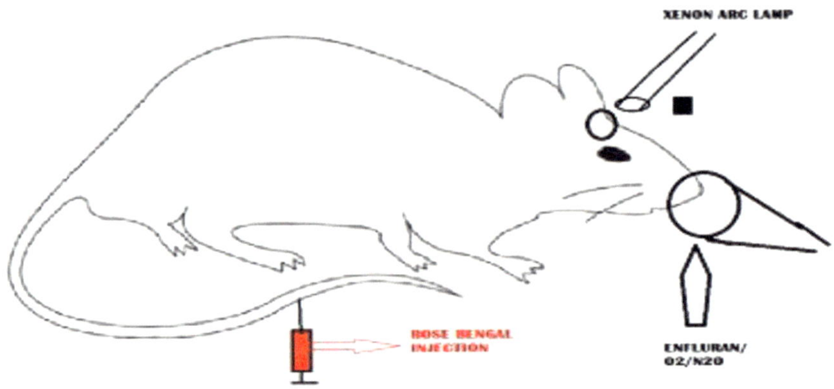

Figure 5.
Photochemical model.

4. Embolic stroke model

This model is widely accepted as clots can be positioned precisely mimicking cerebrovascular clots of humans. Rodents will be anaesthetized using subcutaneous injection of a combination of fentanyl (1 mg/kg) and fluanison (3 mg/kg) followed by subcutaneous injection of atropine(0.015 mg) and intraperitoneal injection of diazepam (2.5 mg/kg). If necessary, continue the anaesthesia with one-third of the initial dose of fentanyl and fluanison. The right femoral artery needs to be catheterized with a polyethene tube to continuously monitor the blood pressure and collect blood samples for estimating blood gases and glucose level. The right femoral vein has to be catheterized for the administration of a drug. Throughout the surgical procedure and for the first 30 min after reversal of the animals' anaesthesia body temperature, it needs to be maintained at 37°C by using a heating lamp connected to a temperature probe in the rectum [42].

Preparation of the emboli: A 1 ml insulin syringe has to be filled with thrombin 60 U/ml saline. Once the femoral arterial catheter was fixed required amount of blood need to be drawn in another insulin syringe; within 20 s, syringes should be connected using a polyethene tube, and the suspension containing thrombin solution and blood in a mixture of 1:4 was moved 70 times from one syringe to the other for 3 min. The syringes should then be left in a standing position with closed compartments for 30 min until embolization.

Carotid operation procedure: The right external carotid artery (ECA) and its branches thyroid, occipital, pterygopalatine arteries need to be exposed and ligated. The catheter has to be inserted into the bifurcation and fixed with ligatures. Throughout the procedure, disturbance to the internal carotid artery's blood flow (ICA) must be avoided to avoid any intima injury. Heparinized saline (5 U/ml) need to be continuously flown in the catheter at a rate of 0.5 ml/h using an infusion pump to avoid clotting.

Merits of embolic stroke model [43]:

- High clinical relevance.
- This procedure does not require craniectomy.
- Large size infarcts can be induced by correctly positioning the clot.
- Infarcts can be induced in the regions of cortical and subcortical regions of the brain.

- It helps in producing neurobehavioural deficits in rodents, similar to that of deficits in humans.

Demerits of emboli stroke model: [44].

- This procedure needs high technical skills as there is a need to place emboli intravascularly.
- Introduction of emboli intravascularly results in multifocal ischemia and produces variable infarct size.
- Brain haemorrhage is commonly observed in this model.
- A high mortality rate is observed in this model compared with other ischemic rodent models.

5. Research envisaged in an embolic stroke model

Martin Andersen, MD et al., studied the effects of the combination of cytidine-59-diphosphocholine (citicoline) and thrombolysis using the embolic stroke model in rodents. Their studies found that the combination of rtPA (Recombinant tissue plasminogen activator) and a low dose of citicoline reduces infarct size in this model. This study also recommends further investigation to check the potential effects of this combination in treating ischemic stroke [45].

Karsten Overgaard et al., studied the effect of delayed thrombolysis with recombinant tissue plasminogen activator in an embolic stroke model. Their study found that infarct volume was significantly reduced by thrombolytic therapy and improved clinical score up to 2 h CAIdelay of treatment. They also found that treatment after 4 hr. may also be beneficial. Thus, delay in treatment may significantly increase the infarct volume and thrombolytic therapy in this model induced recanalization. The most significant advantage of this model was a few hemorrhage complications were seen [46].

D Lekieffre et al., have evaluated the efficacy of eliprodil in combination with the thrombolytic agent, rt-PA, in a rat embolic stroke model. Embolic stroke was induced by intracarotid injection of an arterial blood clot. Their study found that the use of elirodil alone or in combination with a thrombolytic agent reduced the extent of brain damage and neurological deficits in the embolized rat model. This study also confirmed that combined therapy of cytoprotective agent and thrombolytic agent produced effective neuroprotection and would be a new approach to treating stroke in humans [47].

Tomas Sereghy et al., studied the effects of excitatory amino acid receptor antagonist dizocilpine and alteplase and a combination of both in the embolic stroke model. In this model, the carotid artery was embolized using fibrin rich clots. Their research found that treatment with alteplase and dizocilpine reduced infarct volume individually, but combined treatment showed more promising results when compared to individual treatment. Combination treatment significantly reduced neuropathological changes after embolic stroke, and this combination would be a new therapeutic approach in humans for deep brain infarcts [48].

Rasmussen RS et al., studied the effects of D -amphetamine (D -amph) and physical therapy separately and combined on gross motor performance, cognition and acceptable motor performance using the embolic model in rats. Their studies found no significant change in infarct volume, and no significant changes were seen in the gross performance. These results conclude that D -amphetamine (D -amph) improved cognitive functions, and physical therapy improved motor coordination in the embolic stroke model [49].

6. Global cerebral ischemia model

6.1 Two-vessel occlusion model of forebrain ischemia

This model is accepted widely as it mainly focuses on the extent of damage after ischemic stroke and helps understand recovery duration in animals that mimics the common condition in humans. In this model, reversible forebrain ischemia will be produced by occluding the common carotid artery and inducing hypotension to decrease blood flow to the forebrain region. Blood pressure should be reduced to 50 mm Hg by using a specific device [50]. Treatment with phentolamine or trimethaphan can help produce hypotension [51]. Cerebral blood flow (CBF) measured after 15 min shows a reduced flow to the cerebral cortex region, caudoputamen, hippocampus, midbrain, thalamus, and globus pallidus. However, there are variable differences in the CBF in the ischemic region. The two-vessel occlusion model helps understand changes in the selective structures like pyramidal neurons of the hippocampus, neocortex and caudoputamen.

Histopathological reports from studies confirm that the two-vessel occlusion model is associated with neuronal injury to hippocampal pyramidal cells within 2 min. In contrast, injury to caudoputamen happens with 8 min of ischemia and injury to the neocortex takes place in 4 min of ischemia [52]. The two-vessel occlusion model helps study energy metabolism in ischemia, neurotransmitter metabolism, phospholipids, histopathology and effects of cerebral hypothermia [53]. This model will help achieve a good outcome when the blood pressure is regulated correctly at a level of 50 mm Hg without any fluctuations. The two-vessel model has many advantages like producing efficient forebrain ischemia, ease of cerebral recirculation, low experiment failure rate. The disadvantages of two-vessel occlusion are the use of anaesthesia and hypotension induction; these can affect the resulting outcome. In this model, behavioural changes cannot be assessed immediately after occlusion.

Merits of the two-vessel occlusion model

- It helps in studying long term recovery studies as it reverses the condition of ischemia [54].
- It is highly reproducible as it produces more than 90% of ischemic damage that almost mimics ischemic stroke in humans [55].
- Produces consistent brain injury in the regions such as CA1 (Hippocampal Cornu Ammonis)) the region, caudate putamen, hippocampus and the region of the neocortex locations in rats.
- Biochemical and physiological changes can be studied.
- Potential neuroprotective agents can be easily assessed using this model.

Demerits of the two-vessel occlusion model: [55].

- The time frame would be around 10 min beyond which permanent brain damage occurs.
- The high mortality rate.
- Animals would die after 15 min of completion of the experiment.
- Experimental animals develop post-ischemic seizures, the reason for the death of animals.

7. Research envisaged in the two-vessel occlusion model

Máté Marosi et al., have studied oxaloacetate's effect on impaired longterm potentiation induced using a two-vessel occlusion ischemic model in rats. Administration of oxaloacetic acid within 30 min of reperfusion effectively prevented long-term potentiation impairment caused by ischemia. This effect of oxaloacetic acid is because of its blood glutamate scavenging property. Oxaloacetic acid also effectively improves neurological condition after ischemic induced mitochondrial dysfunction [56].

Douglas E. McBean et al. studied the neuroprotective effect of lifarizine using to modified two-vessel occlusion model in rats. Their studies concluded that treatment with lifarizine, a derivative of diphenyl piperazine has effectively produced neuroprotection in a global ischemic rat model. Lifarizine selectively blocks the inactivated sodium channels and decrease the overactivity of the ischemic neuron [57].

Dachun Zhou et al. studied the effect of 2-methoxyestradiol, a HIF-1α inhibitor, by global cerebral ischemia in rats using a two-vessel occlusion model. Hypoxia-inducible factor-1α (HIF-1α) is reported to be protective in focal ischemia. 2-methoxyestradiol, a natural metabolite obtained from oestrogen and inhibitor of HIF-1α found, was tested for its potential use in global ischemia. The studies concluded that 2-methoxyestradiol did significantly inhibit the levels of Hypoxia-inducible factor-1α but did not produce positive results in the treatment but rather worsened the condition [58].

Orsu Prabhakar et al. studied the protective effect of naringin against cerebral infarction induced by ischemic- reperfusion in rats using the two-vessel occlusion model. The study found that increased inflammatory mediators and infiltrating leukocytes play an essential role in the cerebral ischemic-reperfusion injury. Treatment with naringin significantly reduced the infiltrating leukocytes, inflammatory mediators like MPO (Myeloperoxidase), TNF-α (Tumor necrosis factor-α), and IL-6 (Interleukins) and increased anti-inflammatory mediator IL-10 (Interleukins) [59].

Orsu Prabhakar et al. studied the cerebroprotective role of resveratrol through antioxidant and anti-inflammatory effects in diabetic rats. In their study, they found that resveratrol reduced inflammatory mediators and oxidative stress markers like MPO (Myeloperoxidase), TNF-α (Tumor necrosis factor-α) and IL-6 (Interleukins) malondialdehyde and increased levels of anti-inflammatory and antioxidants parameters like IL-10 (Interleukins), superoxide dismutase and catalase [60]. This model is widely accepted as it helps understand the behavioural changes post-ischemic stroke and mimics humans' condition during a stroke. The four-vessel occlusion method is followed in two stages. In the first stage, rats are anaesthetized, and the arterial clasp is fixed around each common carotid artery and exteriorized by an incision through the ventral midline of the neck [61]. A dorsal incision will identify the alar foramina of the first cervical vertebrae. An electrocautery needle is passed through foramina to electro coagulate vertebral arteries [62]. In the recent studies, slight technical modification is recommended that the rat head should be held with stereotactic ear bar and tilted by 30 ° to the horizontal, and the spine should be extended by applying tension on the rats tail so that the alar foramina be brought to the plane and helps in improving visualization. In the second stage, forebrain ischemia is produced after 24 hours of the first stage by tightening the carotid clasps for a moment and later, these clasps are removed for reperfusion.

Studies confirm seizures in animals after 30 min of ischemia. Reports have also confirmed that two-third of animals fail to survive after the first procedure and die within 2–3 min because of respiratory failure [63]. Laboratories have reported variability among different strains of rats show different grades of ischemic effect. Sprague- Dawley rats show respiratory failure; around 50–60% of animals exhibit coma that helps us understand the extent of the strain's ischemic impact. Whereas, in Wistar rats, animals suffer respiratory failure after the first stage of the procedure, and around two-thirds of them die during the first and second stages. This model is used in anaesthetized to investigate morphological and metabolic changes. Histopathological studies also confirm that 10–20 min of ischemia would be sufficient to produce ischemic cell changes in hemispheres and hippocampus regions. The four-vessel occlusion model does not significantly change the neocortical area, even with 30 min of ischemia. Behavioural changes observed in this model confirm that there would be permanent damage to rats' memory, reflecting the hippocampal injury [64]. Though widely used four-vessel occlusion model produces incomplete forebrain ischemia. Its main advantage is that his model can be done both in awake and anaesthetized animals, whereas this model has several limitations in obtaining satisfactory results.

Merits of the four-vessel occlusion model

- Low incidence of seizures.
- An easy surgical procedure to induce occlusion in rodents.
- Minimal use of anaesthesia.
- The regions of the brain targeted are the striatum, the paramedian, hippocampal and posterior neocortex [62].

Demerits of four-vessel occlusion model

- The cell death mechanism involved in the four-vessel occlusion model is not clearly known. It may be due to necrosis or apoptosis.
- Induction in Wistar rats is not possible.
- The mortality rate is high in this model [64].
- Original methodology did not involve the use of anaesthesia, but recent modifications have started using anaesthesia.
- Ischemia cannot be confirmed by precise observation.

8. Research envisaged using the four-vessel occlusion model

Ruchan ergun et al. studied the effect of propofol 2,6-diisopropylphenol following global cerebral ischemia–reperfusion injury using the four-vessel occlusion method. In the present study, malondialdehyde was considered an important marker to estimate lipid peroxidation in ischemic tissue. The reviews concluded that propofol potentially inhibited neuronal death caused by four-vessel occlusion method-induced brain ischemia [65].

Levente Gellert et al. studied the effect of kynurenic acid in global forebrain ischemia insult buy evaluating the loss of CA1 (Hippocampal Cornu Ammonis) hippocampal neurons and long-term potentiation at Schaffer collateral- CA1 (Hippocampal Cornu Ammonis) synapses. The studies showed that kynurenic acid significantly prevented CA1 CA1 (Hippocampal Cornu Ammonis) hippocampal neuronal loss and preserved long-term potentiation expression. The main advantage of using kynurenic acid is that it was effective when used as pre-treatment and during reperfusion [66].

Hui Li et al. studied the Effect of Dehydroepiandrosterone in an animal model of transient severe forebrain ischemia. In this model, forebrain ischemia was induced by a modified four-vessel occlusion model where the occlusion was conducted for 10 min. The studies confirmed that treatment with Dehydroepiandrosterone protected hippocampal CA1 (Hippocampal Cornu Ammonis) area from injury and suggested that NMDA(N-methyl-D-aspartate) may not be the main contributor for hippocampal CA1 (Hippocampal Cornu Ammonis)neuronal cell injury [67].

D shivaraman et al., studied the effect of hemidesmus indicus on cerebral infarct ischemia–reperfusion injury by four-vessel occlusion method. The studies found that hemidesmus indicus significantly improved that neuromuscular, vestibulo-motor, motor action, and decreased lipid peroxidation. Treatment also restored levels of dopamine and serotonin. The above results, it confirmed that hemisesmus indicus produced a neuroprotective effect in ischemic induced brain damage [68].

9. Photochemical stroke model

This model is widely accepted as it helps understand the extent of damage to the brain region by measuring the size of infarcts, which could help estimate human stroke. In this model, rats weighing around 350 g will be selected and anaesthetized using 3% halothane and are maintained with 1.5–2% halothane, 70% nitrous oxide and oxygen. The scalp covering the left hemisphere will be exposed, and the focal infarct would be introduced in rats using the photochemical method. The photosensitizing dye rose bengal (1 mg in 0.133 ml of saline per 100 g body wt) will be injected intravenously, and the rat will be restrained using the stereotactic frame. Light emerging from xenon arc lamp at 560 nm will be focused on to the skull. The light would be focused for a period of 120 sec, and the intensity of light used will be 0.58 W/cm^2. Light penetrating the brain interacts with intravascular photosensitive dye, resulting in oxygen free radicals highly reactive within the blood vessels. These free radicals cause injury to the endothelial cells and initiate the process of platelet aggregation. Once the procedure is completed, animals would be placed back into cages. After 7 days, animals were sacrificed for histopathological evaluation and measuring infarct size. This model is mainly used to study regional cerebral blood flow and to measure infarct size [69].

Merits of focal thrombotic stroke model:

- Helps in developing injury in the regions of the cortical and subcortical region.
- Highly reproducible with minimal surgical procedure.
- Produces cortical lesion that is visible after dissection of cortex region.

- The lesions formed in superficial and deep cortical areas allow easy photoactivation of rose Bengal.
- Easy measurement of cerebral infarcts.
- Histopathological staining with triphenyl-tetrazolium chloride (TTC) or cresyl violet helps measure the infarct size.
- TTC stains regular tissue red and infarcted tissue as a pale colour that accurately measures infarct size [70].

Demerits of focal thrombotic stroke:

- The pattern of stroke slightly differs from a human stroke.
- Some regions of the brain which receive blood by collateral arteries are less affected, and those regions show less death of neuronal cells because of ischemia.
- The pattern of infarction also slightly varies from that of human stroke.
- Formation of vasogenic edema along with ischemic infarction.
- Antithrombotic agents cannot be studied as photothrombotic infarct formation will take place even after blocking platelets [70].

10. Research envisaged using focal thrombotic stroke

Marc De Ryck et al., studies Effect of Flunarizine on Sensorimotor deficits after neocortical infarcts in Rats. After the successful induction of infarcts, rats showed deficits in the proprioceptive placing of hind limbs. Treatment with flunarizine after infarction restored sensorimotor functions in rats [71].

Jens Minnerup et al.studied the effect of intracarotid administration of human bone marrow cells in rats using a photothrombotic ischemia stroke model. Researchers confirmed no significant changes in neurological deficits with human bone marrow cells' treatment after 3 days of stroke induction. This failed neurological activity may be due to a delay in the initiation of treatment as human bone marrow cells have shown significant activity in other stroke models [72].

M De Ryck et al., have studied the lubeluzole's effect on sensorimotor function and infarct size using a photothrombotic stroke model in rats. After successful induction of stroke, it was found that functional deficits like tactile and proprioceptive hindlimb placing and infarcts were observed in the region parietal neocortex region of the brain. Treatment with lubeluzole after 5 min of post-infarct significantly restored all the functional deficits induced by photothrombotic stroke, but the effect seems to be declining with delaying in the initiation of treatment [73].

Boru hou et al.studied the effect of exogenous Neural Stem Cells (NSC) transplantation in Photothrombotic ischemia stroke in mice. After the successful induction of stroke, animals treated with NSC restored all brain functions; this was evident with their performance. Histopathological studies also confirmed that treatment with NSC showed a decline in brain cell damage caused by an ischemic stroke. Immunofluorescent assay for biomarkers revealed NSC's role as they differentiated into neurons and astrocytes to restore brain function [74].

11. Collagenase induced brain hemorrhage model

This method is widely used in understanding the extent of hemorrhage in the brain and mimics the condition of human stroke. In this model, Sprague–Dawley rats are used. Animals will be anaesthetized using 50 mg/kg of pentobarbitol. Once the animals are anaesthetized, they are placed in stereotactic equipment, and a 23-gauge needle will be used to implant the caudate nucleus. Rats will be infused with 2 μl of saline containing (Type VII or Type XI collagenase) for 9 min. After completing the infusion process, the needle is removed, and the wound would be sutured. Rats will be allowed for recovery than will be sacrificed using an intracardiac injection of KCl (Potassium chloride). Brains of the rats will be removed and kept in phosphate-buffered formalin for 24 hours. Later, brains will be sliced, and histopathological changes will be studied [75].

Merits of Collagenase induced brain haemorrhage model [76].

- Highly reproducible for induction of brain haemorrhage.
- Hematoma formation is observed after 10 min of administration of collagenase.
- The brain regions targeted are the lateral striatum, medial striatum and corpus callosum.
- Significant neurological deficits are observed.
- Significant neuronal loss in the region of striatum among all other models of ICH (Intracerebral Hemorrhage).
- Significant reduction in the volume of the corpus callosum.
- The volume of tissue lost increases from 1 to 4 weeks.

Demerits of Collagenase induced brain hemorrhage model [76].

- A high mortality rate is observed with the usage of higher doses of collagenase.
- Hematoma volume found to be low when compared with other ICH (Intracerebral Hemorrhage) models.
- Disruption of the blood–brain barrier was observed in this model.

12. Research envisaged using collagenase induced brain hemorrhage model

N. Kawai et al. studied the effect of recombinant factor VIIa in a collagenase-induced intracerebral hemorrhage model in rats. Early hematoma is the sign associated with neurological deterioration after intracerebral hemorrhage. Two hours after collagenase injection, there was blood accumulation in the striatum region and slowly extended to the thalamus region by 24 h. Thus, administration of recombinant factor VIIa immediately after collagenase injection would help in reducing the average hematoma volume and frequency of hematoma formation [77].

Arne Lauer et al., conducted a comparative study among direct thrombin inhibitor dabigatran etexilate (DE) over anticoagulant warfarin using collagenase induced Intracerebral Hemorrhage. The results found that intracerebral bleeding was severe during warfarin treatment and experimental data also confirms this as severe hematoma expansion. Treatment with dabigatran etexilate did not exaggerate the ongoing process of intracerebral bleeding neither increased hematoma growth. From the above results, we can confirm that cerebral hemorrhage occurring during DE treatment is minimal and harmless compared to warfarin [78].

P.P lema et al., have studied the dexamethasone's effect for treatment of intracerebral hemorrhage using a collagenase-induced intracerebral hematoma model in rats. After the successful induction of intracerebral hemorrhage, animals were evaluated for their neurological evaluation, followed by measurement of hematoma volume and necrotic tissue. Studies revealed that treatment with dexamethasone restored functional deficits, reduced hematoma volume, decreased filtration of neutrophils and astrocytes into hematoma and found to potentially active in the treatment of intracerebral hemorrhage [79].

Marc R. Del Bigio et al., have studied the effect of fucoidan on Collagenase induced intracerebral hemorrhage in rats. After the successful induction of intracerebral hemorrhage, animals were assessed for motor activity and forelimb functioning after six weeks and followed by hematoma evaluation. Animals treated with fucoidan for seven days successfully restored motor and cognitive activity but failed to prevent excess hematoma formation [80].

13. Autologous whole blood induced hemorrhage model

This model is widely used to understand hemorrhagic stroke and mimic a condition similar to that in humans. This model animal will be anaesthetized using an intraperitoneal injection of pentobarbital (50 mg/kg). The animal will be placed on the stereotactic frame, and under aseptic condition, a scalp incision will be made. Further, a hole will be drilled 0.02 mm anterior to the coronal suture and 3 mm lateral to the midline. A 25-gauge needle will be introduced into the cerebral cortex region on the surface of the skull. The rat will receive 50 -μl of autologous whole bold for 5 min. After completing the infusion process, the needle will be kept at the same place for 3 min and later removed. The hole drilled in the skull will be closed using bone wax, and the scalp wound would be sutured [81].

Merits of autologous whole blood induced hemorrhage model [76].

- High reproducibility.
- Hematoma volume found to be higher.
- The brain regions damaged are the medial striatum and corpus callosum.
- Significant reduction in the volume of the corpus callosum.
- The blood–brain barrier is not much affected.
- Neurological deficits can be observed.

Demerits of autologous whole blood induced hemorrhage model [76].

1. No significant neuronal loss found in the regions of the striatum.

2. No significant increase in the volume of tissue lost from 1 to 4 weeks.

3. Quick recovery of animals from neurological deficits.

14. Research envisaged using autologous whole blood induced haemorrhage model

Takehiro Nakamura, MD et al., have studied the effect of Deferoxamine an iron chelator, on brain edema and neurological deficits induced by autologous whole blood intracerebral haemorrhage model in rats. The effect of Deferoxamine was assessed by measuring edema formation in the brain, and neurological deficits were studies using functional tests. 8-hydroxyl-2-deoxyguanosine (8-OHdG), a marker to check the oxidative DNA damage, was estimated using immunohistochemical analysis followed by a western blot test to estimate the amount of redox effector factor–1 and apurinic/apyrimidinic endonuclease (Ref-1/APE) to assess DNA oxidative damage. Treatment

Model	The affected region of the brain	Mortality rate	Significance	Key limitation
MCAo (intra-arterial suture occlusion of the middle cerebral artery)	Cortex	+	Formation of cerebral edema which resembles a human stroke	Dimensions of filament affect final results
Emboli Stroke Model	Cortical and subcortical regions of the brain	+++	Neurobehavioral deficits are similar to that of humans	Brain hemorrhage
Two vessel occlusion model	CA1 (Hippocampal Cornu Ammonis) region, caudate-putamen, hippocampus, and the region of neocortex	++	Useful in studying long term recovery studies	Postischemic seizures
Four-Vessel Occlusion Model	The striatum, paramedian, hippocampal, and posterior neocortex	+++	Neuronal damage produced is similar to that in humans	The cell death mechanism is still unclear whether it is necrosis or apoptosis
Focal thrombotic stroke model	cortical and subcortical regions.	+	Easy measurement of cerebral infracts	Formation of vasogenic edema
Collagenase induced brain hemorrhage model	lateral striatum, medial striatum and corpus callosum.	+++	Assess long term functional outcomes.	Neurotoxicity of collagenase
Autologous whole blood induced hemorrhage model	Medial striatum and corpus callosum	+++	Produces consistent hemorrhage volume	Evaluation of microvascular breakdown cannot be done.

Mortality rate: "+" Low, "++" Medium, "+++" High.

Table 1.
Comparision between invivo cerebral ischemic models.

with deferoxamine inherited brain edema formation, restored all neurological deficits, and prevented intracerebral haemorrhage-induced changes in 8-OHdG and Ref-1/APE. The results confirmed that deferoxamine might have potential use in decreasing oxidative stress caused by hematoma [82].

Takehiro Nakamura MD has studied the effect of nafamostat mesylate (FUT), a serine protease inhibitor, on brain injury and edema formation using intracerebral haemorrhage model rats. FUT was injected intraperitoneally after 6 hr. of intracerebral haemorrhage. Treatment with FUT reduced brain water content in the basal ganglia region and inhibited 8-hydroxyl-2-deoxyguanosine changes; thus, FUT would be a potential component to treat intracerebral haemorrhage [83].

Takehiro Nakamura, MD et al., have studied the effect of edaravone on brain edema and neurologic deficits using the Intracerebral haemorrhage model in rats. The model was adapted to measure edema size and neurological deficits, and oxidative markers to estimate brain injury. Treatment with edaravone after 2 hr. of ICH (Intracerebral Hemorrhage) successfully ameliorated the formation of brain edema and reduced impact on neurological activity. It also inhibited ICH (Intracerebral Hemorrhage) induced changes in oxidative biomarkers and prevented an oxidative injury. These results recommend Edaravone as an active component in treating ICH (Intracerebral Hemorrhage) [84].

T. Nakamura et al., have studied the effects of endogenous and exogenous estrogen on intracerebral haemorrhage ICH (Intracerebral Hemorrhage) induced brain damage in male and female rats. In the study impact of delayed administration of estradiol on ICH (Intracerebral Hemorrhage) induced brain injury was examined along with dependence on the estrogen receptor. The effect of estradiol on neuronal deficits and brain edema was estimated 24 h after ICH (Intracerebral Hemorrhage) induction. Formation of brain edema was evident in male rats when compared with that of female rats. Estrogen receptor activation takes place in a female after ICH (Intracerebral Hemorrhage). After 2 hr. of ICH (Intracerebral Hemorrhage), estradiol administration to male rats restored neurological deficits, reduced edema formation, and increased Heme oxygenase-1. Treatment with estradiol in male rats was adequate compared to female rats and could be accepted as a potential component in ICH treatment (Intracerebral Hemorrhage) (**Table 1**) [85].

15. Conclusion

In vivo experimental model are used widely to understand the underlying physiology involved in different types of human stroke. The pattern of ischemic injury involved would vary in each model. The pathophysiological changes in rodents post-ischemic injury can be compared to that of injury pattern in human stroke. There are several other stroke models, but we have explained the most commonly used methods in this chapter. Based on the investigator's interest, a suitable model can be used to study different types of ischemic strokes.

Author details

Prabhakar Orsu* and Y. Srihari
GITAM Institute of Pharmacy, GITAM Deemed to be University,
Visakhapatnam, India

*Address all correspondence to: orsuprabhakar@gmail.com

References

[1] Lin L, Wang X, Yu Z. Ischemia-reperfusion injury in the brain: mechanisms and potential therapeutic strategies. Biochemistry & pharmacology: open access. 2016;5(4).

[2] Pan J, Konstas AA, Bateman B, Ortolano GA, Pile-Spellman J. Reperfusion injury following cerebral ischemia: pathophysiology, MR imaging, and potential therapies. Neuroradiology. 2007 Feb 1;49(2):93-102.

[3] World Health Organization. The World Health Report: 2002: Reducing risks, promoting healthy life. 2002. World Health Organization.

[4] Townsend N, NICH (Intracerebral hemorrhage)ols M, Scarborough P, et al. Cardiovascular disease in Europe--epidemiological update 2015. Eur Heart J 2015;36:2696-705.

[5] Mozaffarian D, Benjamin EJ, Go AS, et al., American Heart Association Statistics Committee and Stroke Statistics Subcommittee. Heart disease and stroke statistics – 2015 update a report from the American Heart Association. Circulation. 2015;131(4):e29–e322.

[6] Toyoda K, Ninomiya T. Stroke and cerebrovascular diseases in patients with chronic kidney disease. *Lancet Neurol*. 2014;13(8):823-833. doi:10.1016/S1474-4422(14)70026-2

[7] Banerjee AK. CEREBROVASCULAR DISEASES IN INDIA—A PATHOLOGISTS VIEWPOINT. Medical journal, Armed Forces India. 1996 Apr;52(2):116

[8] Marmot MG and Poulter NR. Primary prevention of stroke. Lancet 339, 344-347. 1992.

[9] Dunbabin DW and Sandercock P. Preventing stroke by the modification of risk factors. Stroke 21;suppl IV, 36-39. 1990

[10] Shinton R and Beevers G. Meta-analysis of relation between cigarette smoking and stroke. BMJ 298, 789-795. 1989.

[11] Koizumi J, Yoshida Y, Nakazawa T, Ooneda G. Experimental studies of ischemic brain edema. I. A new experimental model of cerebral embolism in whICH (Intracerebral hemorrhage) recirculation can introduced into the ischemic area. Jpn J Stroke 8:108, 1986.

[12] Belayev L, Alonso OF, Busto R, Zhao W, Ginsberg MD. Middle cerebral artery occlusion in the rat by intraluminal suture. Neurological and pathological evaluation of an improved model. Stroke 27:1616-622, 1996.

[13] Schmid-Elsaesser R, Zausinger S, Hungerhuber E, Baethmann A, Reulen HJ. A critical reevaluation of the intraluminal thread model of focal cerebral ischemia: evidence of inadvertent premature reperfusion and subarachnoid hemorrhage in rats by laser doppler flowmetry. Stroke 29:2162-2170, 1998.

[14] Chen TY, Goyagi T, Toung TJ, Kirsch JR, Hurn PD, Koehler RC, et al. Prolonged opportunity for ischemic neuroprotection with selective -opioid receptor agonist in rats. Stroke 35:1180-1185, 2004.

[15] Dittmar M, Spruss T, Schuierer G, Horn M. External carotid artery territory ischemia impairs outcome in the endovascular filament model of middle cerebral artery occlusion in rats. Stroke 34:2252-2257, 2003.

[16] Garcia JH, Liu KF, Ho KL. Neuronal necrosis after middle cerebral artery occlusion in Wistar rats progresses at

different time intervals in the caudoputamen and the cortex. Stroke 26:636– 642, 1995.

[17] Kanemitsu H, Nakagomi T, Tamura A, Tsuchiya T, Kono G, Sano K. Differences in the extent of primary ischemic damage between middle cerebral artery coagulation and intraluminal occlusion models. J Cereb Blood Flow Metab 22:1196-1204, 2002.

[18] Williams AJ, Berti R, Dave JR, Elliot PJ, Adams J, Tortella FC. Delayed treatment of ischemia/reperfusion brain injury: extended therapeutic window with the proteosome inhibitor MLN519. Stroke 35:1186-1191, 2004.

[19] Li F, Omae T, Fisher M. Spontaneous hyperthermia and its mechanism in the intraluminal suture middle cerebral artery occlusion model of the rat. Stroke 30:2464-2471, 1999.

[20] Yamashita K, Busch E, Wiessner C, Hossmann KA. Thread occlusion but not electrocoagulation of the middle cerebral artery causes hypothalamic damage with subsequent hyperthermia. Neurol Med Chir (Tokyo) 37:723-727, 1997.

[21] Reglodi D, Somogyvari-Vigh A, Maderdrut JL, Vigh S, Arimura A. Postischemic spontaneous hyperthermia and its effects in middle cerebral artery occlusion in the rat. Exp Neurol 163:399-407, 2000.

[22] Li Y, Chopp M, Jiang N, Zhang ZG, Zaloga C. Induction of DNA fragmentation after 10 to 120 minutes of focal cerebral ischemia in rats. Stroke 26:1252-1257, 1995.

[23] Mohamed AA, Gotoh O, Graham DI, Osborne KA, McCulloch J, Mendelow AD, et al. effect of pretreatment with the calcium antagonist nimodipine on local cerebral blood flow and histopathology after middle cerebral artery occlusion. Ann Neurol 18: 705-711, 1985

[24] Buchan AM, Xue D, Huang ZG, Smith KH Lesiuk H. Delayed AMPA receptor blockade reduces cerebral infarction induced by focal ischemia. Neuroreport 2:473-476, 1991

[25] Sydserff SG, Borelli AR, Green AR, Cross AJ. Effect of NXY059 on infarct volume after transient or permanent middle cerebral artery occlusion in the rat; studies on a dose, plasma concentration and therapeutic time window. Br J Pharmacol 135:103–112, 2002.

[26] Minematsu K, Fisher M, Li L, Davis MA, Knapp AG, Cotter RE, McBurney RN, et al. Effects of a novel NMDA antagonist on experimental stroke rapidly and quantitatively assessed by diffusion-weighted MRI. Neurology 43:397-403, 1993.

[27] Yrjanheikki J, Tikka T, Keinanen R, Goldsteins G, Chan PH, Koistinaho J. A tetracycline derivative, minocycline, reduces inflammation and protects against focal cerebral ischemia with a wide therapeutic window. Proc Natl Acad Sci USA 96:13496– 13500, 1999.

[28] Linnik MD, Miller JA, Sprinkle-Cavallo J, Mason PJ, Thompson FY, Montgomery LR, et al. Apoptotic DNA fragmentation in the rat cerebral cortex induced by permanent middle cerebral artery occlusion. Brain Res Mol Brain Res 32:116-124, 1995.

[29] Li Y, Chopp M, Jiang N, Yao F, Zaloga C. Temporal profile of in situ DNA fragmentation after transient middle cerebral artery occlusion in the rat. J Cereb Blood Flow Metab 15:389-397, 1995.

[30] Takagi K, Zhao W, Busto R, Ginsberg MD. Local hemodynamic changes during transient middle cerebral artery occlusion and

recirculation in the rat: an [14C] iodoantipyrine autoradiographic study. Brain Res 691:160-168, 1995.

[31] Nagayama T, Lan J, Henshall DC, Chen D, O'Horo C, Simon RP, Chen J Induction of oxidative DNA damage in the peri-infarct region after permanent focal cerebral ischemia. J Neurochem 75:1716-1728, 2000.

[32] Gladstone DJ, Black SE, Hakim AM. Heart and Stroke Foundation of Ontario Centre of Excellence in Stroke Recovery. Toward wisdom from failure: lessons from neuroprotective stroke trials and new therapeutic directions. Stroke 33:2123-2236, 2003.

[33] Cheng YD, Al-Khoury L, Zivin JA. Neuroprotection for ischemic stroke: two decades of success and failure. NeuroRx 1:36-45, 2004.

[34] Tamura A, Graham DI, Mcculloch J, Teasdale GM: Focal cerebral ischemia in the rat. I: Description of technique and early neuropathological consequences following middle cerebral artery occlusion. J Cereb Blood Flow Metabol 1: 53-60, 1981

[35] Tamura A, Graham DI, McCulloch J, Teasdale GM: Focal cerebral ischemia in the rat. 2. Regional cerebral blood flow determined by (I4C) iodoantipyrine autoradiography following middle cerebral artery occlusion. J Cereb Blood Flow Metabol 1: 61-69, 1981

[36] Gotoh O, Asano T, Koide T, Takakura K. Ischemic brain edema following occlusion of the middle cerebral artery in the rat. I: The time courses of the brain water, sodium and potassium contents and blood-brain barrier permeability to 125I-albumin. Stroke. 1985 Jan;16(1):101-9.

[37] Macrae IM. Preclinical stroke research–advantages and disadvantages of the most common rodent models of focal ischaemia. British journal of pharmacology. 2011 Oct;164(4):1062-78.

[38] Chopp M, Zhang RL, Chen H, Li Y, Jiang N, Rusche JR. Postischemic administration of an anti-Mac-1 antibody reduces ischemic cell damage after transient middle cerebral artery occlusion in rats. Stroke. 1994 Apr;25(4):869-75.

[39] Simpkins JW, Rajakumar G, Zhang YQ, Simpkins CE, Greenwald D, Chun JY, Bodor N, Day AL. Estrogens may reduce mortality and ischemic damage caused by middle cerebral artery occlusion in the female rat. Journal of neurosurgery. 1997 Nov 1;87(5):724-30.

[40] Thiyagarajan M, Sharma SS. Neuroprotective effect of curcumin in middle cerebral artery occlusion induced focal cerebral ischemia in rats. Life sciences. 2004 Jan 9;74(8):969-85.

[41] Kurozumi K, Nakamura K, Tamiya T, Kawano Y, Ishii K, Kobune M, Hirai S, Uchida H, Sasaki K, Ito Y, Kato K. Mesenchymal stem cells that produce neurotrophic factors reduce ischemic damage in the rat middle cerebral artery occlusion model. Molecular Therapy. 2005 Jan 1;11(1):96-104.

[42] Overgaard K, Sereghy T, Boysen G, Pedersen H, Høyer S, Diemer NH. A rat model of reproducible cerebral infarction using thrombotic blood clot emboli. J Cereb Blood Flow Metab. 1992;12:484-490.

[43] Perel P, Roberts I, Sena E, Wheble P, Briscoe C, Sandercock P et al. (2007). Comparison of treatment effects between animal experiments and clinical trials: a systematic review. BMJ 334: 197.

[44] Busch E, Krüger K, Hossmann K-A (1997). An improved model of thromboembolic stroke and rt-PA

induced reperfusion in the rat. Brain Res 778: 16-24.

[45] Andersen M, Overgaard K, Meden P, Boysen G, Choi SC. Effects of citicoline combined with thrombolytic therapy in a rat embolic stroke model. Stroke. 1999 Jul 1;30:1464-70.

[46] Overgaard K, Sereghy T, Pedersen H, Boysen G. Effect of delayed thrombolysis with rt-PA in a rat embolic stroke model. Journal of Cerebral Blood Flow & Metabolism. 1994 May;14(3):472-7.

[47] Lekieffre D, Benavides J, Scatton B, Nowicki JP. Neuroprotection afforded by a combination of eliprodil and a thrombolytic agent, rt-PA, in a rat thromboembolic stroke model. Brain research. 1997 Nov 21;776(1-2):88-95.

[48] Sereghy T, Overgaard K, Boysen G. Neuroprotection by excitatory amino acid antagonist augments the benefit of thrombolysis in embolic stroke in rats. Stroke. 1993 Nov;24(11):1702-8.

[49] Rasmussen RS, Overgaard K, Hildebrandt-Eriksen ES, Boysen G. d-Amphetamine improves cognitive deficits, and physical therapy promotes fine motor rehabilitation in a rat embolic stroke model. Acta neurologica scandinavica. 2006 Mar;113(3):189-98.

[50] Kagstrom E, Smith M-L, Siesjo BK: Cerebral circulatory responses to hypercapnia and hypoxia in the recovery Ginsberg and Busto Rodent Models of Cerebral Ischemia period following complete and incomplete cerebral ischemia in the rat. Ada Physiol Scand 1983;118:281-291

[51] Smith M-L, Bendek G, Dahlgren N, Rosen I, Wieloch T, Siesjo BK: Models for studying long-term recovery following forebrain ischemia in the rat. 2. A 2-vessel occlusion model. Ada Neurol Scand 1984;69:385-401

[52] Smith M-L, Auer RN, Siesjo BK: The density and distribution of ischemic brain injury in the rat following 2-10 min of forebrain ischemia. Ada Neuropathol (Berl) 1984; 64:319-332

[53] Busto R, DietrICH (Intracerebral hemorrhage) WD, Globus MY-T, Ginsberg MD: Postischemic moderate hypothermia inhibits CA1 (HIPPOCAMPAL CORNU AMMONIS)) hippo- 37. campal ischemic neuronal injury. Neurosci Lett 1989; 101:299-304

[54] Smith ML, Bendek G, Dahlgren N, Rosén I, Wieloch T, Siesjö BK. Models for studying long-term recovery following forebrain ischemia in the rat. 2. A 2-vessel occlusion model. Acta neurologica Scandinavica. 1984 Jun;69(6):385-401.

[55] Raval AP, Liu C, Hu BR. A rat model of global cerebral ischemia: the two-vessel occlusion (2VO) model of forebrain ischemia. InAnimal Models of Acute Neurological Injuries in 2009 (pp. 77-86). Humana Press.

[56] Marosi M, Fuzik J, Nagy D, Rákos G, Kis Z, Vécsei L, Toldi J, Ruban-Matuzani A, TeICH (Intracerebral hemorrhage)berg VI, Farkas T. Oxaloacetate restores the long-term potentiation impaired in rat hippocampus CA1 (HIPPOCAMPAL CORNU AMMONIS)) region by 2-vessel occlusion. European journal of pharmacology. 2009 Feb 14;604(1-3):51-7.

[57] McBean DE, Winters V, Wilson AD, Oswald CB, Alps BJ, Armstrong JM. Neuroprotective efficacy of lifarizine (RS-87476) in a simplified rat survival model of 2 vessel occlusion. British journal of pharmacology. 1995 Dec;116(8):3093-8.

[58] Zhou D, Matchett GA, Jadhav V, Dach N, Zhang JH. The effect of 2-methoxyestradiol, a HIF-1 α inhibitor,

in global cerebral ischemia in rats. Neurological research. 2008 Apr 1;30(3):268-71.

[59] Prabhakar O, Arun K and Naveen Y: Protective effect of naringin against cerebral infarction induced by ischemic-reperfusion in rats. Int J Pharm Sci & Res 2020; 11(11): 5497-01. doi: 10.13040/IJPSR.0975-8232.11(11). 5497-01.

[60] Prabhakar, O. Cerebroprotective effect of resveratrol through antioxidant and anti-inflammatory effects in diabetic rats. *Naunyn-Schmiedeberg's Arch Pharmacol* 386, 705-710 (2013). https://doi.org/10.1007/s00210-013-0871-2

[61] Brown AW, Brierley JB: The nature, distribution and earliest stages of anoxic-ischemic nerve cell damage in the rat brain as defined by the optical microscope. Br J Exp 41. Pathol 1968;49:87-106

[62] Pulsinelli WA, Brierley JB: A new model of bilateral hemispheric ischemia in the unanesthetized rat. Stroke 1979;10:267-272

[63] Volpe BT, Pulsinelli WA, Tribuna J, Davis HP: Behavioral performance of rats following transient forebrain ischemia. Stroke 1984;15:558-562.

[64] O'Neill, MICH (Intracerebral hemorrhage)all J., and James *A. Clemens*. "Rodent models of focal cerebral ischemia." Current protocols in neuroscience 12.1 (2000): 9-6.

[65] Ergün R, Akdemir G, Şen S, Taşçı A, Ergüngör F. Neuroprotective effects of propofol following global cerebral ischemia in rats. Neurosurgical review. 2002 Mar 1;25(1-2):95-8.

[66] Gellért L, Fuzik J, Göblös A, Sárközi K, Marosi M, Kis Z, Farkas T, Szatmári I, Fülöp F, Vécsei L, Toldi J. Neuroprotection with a new kynurenic acid analog in the four-vessel occlusion model of ischemia. European journal of pharmacology. 2011 Sep 30;667(1-3):182-7.

[67] Li H, Klein G, Sun P, Buchan AM. Dehydroepiandrosterone (DHEA) reduces neuronal injury in a rat model of global cerebral ischemia. Brain research. 2001 Jan 12;888(2):263-6.

[68] Sivaraman D, Kumar PS, Muralidharan P, Rahman H, Nagar I, Thoraipakkam C. Effect of Hemidesmus indicus on cerebral infarct Ischemia-reperfusion injured rats by four-vessel occlusion method. Pharmacologia. 2012;3(4):91-102.

[69] Ginsberg MD, Prado R, DietrICH (Intracerebral hemorrhage) WD, Busto R, Watson BD. Hyperglycemia reduces the extent of cerebral infarction in rats. Stroke. 1987 May;18(3):570-4

[70] Labat-gest V, Tomasi S. Photothrombotic ischemia: a minimally invasive and reproducible photochemical cortical lesion model for mouse stroke studies. JoVE (Journal of Visualized Experiments). 2013 Jun 9(76):e50370.

[71] De Ryck M, Van Reempts J, Borgers M, Wauquier A, Janssen PA. Photochemical stroke model: flunarizine prevents sensorimotor deficits after neocortical infarcts in rats. Stroke. 1989 Oct;20(10):1383-90.

[72] Minnerup J, Seeger FH, Kuhnert K, DiederICH (Intracerebral hemorrhage) K, Schilling M, Dimmeler S, Schäbitz WR. Intracarotid administration of human bone marrow mononuclear cells in rat photothrombotic ischemia. Experimental & translational stroke medicine. 2010 Dec 1;2(1):3.

[73] De Ryck M, Keersmaekers R, Duytschaever H, Claes C, Clincke G, Janssen M, Van Reet G. Lubeluzole

protects sensorimotor function and reduces infarct size in a photochemical stroke model in rats. Journal of Pharmacology and Experimental Therapeutics. 1996 Nov 1;279(2):748-58.

[74] Hou B, Ma J, Guo X, Ju F, Gao J, Wang D, Liu J, Li X, Zhang S, Ren H. Exogenous neural stem cells transplantation as a potential therapy for photothrombotic ischemia stroke in kunming mice model. Molecular neurobiology. 2017 Mar 1;54(2):1254-62.

[75] Rosenberg GA, Mun-Bryce S, Wesley M, Kornfeld M. Collagenase-induced intracerebral hemorrhage in rats. Stroke. 1990 May;21(5):801-7.

[76] MacLellan CL, Silasi G, Poon CC, Edmundson CL, Buist R, Peeling J, Colbourne F. Intracerebral hemorrhage models in the rat: comparing collagenase to blood infusion. Journal of Cerebral Blood Flow & Metabolism. 2008 Mar;28(3):516-25.

[77] Kawai N, Nakamura T, Nagao S. Early hemostatic therapy using recombinant factor VIIa in a collagenase-induced intracerebral hemorrhage model in rats. InBrain Edema XIII 2006 (pp. 212-217). Springer, Vienna.

[78] Lauer A, Cianchetti FA, Van Cott EM, Schlunk F, Schulz E, Pfeilschifter W, Steinmetz H, Schaffer CB, Lo EH, Foerch C. Anticoagulation with the oral direct thrombin inhibitor dabigatran does not enlarge hematoma volume in experimental intracerebral hemorrhage. Circulation. 2011 Oct 11;124(15):1654-62.

[79] Lema PP, Girard C, Vachon P. Evaluation of dexamethasone for the treatment of intracerebral hemorrhage using a collagenase-induced intracerebral hematoma model in rats. Journal of veterinary pharmacology and therapeutics. 2004 Oct;27(5):321-8.

[80] Del Bigio MR, Jin Yan H, Campbell TM, Peeling J. Effect of fucoidan treatment on collagenase-induced intracerebral hemorrhage in rats. Neurological research. 1999 Jun 1;21(4):415-9.

[81] JXue M, Del—Bigio MR. Intracortical hemorrhage injury in rats; the relationship between blood fractions and brain cell death cell death. Stroke. 2000;3(1):172l-7.

[82] Nakamura T, Keep RF, Hua Y, Schallert T, Hoff JT, Xi G. Deferoxamine-induced attenuation of brain edema and neurological deficits in a rat model of intracerebral hemorrhage. Journal of neurosurgery. 2004 Apr 1;100(4):672-8.

[83] Nakamura T, Kuroda Y, Hosomi N, Okabe N, Kawai N, Tamiya T, Xi G, Keep RF, Itano T. Serine protease inhibitor attenuates intracerebral hemorrhage-induced brain injury and edema formation in the rat. In Brain Edema XIV 2010 (pp. 307-310). Springer, Vienna.

[84] Nakamura T, Kuroda Y, Yamashita S, Zhang X, Miyamoto O, Tamiya T, Nagao S, Xi G, Keep RF, Itano T. Edaravone attenuates brain edema and neurologic deficits in a rat model of acute intracerebral hemorrhage. Stroke. 2008 Feb 1;39(2):463-9.

[85] Nakamura T, Xi G, Keep RF, Wang M, Nagao S, Hoff JT, Hua Y. Effects of endogenous and exogenous estrogen on intracerebral hemorrhage-induced brain damage in rats. InBrain Edema XIII 2006 (pp. 218-221). Springer, Vienna.

Chapter 7

Mouse Models of Acute Kidney Injury

Navjot Pabla, Yogesh Scindia, Joseph Gigliotti and Amandeep Bajwa

Abstract

Acute Kidney Injury (AKI) is a poor prognosis in hospitalized patients that is associated with high degree of mortality. AKI is also a major risk factor for development of chronic kidney disease. Despite these serious complications associated with AKI there has not been a great amount of progress made over the last half-century. Here we have outlined and provided details on variety of mouse models of AKI. Some of the mouse models of AKI are renal pedicle clamping (ischemia reperfusion injury), Cisplatin induced nephrotoxicity, sepsis (LPS, cecal slurry, and cecal ligation and puncture), folic acid, and rhabdomyolysis. In this chapter we describe in detail the protocols that are used in our laboratories.

Keywords: ischemia reperfusion injury, cecal ligation and puncture, cecal slurry, sepsis, LPS, kidney, inflammation, immune cells, cisplatin, folic Acid, rhabdomyolysis, acute kidney injury, nephropathy

1. Introduction

Acute kidney injury (AKI) is a common clinical disorder characterized by a precipitous decline in renal function [1]. AKI is particularly prevalent in hospitalized patients and is associated with varied underlying etiologies, such as sepsis [2], cardiac surgery [3], rhabdomyolysis [4], and drug toxicity [5]. Patient outcomes are varied and depend partly on severity, with higher mortality seen in critically ill patients [1]. Importantly, patients who survive an episode of AKI are at increased risk for major adverse cardiovascular events, as well as for progression to chronic kidney disease (CKD) and end-stage renal disease (ESRD) [6]. Despite our growing understanding of the causes and mechanisms of AKI, as well as an effort to develop better diagnostic strategies, few preventive or therapeutic options exist.

Therefore, animal models of AKI are essential for identifying mechanisms of renal dysfunction and for development of therapeutic and diagnostic strategies [7]. To this end, mice have been the main experimental organisms for studying AKI. Since the underlying causes of AKI are varied, several murine animal models have been established. These animal models recapitulate several pathophysiological features of AKI, such as endothelial dysfunction [8], epithelial cell death [9], and immune cell infiltration [10] (**Figure 1**). In the current chapter, we provide an overview of the methods and highlight issues that are critical in establishing various murine models of AKI.

IntechOpen

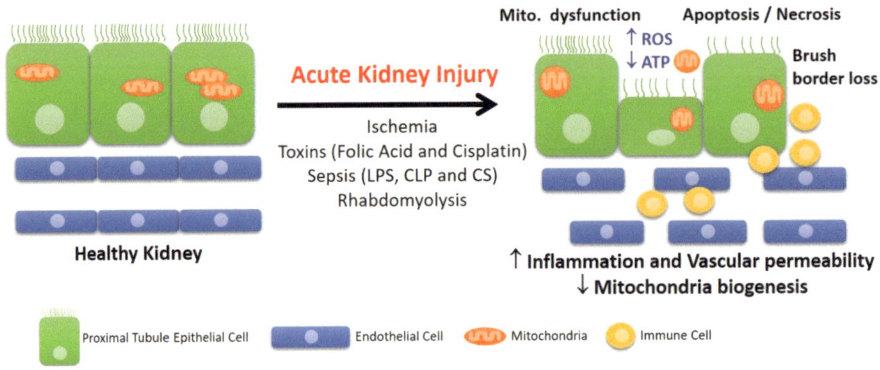

Figure 1.
Complex pathophysiology of AKI: Involvement of endothelium, renal tubules (specifically proximal tubule (PT) segment) and immune cells. Compared to normal/healthy kidney, various AKI insults result in overall decrease in ATP, loss of PT brush border, increase in vascular permeability and inflammation ultimately resulting in apoptosis and necrosis.

2. Ischemia reperfusion injury (IRI) model of acute kidney injury

2.1 Background

Mouse Model of Kidney Ischemia Reperfusion Injury: Warm ischemia and reperfusion injury models is the most widely used model of AKI, in rodents the renal blood flow is temporarily interrupted for a various time periods ranging from 20 to 45 minutes followed by varied amounts of reperfusion. In our laboratory we use a standard clamp time of 26 minutes followed by 24 hours of reperfusion. The IRI model of AKI can be further divided into bilateral, unilateral, and unilateral with simultaneous nephrectomy depending on the questions or therapeutic tested. In bilateral both renal pedicles are clamped, whereas unilateral with simultaneous nephrectomy can be utilized to reduce the variability that can be observed. However, in unilateral either left or right pedicle is clamped without disturbing the contralateral control kidney, ideally the unilateral IRI model is used for studies that have interest in evaluating progression to chronic kidney disease or fibrosis.

2.2 Methods

1. We routinely use 10–12 weeks old C57BL/6 male mice or either commercially purchased from vendor (Jackson Laboratories or NCI) or bred in house. The commercially purchased animals acclimate for one week in a 12-hour dark and 12-hour light cycle room prior to undergoing any surgeries. If using female or other strains (BALB/c or FVB) the ischemia time can be adjusted, ideally, we have established that 26-minutes of clamp time for C57BL/6 male mice and 28-minutes for BALB/c [11–13] or female C57BL/6 mice (unpublished observations) results in similar ischemic injury in our laboratory.

2. All surgical tools are sterilized by autoclaving before each experiment and between mice a hot bead sterilizer is used.

3. The mice are anesthetized with a mixture of Ketamine/Xylazine (120/12 mg/kg, Intraperitoneal injection) and as analgesic buprenorphine (0.15 mg/kg, subcutaneous injection) prior to placing on a warm pad (pad temperature is set to 34.6°C). Additionally, ophthalmic ointment is applied to the eyes following induction of anesthesia to prevent corneal drying.

4. The surgical site is shaved and cleaned by alternating between 70% ethanol and betadine (minimum 3 times).

5. Prior to any surgical procedure the mouse body temperature needs to reach 34°C (this will reduce overall variability in injury).

6. Bilateral flank incisions are made, and the renal pedicle (vein and artery) on both sides are clamped using micro-serrefine atraumatic vascular clamps (Fine Science Tools, 18055–02) for bilateral IRI. If mice are used for chronic studies, only clamp one side (we usually clamp the right pedicle as it is easier to perform nephrectomy on left contralateral control kidney 1 day before terminating studies, usually day 13) [14]. An alternative here can be to have surgical mice undergo simultaneous nephrectomy of contralateral control kidney. We do not practice this protocol in our lab as this could lead to a more severe kidney injury with standard clamp time of 26 minutes.

7. Sham mice will undergo the same procedure (steps 3-step 6) without applying the clamps to induce ischemia.

8. The mouse body temperature is checked intermittently during ischemia using rectal probe and maintained to be above 34°C along with visual confirmation of clamped kidneys (dark purple color).

9. The atraumatic clamps are removed and reperfusion on both sides is confirmed by checking the kidney color (changes from dark purple to pink). Both incision sites are closed with a 4.0 vicryl suture.

10. The mice recover from anesthesia on heating pad are returned to cages once awake and kept in a home-made chamber with a heating lamp to maintain chamber temperatures to around 30–33°C.

11. Depending on the protocol need for experiments, surgical mice will undergo reperfusion for 24–72 hours.

12. Kidney function can be rapidly assessed by measuring changes in plasma creatinine (Diazyme Laboratories) [11, 12, 14–16] and BUN. Histological changes are usually determined by analyzing hematoxylin and eosin (H&E) or periodic-acid Schiff (PAS) staining. All histology samples are scored for acute tubular necrosis (ATN). For quantification of tubular injury score, sections are assessed by counting the percentage of tubules that display cell necrosis, loss of brush border, cast formation, and tubule dilation as follows: 0 = normal; 1 = <10%; 2 = 10 to 25%; 3 = 26 to 50%; 4 = 51 to 75%; 5 = >75%. Five to 10 fields from each outer medulla are evaluated and scored in a blinded manner. The histological changes are expressed as ATN, scored as previously described [12, 17].

2.3 Critical notes

1. The IRI protocol in mice is not very technically challenging but does require some expertise. Some of the alternatives that can be used for a beginner is to do a midline laparotomy to have a better visual of the kidneys (step 6) or using flank incision gently pop each of the kidney out of the body cavity to have a better visual of the renal pedicle.

2. The clamping or ischemia times (20–45 minutes) may need to be changed if other anesthetic (pentobarbital sodium or isoflurane) is used.

3. The sex and age of mice also can contribute to the level of injury. Older mice and rats [18] are more susceptible to IRI induced AKI and it is also well-known and accepted that female [7, 19] mice are less susceptible compared to age matched male mice.

4. The type of mouse strain is also a critical variable that needs to be documented. Our recent unpublished work using C57BL/6 and DBA/2 J mice demonstrated that compared to C57BL/6 mice DBA/2 J mice are significantly protected from 26 minutes of bilateral IRI. Furthermore, these mice were also protected with cisplatin induce AKI. These preliminary observations from the Bajwa and Pabla labs indicate that strain of animals is a very important variable that needs to be considered in preclinical models of AKI.

5. In many of the studies all post-operative mice are supplemented with 0.5–1 ml of saline as a subcutaneous injection. This additional procedure can be applied depending on the protocols approved in your institution.

3. Cisplatin associated acute kidney injury

3.1 Background

Due to their role in the metabolism and excretion of xenobiotics, kidneys are particularly vulnerable to drug-induced toxicities [1]. The renal tubular epithelial cells have significant capacity for uptake of drugs, and this can result in high intracellular concentrations, which can lead to toxicities and development of acute kidney injury. Cisplatin is a widely used chemotherapy drug that accumulates in renal tubular cells causing acute kidney injury [5]. Cisplatin is used as part of chemotherapy regimens for the treatment of a wide spectrum of malignancies such as testicular, head and neck, ovarian, lung, cervical, and bladder cancers. Cisplatin accumulates in the tubular epithelial cells through organic cation [20] and copper transporters [21], which in turn activates a plethora of signaling pathways that culminate in epithelial cell death, inflammation, and kidney injury [5]. Tubulointerstitial injury is the predominant lesion observed during cisplatin nephrotoxicity, wherein both proximal and distal tubules are affected and display significant necrosis. It is observed that renal function improves in most patients, however a subset of patients can develop chronic renal impairment [22].

Cisplatin nephrotoxicity can be mimicked in murine models through single [16, 23] or multiple [24] injections. The single injection induced AKI is the most widely used model of cisplatin nephrotoxicity. In this model, a single intraperitoneal injection (10–30 mg/kg) results in development of AKI within 2–3 days.

3.2 Methods

1. Prepare a 1 mg/mL solution by dissolving cisplatin in normal saline (0.9% NaCl). To this end, add cisplatin to pre-warmed normal saline (37°C), followed by transferring the tube to a shaker at room temperature for 1 hour, along with intermittent vortexing. While this solution can be stored at room temperature (dark) and used for up to two weeks, preparing fresh solution on the day of injection generally leads to more consistent injury.

2. Inject cisplatin intraperitoneally using a 1 ml syringe with 26 G needle at a dose of 10–30 mg/kg body weight. We have found that dosing the mice in the

afternoon (2 PM) leads to more consistent injury and this might be related to the circadian regulation of organic cation transporters that are involved in renal uptake of cisplatin [25].

3. On day three post-cisplatin injection, sacrifice the mice by carbon dioxide euthanasia followed by serum and renal tissue collection for further analysis. Kidney injury can then be evaluated by serum analysis [blood urea nitrogen (BUN) and creatinine], histological analysis [hematoxylin–eosin (H&E) staining], and examination of renal expression of injury biomarkers [kidney injury molecule-1 (KIM1) and neutrophil gelatinase-associated lipocalin (NGAL)] [26, 27]. Blood urine nitrogen and enzymatic assay-based creatinine measurements can be performed in serum or plasma samples using commercially available kits. For histological analysis, mouse kidneys are harvested and embedded in paraffin and tissue sections (4–5 μm) are stained with H&E using standard methods. Histopathological scoring can be conducted by examining 10 consecutive ×100 fields per section from at least 3 mice/group. Tubular damage is then scored by calculating the percentage of tubules that showed dilation, epithelium flattening, cast formation, loss of brush border and nuclei, and denudation of the basement membrane using a previously [28] described injury scale: 0, no damage; 1, <25%; 2, 25–50%; 3, 50–75%; and 4, >75%.

3.3 Critical notes

1. The severity of cisplatin nephrotoxicity is strain dependent and hence the dose used may have to be identified through preliminary dose–response experiments. For example, the FVB/NJ mice [28] are more sensitive to cisplatin nephrotoxicity than C57BL/6 J mice [23].

2. Female mice display more variability and are in general more sensitive to cisplatin nephrotoxicity [26].

3. 8–12-week-old male mice are ideal for cisplatin nephrotoxicity experiments.

4. It has been shown that DMSO can inactivate cisplatin [29], hence it should be avoided for preparing cisplatin or for preparation of other drugs used in combination with cisplatin.

4. Rhabdomyolysis associated acute kidney injury

4.1 Background

AKI is the most serious complication of rhabdomyolysis, representing up to 10% of all cases of AKI [4]. Although the exact mechanisms remain unknown, hypovolemia, myoglobinuria, and metabolic acidosis contribute to the pathogenesis of rhabdomyolysis-associated AKI. Importantly, myoglobinuria is likely initiating factor. Myoglobin is a 17.8-kDa iron- and oxygen-binding protein found in the skeletal muscle cells [4]. During rhabdomyolysis, myoglobin is released into the circulation, and since it is freely filtered by the glomerulus, it then enters the tubule epithelial cell through endocytosis. Traditionally, it has been believed that heme and free iron-driven hydroxyl radicals associated with myoglobin contribute to tubular damage through oxidative stress linked mechanisms [30]. Interestingly, it has been suggested recently that myoglobin can also directly promote oxidation of biomolecules, lipid peroxidation, and the generation of isoprostanes through its peroxidase-like enzyme activity [31].

Rhabdomyolysis-associated AKI can be mimicked in murine models through glycerol injection in the hind-leg muscles [27]. In this model, a single bilateral intramuscular injection (7.5 mL/kg 50% glycerol) results in development of AKI within 24 hours.

4.2 Methods

1. Prepare a 50% glycerol solution in normal saline (0.9% NaCl) followed by transferring the tube to a shaker at room temperature for 15 minutes to mix the solution. Prepare fresh solution on the day of injection.

2. Administer 50% glycerol by intramuscular injection using a 1 ml syringe with 26G needle to both the hindlimbs (once for each hindlimb). During glycerol injection, the mice are anesthetized by isoflurane administration (inhalation) before and throughout the glycerol administration procedure.

3. Immediately following glycerol injection, isoflurane inhalation is stopped, and mice are allowed to recover, followed by transfer to regular cages. Since the mice will have severe muscle injury, food, water, and painkillers (e.g., Caprofen) are provided in 1–2 oz. gel cup for up to 5 mice per cage.

4. The mice will develop AKI within 24–48 hours and at these time-points, mice can be euthanized by carbon dioxide euthanasia followed by serum and tissue collection [27]. Kidney injury can then be evaluated by biochemical analysis [blood urea nitrogen (BUN) and creatinine], histological examination [hematoxylin–eosin (H&E) staining], and analysis of renal expression of injury biomarkers such as kidney injury molecule-1 (KIM1) and neutrophil gelatinase-associated lipocalin (NGAL) [32]. Blood urine nitrogen and enzymatic assay-based creatinine measurements can be performed in serum or plasma samples using commercially available kits. For histological analysis, mouse kidneys are harvested and embedded in paraffin and tissue sections (4–5 µm) are stained with H&E using standard methods. Histopathological scoring can be conducted by examining 10 consecutive ×100 fields per section from at least 3 mice/group. Tubular damage is then scored by calculating the percentage of tubules that showed dilation, epithelium flattening, cast formation, loss of brush border and nuclei, and denudation of the basement membrane using a previously described [28] injury scale: 0, no damage; 1, <25%; 2, 25–50%; 3, 50–75%; and 4, >75%.

4.3 Critical notes

1. The severity of rhabdomyolysis-associated AKI is strain dependent and hence the dose used may have to be identified through preliminary dose–response experiments. For example, the FVB/NJ mice are more sensitive than C57BL/6 J mice to rhabdomyolysis associated AKI.

2. Due to lower muscle mass, it is technically challenging to induce rhabdomyolysis associated AKI in female mice.

3. 8–12-week-old male mice are ideal for rhabdomyolysis experiments.

4. We have found no circadian related differences in severity of rhabdomyolysis associated AKI and hence glycerol can be injected at any time to initiate injury.

5. Folic acid-induced nephropathy

5.1 Background

It was reported in the late 60's that a single bolus injection of high-dose (250 mg/kg body weight) induced rampant renal hypertrophy and cell proliferation [33]. A large increase in the number of dividing cells was reported within 18 hours, with the maximum division of cells within the renal medulla occurring at 24-hours post FAN whereas the cortex reached its peak at 26 hours. This appears to be due to renal tubular epithelial damage that appear to be mediated by both the deposition of folic acid crystals and subsequent tubular obstruction as well as direct nephrotoxicity due to high-dose FAN [34]. The histological evidence of tubular injury is accompanied by reduced renal function as measured by circulating creatinine and blood urea nitrogen levels. Both increase in proportion to the dose of FAN, with the 250 mg/kg dose resulting in severe acute kidney injury with significant increase (greater than double) in circulating markers and histological evidence of acute tubular necrosis at 48 hours post injection. If the animals survive, the FAN model is also commonly used to study renal fibrosis (key finding in chronic kidney disease) that develops 7–14 days after injection [14, 35] and continues to progress weeks thereafter and can be exacerbated with repeated administration of FA [36, 37].

5.2 Methods

1. Weigh mice and calculate the amount of folic acid needed to achieve a 250 mg/kg body weight dose.

2. Dissolve the folic acid into 500 μL of 0.3 mM sodium bicarbonate for each mouse to be injected.

3. Anesthetize the animal (3% isoflurane in 100% oxygen) and sterilize the abdomen with repeated 70% ethanol/betadine wipes.

4. Invert the FA solution several times and then inject the 500 μL of the folic acid/0.3 mM FA solution into the peritoneal cavity, being careful not to puncture the gastrointestinal tract.

    a. Larger gauge needle (18-24G) will allow for easier injection as the folic acid may clog smaller needles.

    b. 500 μL of 0.3 mM sodium bicarbonate can be used as the vehicle control.

5. Allow the animals to recover from anesthesia and return to original housing once consciousness is retained.

6. Disease is evident after 24 hours, with peak evidence of kidney dysfunction occurring 36–48 hours post injection.

    a. In our experience, this is when animal mortality begins to occur.

7. 36–48 hours after injection, blood can be collected, and the animals euthanized (order depending on method of blood collected). Kidneys can be collected for quantification of tissue injury by histology or a variety of other methods. Blood can be processed to plasma or serum and used to quantify creatinine or blood urea nitrogen using commercially available assays.

5.3 Critical notes

1. This method will result in robust kidney injury in 8–12-week-old male mice of the C57BL/6 J strain (~25 grams of body weight).

2. If using females, a different strain, or older mice it is recommended to perform a pilot study to determine optimal dose.

   a. Similar protocols have been employed to induce kidney injury in rats.

   b. Older mice will develop more severe injury so a reduced dose of folic acid may be needed to assess treatment effects or avoid unintentional mortality.

3. If mice differ in body weights, it may be of value to apply the same dose (based on the animal with the smallest body weight) to avoid differences in absolute amount of folic acid administered.

   a. As an example, for more obese animals in different dietary groups

6. Sepsis and sepsis-associated AKI

6.1 Background

Sepsis is characterized by a severe inflammatory response to infection, and one of its complications is acute kidney injury. Animal models that mimic the pathophysiology of human sepsis and associated acute kidney injury are valuable because they aid in identifying molecular targets and in developing therapeutics. Too often, animal models do not properly mimic human disease. In this chapter, we describe the three commonly used approaches that have resulted in improved animal models to study sepsis.

Sepsis is a complex condition that results in a dysregulated host response to an infection and is associated with unacceptably high mortality [38]. Sepsis-associated acute kidney injury (S-AKI) is a common end organ manifestation in hospitalized and critically ill patients and is associated with high mortality and increased risk of developing chronic comorbidities [39, 40]. As individual syndromes, sepsis and AKI render the host susceptible to each other. Sepsis has a complex and unique pathophysiology, which makes S-AKI a distinct syndrome from any other phenotype of AKI. Identifying the exact onset of AKI in sepsis is nearly impossible, leading to difficulty in timely intervention for prevention of renal injury. This has limited our understanding of pathophysiologic mechanisms and precluded the development of effective therapies. The pathogenesis of S-AKI is multifactorial and involves systemic cytokine storm, hypoxia, mitochondrial dysfunction, tubular epithelial cell injury, and endothelial dysfunction [41, 42].

Local mechanisms cannot be identified and studied in humans, and hence the use of relevant animal models is paramount to eventually identify new therapeutic target to treat a syndrome still mainly managed by antibiotics and fluid resuscitations. Animal models of sepsis need to reproduce the complexity and severity of human sepsis, mimic the key hemodynamic and immunologic (proinflammatory stimulation, anti-inflammatory counter regulation, i.e., immune depression) stages as well as the modest histological findings. The sepsis inducing procedure should result in toxicity and bacteremia and should result as metabolic and physiologic changes. Furthermore, the septic insult should manifest over sufficient length of time to allow the study of its evolution and finally the model should be reproducible and inexpensive.

Below we discuss the three commonly used animal models of sepsis and S-AKI and summarize the advantage and shortcomings of each.

7. Lipopolysaccharide injection: A model of Endotoxemia

Probably the most extensively studied animal model of sepsis is based on the intraperitoneal injection of lipopolysaccharide (LPS) [43, 44]. LPS is the major outer surface membrane component present in almost all Gram-negative bacteria and act as extremely strong stimulators of innate [45]. Although this model is simple to learn and perform, it has inherent limitations. The primary ones being that it neglects the direct host-pathogen interactions and is limited to Gram negative organism-induced sepsis. A bolus administration of LPS is essentially a model of severe inflammatory response syndrome (SIRS), rather than a true septic mimetic [46] and there is no microbial source for ongoing LPS, or pathogen associated pattern (PAMP) release. Key to the optimal success of this septic AKI model is amongst others, the use of the proper serology of LPS (E Coli. O111.B4), age of mice [43] and fluid resuscitation [47]. Compared to true human sepsis, endotoxemia results in a rapid and exponential spike in plasma inflammatory cytokines, and this SIRS like condition resolves rapidly [48–50]. This model is of scientific utility in interrogating specific biological mechanisms and pathways, such as the immune response to prototypical stimuli of specific toll-like receptor (TLR) pathways, TLR4.

7.1 Methods

1. Prepare a 1 mg/mL stock solution of LPS in sterile PBS or normal saline (0.9%NaCL). For consistent results use the same serology of LPS (*E. coli* O111. B4). If not being used immediately, aliquot and stored in - 80°C for up to 6 months. Avoid repeated freeze thaw.

2. Generally male mice between 8 and 12 weeks are used in this model, unless the effect of aging is a study parameter. Aged mice are more suspectable to LPS-induced injury. To inject mice, bring to room temperature and inject based on your experimental requirements. Dilute if required using PBS or normal saline. A low dose 1 mg/kg, intraperitoneal injection causes mild to no AKI, whereas 5 mg/kg and above results in severe SIRS and resultant AKI.

3. Depending upon the dose a spike in TNF-alpha is observed within an hour which subsequently subsides with time (at 24 hours, no to little TNF alpha is observed in the serum). Other key cytokines like IL-6 also go up by 3–4 hours. In the kidney, local changes can be observed at microscopic levels, but no signs of AKI are seen.

4. Even with the high dose of LPS, the mice look healthy and move around freely during the first 3–4 hours. However, 6 hours post treatment, mice start to assume a hunched posture, lack of movement is obvious. Clinical indicators of AKI like blood urea nitrogen (BUN) are measurable. If liquid (PBS) resuscitation is given (intradermal PBS, up to 700 μL), mice recovery and progression of AKI is mitigated.

5. 16–18 hours post high dose LPS injection, mice look morbidant and are hypothermic. Clinical measurements like glomerular filtration rate drop. Mice can be sacrificed by carbon dioxide inhalation and the serum and renal tissue can be harvested for further analysis. Kidney injury can then be evaluated by serum analysis [blood urea nitrogen (BUN) and creatinine] and examination of renal expression of injury biomarkers like kidney injury molecule-1 (KIM1) and neutrophil gelatinase-associated lipocalin (NGAL). Blood urine nitrogen and enzymatic assay-based creatinine measurements can be performed in serum or plasma samples using commercially available kits.

6. Overall changes in histology are minimal. Even in severe sepsis, AKI can develop in the absence of overt histological or immune-histological changes and may be functional in nature. LPS-induced endotoxemia affects renal mitochondrial function and reduces PPARγ coactivator-1α (PGC-1α), the master regulator of mitochondrial biogenesis and metabolism and are excellent read outs for kidney pathology in this model.

7.2 Key notes

An increase in LPS-induced TNFα and TNFR1 directly damages the glomerular endothelial cell fenestrae and the glomerular endothelial surface layer [8]. We have shown that not only does LPS-induce AKI in mice, but the serum of mice injected with LPS also contains cytotoxic milieu that can directly cause renal epithelial cell death [51, 52]. Overall, these studies suggest that LPS-induced AKI can be an effect of direct activity of LPS on renal parenchyma and in parallel the SIRS like condition can result in cytokine driven renal parenchymal damage to collectively worsen outcomes. Given the dependency of this model on above mentioned variables, emphasis on the importance of testing in multiple, different animal models prior to advancing therapeutic agents into clinical trials is warranted.

8. Cecal-ligation and puncture (CLP)

Cecal ligation and puncture (CLP) is considered the gold standard model for sepsis research and one of the most frequently used procedures to induce experimental sepsis in laboratory settings [53, 54]. Unlike in LPS model, endotoxic shocks are rare in humans and sepsis origin is often localized and the CLP model mimics the nature and evolution of human sepsis [55]. After a simple procedure, CLP induces sepsis secondary to a stercoral peritonitis. This is followed by bacteremia with an early inflammatory phase, followed by an anti-inflammatory response [53]. However, significant variability in mortality from one experimental protocol to another can lead to differing interpretations of the results and S-AKI.

8.1 Methods

1. Majority of the studies in this model have been performed using male mice between 8 and 12 weeks of age. Age plays a critical role in susceptibility to injury in this model and the researchers should use appropriately aged mice depending upon their research questions.

2. Anesthetize the mice by intraperitoneal injection of a mixture of ketamine/xylazine. Isoflurane at a concentration between 3.5 to 4.5% with O_2 flow at 2 L/min can also be used. Scruff the mouse and shave the lower half of their

abdomen. Wipe done the shaved area 3 times alternating between 10% iodine and 70% ethanol. After the final ethanol wash, using either straight-edge or iris scissors, make a 1.5 cm midline cut into the skin only, approximately 0.5–1 cm away from xiphoid process.

3. Identify the abdominal wall and make another 1 cm midline cut into the peritoneum. In most instances, the cecum will be located directly under the incision. Exteriorize the cecum, align it and ligate it with a 2–0 silk suture. The cecum can be ligated at 5, 20 or 100% distal to the ileocecal valve. The ligation length is a major severity factor in CLP as the extent of the septic shock and hypotension, pro-inflammatory status, organ dysfunction, and hyperlactatemia are directly proportional to ligation length [56]. Following ligation, the cecum is punctured with a needle (generally 20–21 g) leading to leakage of fecal contents into the peritoneum. The puncture needs to be made in one pass, through and through both sides of the bowel wall. Some researchers apply pressure to release cecal contents into the peritoneal cavity. This part of the surgical manipulation is operator dependent and not well standardized across labs, resulting in differences in extent of injury and interpretation of outcomes.

4. Replace the ligated and punctured cecum into the abdomen. Close the abdominal wall with two 3–0 absorbable polyfilament interrupted sutures. Subsequently, approximate the skin using an auto-stapler. This part of the surgical manipulation is operator dependent and not well standardized across labs, resulting in differences in extent of injury and interpretation of outcomes. Inject 1 mL of saline/buprenorphine mix into the scruff of the animal's neck subcutaneously. Supportive treatment with fluids and antibiotics is too a variable and adds a new level of complexity [57]. Return the animals to their cages after they awaken from anesthesia.

5. With time, both Gram positive and negative bacterial species invade the blood stream, leading to a progressive systemic inflammatory response syndrome followed by septic shock and multiorgan injury including S-AKI [58, 59]. CLP-induced sepsis shows a cytokine profile like that observed in human sepsis [46, 60].

8.2 Key notes

CLP-induced sepsis increases lymphocyte apoptosis, which mimics immunosuppression during the late stage of human sepsis [61, 62]. In this respect, CLP-induced sepsis is completely different from LPS-induced sepsis and more closely mimics human sepsis. While we and others have reported that the CLP model can result in S-AKI [52, 63–66], AKI as measured by changes in BUN and creatinine is not always detected in this model [67, 68]. Thus, the standard CLP model amalgamates the common clinical features of human sepsis than the LPS model but misses some key features, especially acute lung injury [69] and variability in development of AKI.

9. Cecal slurry-induced peritonitis

Given the short comings and technical difficulties associated with existing models of sepsis, Gonnert *et. al* [70], developed a new model of sepsis by transferring human fecal matter into rats. This model, termed cecal slurry-induced sepsis

(CS) has since been adapted in both mice and rats, wherein the contents from the cecum of unmanipulated animals are suspended in liquid form and injected into the abdominal cavity of other animals to induce polymicrobial sepsis [71–73]. The CS model of sepsis was initially limited to those who study sepsis in neonatal mice [74], but now is also utilized to study the pathogenesis of sepsis in adult and old mice [75].

9.1 Methods

1. Generate sufficient cecal slurry by collecting cecal content from donor 16-week-old C57BL/6 mice was mixed with sterile water (0.5 mL per 100 mg cecal content). This is achieved by euthanizing the mouse by method of choice and collecting the entire cecal contents using sterile forceps and spatula. The collected cecal contents are combined, weighed, and mixed with sterile water at a ratio of 0.5 ml of water for 100 mg of cecal content. This slurry was sequentially filtered through 860-μm, 190-μm, and 70 μm mesh strainer without loss of bacteria. The filtered slurry was then mixed with an equal volume of 30% glycerol in phosphate buffered saline (PBS), resulting in a final CS stock solution in 15% glycerol.

2. Immediately after preparation of CS stock, an aliquot of CS should be serially diluted with sterile saline and plated onto multiple agar plates containing 3.7% w/v brain- heart infusion broth and 0.15% w/v agar to assess bacterial viability.

3. To induce polymicrobial sepsis using CS, mice (12–14 weeks) are used. The extent of sepsis induced is dependent on the CFU injected (from 4 to 6 X10 [4]) and age of the mice. 100 μL of CS, injected intraperitoneally is non-lethal to young and middle-aged mice but resulted in only 50% survival in aged mice [75]. The mortality increases with the volume injected. Since this model involves only a peritoneal injection, it is easy to perform and has less operator variability. Circulating bacteria levels strongly correlate with mortality in this model, suggesting an infection-mediated death.

9.2 Key notes

This model shows similar hemodynamic and physiological changes to those in human sepsis, is reproducible, and is operator-independent [76]. The development of S-AKI in this model is still understudied [77] and the induction of peritonitis by this model may not always induce kidney injury as shown recently by Shaver *et. al*[78]. However, since degree of early inflammation associated with this model is mild, it allows us to introduce other confounding like hemorrhage and investigate the finer mechanisms that can lead to S-AKI [78].

The principal reason for investigating different animal models of abdominal sepsis and its progression to S-AKI is eventually to develop therapies to treat sepsis and associated morbidities in a clinical setting. Therefore, the choice of animal model should incorporate and account for clinical caveats. Animal models of sepsis and S-AKI are essential for scientific understanding of human disease, but if they are not well characterized and understood, erroneous conclusions may be drawn, which can hinder scientific progress. A well-designed septic animal model requires a thorough understanding of the similarities and differences in the physiology of humans. To that end, the information presented in this chapter provides a systematic basis for the development of animal models for abdominal sepsis research. A perfect murine model of sepsis does not exist. While none of the current animal models manifest and replicate the intricacies of human sepsis and S-AKI, they provide a platform for sophisticated testing that is far beyond that of cell and tissue culture.

10. Conclusions

The pathophysiology of AKI is remarkably complex, due to the involvement of multiple cells types in the endothelium, renal tubules, and the immune system. To add to this complexity, AKI occurs in the setting of other diseases such as sepsis, rhabdomyolysis, cancer, and cardiovascular disorders, wherein the underlying disease or related therapies trigger renal dysfunction through complex mechanisms that remain incompletely understood. The animal models described in the current chapter reflect and recapitulate the complexities associated with AKI and are essential tools for studying the pathophysiological mechanisms that drive acute kidney injury.

Author details

Navjot Pabla[1], Yogesh Scindia[2], Joseph Gigliotti[3] and Amandeep Bajwa[4*]

1 Division of Pharmaceutics and Pharmacology, College of Pharmacy and Comprehensive Cancer Center, The Ohio State University, Columbus, Ohio, United States

2 Department of Medicine, University of Florida, Gainesville, Florida, United States

3 Department of Integrated Physiology and Pharmacology, College of Osteopathic Medicine, Liberty University, Lynchburg, Virginia, United States

4 Department of Surgery, Transplant Research Institute, James D. Eason Transplant Institute, Department of Microbiology, Immunology, and Biochemistry; Department of Genetics, Genomics, and Informatics; College of Medicine, The University of Tennessee Health Science Center, Memphis, Tennessee, United States

*Address all correspondence to: abajwa@uthsc.edu

References

[1] Zuk A, Bonventre JV: Acute Kidney Injury. Annu Rev Med 2016, 67:293-307.

[2] Bonventre JV, Yang L: Cellular pathophysiology of ischemic acute kidney injury. J Clin Invest 2011, 121:4210-21.

[3] Rosner MH, Okusa MD: Acute kidney injury associated with cardiac surgery. Clin J Am Soc Nephrol 2006, 1:19-32.

[4] Bosch X, Poch E, Grau JM: Rhabdomyolysis and acute kidney injury. N Engl J Med 2009, 361:62-72.

[5] Pabla N, Dong Z: Cisplatin nephrotoxicity: mechanisms and renoprotective strategies. Kidney Int 2008, 73:994-1007.

[6] Basile DP, Bonventre JV, Mehta R, Nangaku M, Unwin R, Rosner MH, Kellum JA, Ronco C, Group AXW: Progression after AKI: Understanding Maladaptive Repair Processes to Predict and Identify Therapeutic Treatments. J Am Soc Nephrol 2016, 27:687-97.

[7] de Caestecker M, Humphreys BD, Liu KD, Fissell WH, Cerda J, Nolin TD, Askenazi D, Mour G, Harrell FE, Jr., Pullen N, Okusa MD, Faubel S, Group AAA: Bridging Translation by Improving Preclinical Study Design in AKI. J Am Soc Nephrol 2015, 26:2905-16.

[8] Xu C, Chang A, Hack BK, Eadon MT, Alper SL, Cunningham PN: TNF-mediated damage to glomerular endothelium is an important determinant of acute kidney injury in sepsis. Kidney Int 2014, 85:72-81.

[9] Bonventre JV, Weinberg JM: Recent advances in the pathophysiology of ischemic acute renal failure. J Am Soc Nephrol 2003, 14:2199-210.

[10] Okusa MD: The inflammatory cascade in acute ischemic renal failure. Nephron 2002, 90:133-8.

[11] Bajwa A, Huang L, Kurmaeva E, Gigliotti JC, Ye H, Miller J, Rosin DL, Lobo PI, Okusa MD: Sphingosine 1-Phosphate Receptor 3-Deficient Dendritic Cells Modulate Splenic Responses to Ischemia-Reperfusion Injury. J Am Soc Nephrol 2015.

[12] Bajwa A, Huang L, Ye H, Dondeti K, Song S, Rosin DL, Lynch KR, Lobo PI, Li L, Okusa MD: Dendritic cell sphingosine 1-phosphate receptor-3 regulates Th1-Th2 polarity in kidney ischemia-reperfusion injury. J Immunol 2012, 189:2584-96.

[13] Rousselle TV, Kuscu C, Kuscu C, Schlegel K, Huang L, Namwanje M, Eason JD, Makowski L, Maluf D, Mas V, Bajwa A: FTY720 Regulates Mitochondria Biogenesis in Dendritic Cells to Prevent Kidney Ischemic Reperfusion Injury. Front Immunol 2020, 11:1278.

[14] Bajwa A, Huang L, Kurmaeva E, Ye H, Dondeti KR, Chroscicki P, Foley LS, Balogun ZA, Alexander KJ, Park H, Lynch KR, Rosin DL, Okusa MD: Sphingosine Kinase 2 Deficiency Attenuates Kidney Fibrosis via IFN-gamma. J Am Soc Nephrol 2017, 28:1145-61.

[15] Bajwa A, Jo SK, Ye H, Huang L, Dondeti KR, Rosin DL, Haase VH, Macdonald TL, Lynch KR, Okusa MD: Activation of sphingosine-1-phosphate 1 receptor in the proximal tubule protects against ischemia-reperfusion injury. J Am Soc Nephrol 2010, 21:955-65.

[16] Bajwa A, Rosin DL, Chroscicki P, Lee S, Dondeti K, Ye H, Kinsey GR, Stevens BK, Jobin K, Kenwood BM,

Hoehn KL, Lynch KR, Okusa MD: Sphingosine 1-phosphate receptor-1 enhances mitochondrial function and reduces cisplatin-induced tubule injury. J Am Soc Nephrol 2015, 26:908-25.

[17] Awad AS, Ye H, Huang L, Li L, Foss FW, Jr., Macdonald TL, Lynch KR, Okusa MD: Selective sphingosine 1-phosphate 1 receptor activation reduces ischemia-reperfusion injury in mouse kidney. Am J Physiol Renal Physiol 2006, 290:F1516-24.

[18] Xu X, Fan M, He X, Liu J, Qin J, Ye J: Aging aggravates long-term renal ischemia-reperfusion injury in a rat model. J Surg Res 2014, 187:289-96.

[19] Park KM, Kim JI, Ahn Y, Bonventre AJ, Bonventre JV: Testosterone is responsible for enhanced susceptibility of males to ischemic renal injury. J Biol Chem 2004, 279:52282-92.

[20] Filipski KK, Mathijssen RH, Mikkelsen TS, Schinkel AH, Sparreboom A: Contribution of organic cation transporter 2 (OCT2) to cisplatin-induced nephrotoxicity. Clin Pharmacol Ther 2009, 86:396-402.

[21] Pabla N, Murphy RF, Liu K, Dong Z: The copper transporter Ctr1 contributes to cisplatin uptake by renal tubular cells during cisplatin nephrotoxicity. Am J Physiol Renal Physiol 2009, 296:F505-11.

[22] Lam AQ, Humphreys BD: Onco-nephrology: AKI in the cancer patient. Clin J Am Soc Nephrol 2012, 7:1692-700.

[23] Pabla N, Dong G, Jiang M, Huang S, Kumar MV, Messing RO, Dong Z: Inhibition of PKCdelta reduces cisplatin-induced nephrotoxicity without blocking chemotherapeutic efficacy in mouse models of cancer. J Clin Invest 2011, 121:2709-22.

[24] Perse M, Veceric-Haler Z: Cisplatin-Induced Rodent Model of Kidney Injury: Characteristics and Challenges. Biomed Res Int 2018, 2018:1462802.

[25] Oda M, Koyanagi S, Tsurudome Y, Kanemitsu T, Matsunaga N, Ohdo S: Renal circadian clock regulates the dosing-time dependency of cisplatin-induced nephrotoxicity in mice. Mol Pharmacol 2014, 85:715-22.

[26] Kim JY, Bai Y, Jayne LA, Hector RD, Persaud AK, Ong SS, Rojesh S, Raj R, Feng M, Chung S, Cianciolo RE, Christman JW, Campbell MJ, Gardner DS, Baker SD, Sparreboom A, Govindarajan R, Singh H, Chen T, Poi M, Susztak K, Cobb SR, Pabla NS: A kinome-wide screen identifies a CDKL5-SOX9 regulatory axis in epithelial cell death and kidney injury. Nat Commun 2020, 11:1924.

[27] Kim JY, Bai Y, Jayne LA, Abdulkader F, Gandhi M, Perreau T, Parikh SV, Gardner DS, Davidson AJ, Sander V, Song MA, Bajwa A, Pabla NS: SOX9 promotes stress-responsive transcription of VGF nerve growth factor inducible gene in renal tubular epithelial cells. J Biol Chem 2020.

[28] Pabla N, Gibson AA, Buege M, Ong SS, Li L, Hu S, Du G, Sprowl JA, Vasilyeva A, Janke LJ, Schlatter E, Chen T, Ciarimboli G, Sparreboom A: Mitigation of acute kidney injury by cell-cycle inhibitors that suppress both CDK4/6 and OCT2 functions. Proc Natl Acad Sci U S A 2015, 112:5231-6.

[29] Hall MD, Telma KA, Chang KE, Lee TD, Madigan JP, Lloyd JR, Goldlust IS, Hoeschele JD, Gottesman MM: Say no to DMSO: dimethylsulfoxide inactivates cisplatin, carboplatin, and other platinum complexes. Cancer Res 2014, 74:3913-22.

[30] Plotnikov EY, Chupyrkina AA, Pevzner IB, Isaev NK, Zorov DB: Myoglobin causes oxidative stress, increase of NO production and

dysfunction of kidney's mitochondria. Biochim Biophys Acta 2009, 1792:796-803.

[31] Moore KP, Holt SG, Patel RP, Svistunenko DA, Zackert W, Goodier D, Reeder BJ, Clozel M, Anand R, Cooper CE, Morrow JD, Wilson MT, Darley-Usmar V, Roberts LJ, 2nd: A causative role for redox cycling of myoglobin and its inhibition by alkalinization in the pathogenesis and treatment of rhabdomyolysis-induced renal failure. J Biol Chem 1998, 273:31731-7.

[32] Kim JY, Bai Y, Jayne LA, Cianciolo RE, Bajwa A, Pabla NS: Involvement of the CDKL5-SOX9 signaling axis in rhabdomyolysis-associated acute kidney injury. 0:null.

[33] Baserga R, Thatcher D, Marzi D: Cell proliferation in mouse kidney after a single injection of folic acid. Lab Invest 1968, 19:92-6.

[34] Fink M, Henry M, Tange JD: Experimental folic acid nephropathy. Pathology 1987, 19:143-9.

[35] Shen Y, Jiang L, Wen P, Ye Y, Zhang Y, Ding H, Luo J, Xu L, Zen K, Zhou Y, Yang J: Tubule-derived lactate is required for fibroblast activation in acute kidney injury. Am J Physiol Renal Physiol 2020, 318:F689-F701.

[36] Xiao W, E J, Bao L, Fan Y, Jin Y, Wang A, Bauman D, Li Z, Zheng YL, Liu R, Lee K, He JC: Tubular HIPK2 is a key contributor to renal fibrosis. JCI Insight 2020, 5.

[37] Newbury LJ, Wang JH, Hung G, Hendry BM, Sharpe CC: Inhibition of Kirsten-Ras reduces fibrosis and protects against renal dysfunction in a mouse model of chronic folic acid nephropathy. Sci Rep 2019, 9:14010.

[38] Fleischmann C, Scherag A, Adhikari NK, Hartog CS, Tsaganos T, Schlattmann P, Angus DC, Reinhart K, International Forum of Acute Care T: Assessment of Global Incidence and Mortality of Hospital-treated Sepsis. Current Estimates and Limitations. Am J Respir Crit Care Med 2016, 193:259-72.

[39] Uchino S, Kellum JA, Bellomo R, Doig GS, Morimatsu H, Morgera S, Schetz M, Tan I, Bouman C, Macedo E, Gibney N, Tolwani A, Ronco C, Beginning, Ending Supportive Therapy for the Kidney I: Acute renal failure in critically ill patients: a multinational, multicenter study. JAMA 2005, 294:813-8.

[40] Bagshaw SM, Uchino S, Bellomo R, Morimatsu H, Morgera S, Schetz M, Tan I, Bouman C, Macedo E, Gibney N, Tolwani A, Oudemans-van Straaten HM, Ronco C, Kellum JA, Beginning, Ending Supportive Therapy for the Kidney I: Septic acute kidney injury in critically ill patients: clinical characteristics and outcomes. Clin J Am Soc Nephrol 2007, 2:431-9.

[41] Havasi A, Borkan SC: Apoptosis and acute kidney injury. Kidney Int 2011, 80:29-40.

[42] Zarjou A, Agarwal A: Sepsis and acute kidney injury. J Am Soc Nephrol 2011, 22:999-1006.

[43] Doi K, Leelahavanichkul A, Yuen PS, Star RA: Animal models of sepsis and sepsis-induced kidney injury. J Clin Invest 2009, 119:2868-78.

[44] Fink MP: Animal models of sepsis and its complications. Kidney Int 2008, 74:991-3.

[45] Poli-de-Figueiredo LF, Garrido AG, Nakagawa N, Sannomiya P: Experimental models of sepsis and their clinical relevance. Shock 2008, 30 Suppl 1:53-9.

[46] Remick DG, Ward PA: Evaluation of endotoxin models for the study of sepsis. Shock 2005, 24 Suppl 1:7-11.

[47] Nakano D, Kitada K, Wan N, Zhang Y, Wiig H, Wararat K, Yanagita M, Lee S, Jia L, Titze JM, Nishiyama A: Lipopolysaccharide induces filtrate leakage from renal tubular lumina into the interstitial space via a proximal tubular Toll-like receptor 4-dependent pathway and limits sensitivity to fluid therapy in mice. Kidney Int 2020, 97:904-12.

[48] Chen P, Stanojcic M, Jeschke MG: Differences between murine and human sepsis. Surg Clin North Am 2014, 94:1135-49.

[49] Deitch EA: Animal models of sepsis and shock: a review and lessons learned. Shock 1998, 9:1-11.

[50] Rittirsch D, Hoesel LM, Ward PA: The disconnect between animal models of sepsis and human sepsis. J Leukoc Biol 2007, 81:137-43.

[51] Leeds J, Scindia Y, Loi V, Wlazlo E, Ghias E, Cechova S, Portilla D, Ledesma J, Swaminathan S: Protective role of DJ-1 in endotoxin-induced acute kidney injury. Am J Physiol Renal Physiol 2020, 319:F654-F63.

[52] Scindia Y, Wlazlo E, Leeds J, Loi V, Ledesma J, Cechova S, Ghias E, Swaminathan S: Protective Role of Hepcidin in Polymicrobial Sepsis and Acute Kidney Injury. Front Pharmacol 2019, 10:615.

[53] Dejager L, Pinheiro I, Dejonckheere E, Libert C: Cecal ligation and puncture: the gold standard model for polymicrobial sepsis? Trends Microbiol 2011, 19:198-208.

[54] Mishra SK, Choudhury S: Experimental Protocol for Cecal Ligation and Puncture Model of Polymicrobial Sepsis and Assessment of Vascular Functions in Mice. Methods Mol Biol 2018, 1717:161-87.

[55] Hubbard WJ, Choudhry M, Schwacha MG, Kerby JD, Rue LW, 3rd, Bland KI, Chaudry IH: Cecal ligation and puncture. Shock 2005, 24 Suppl 1:52-7.

[56] Ruiz S, Vardon-Bounes F, Merlet-Dupuy V, Conil JM, Buleon M, Fourcade O, Tack I, Minville V: Sepsis modeling in mice: ligation length is a major severity factor in cecal ligation and puncture. Intensive Care Med Exp 2016, 4:22.

[57] Freise H, Bruckner UB, Spiegel HU: Animal models of sepsis. J Invest Surg 2001, 14:195-212.

[58] Ertel W, Morrison MH, Wang P, Ba ZF, Ayala A, Chaudry IH: The complex pattern of cytokines in sepsis. Association between prostaglandins, cachectin, and interleukins. Ann Surg 1991, 214:141-8.

[59] Holly MK, Dear JW, Hu X, Schechter AN, Gladwin MT, Hewitt SM, Yuen PS, Star RA: Biomarker and drug-target discovery using proteomics in a new rat model of sepsis-induced acute renal failure. Kidney Int 2006, 70:496-506.

[60] Eskandari MK, Bolgos G, Miller C, Nguyen DT, DeForge LE, Remick DG: Anti-tumor necrosis factor antibody therapy fails to prevent lethality after cecal ligation and puncture or endotoxemia. J Immunol 1992, 148:2724-30.

[61] Ayala A, Chaudry IH: Immune dysfunction in murine polymicrobial sepsis: mediators, macrophages, lymphocytes and apoptosis. Shock 1996, 6 Suppl 1:S27-38.

[62] Drewry AM, Samra N, Skrupky LP, Fuller BM, Compton SM, Hotchkiss RS: Persistent lymphopenia after diagnosis of sepsis predicts mortality. Shock 2014, 42:383-91.

[63] Haybron DM, Townsend MC, Hampton WW, Schirmer WJ,

Schirmer JM, Fry DE: Alterations in renal perfusion and renal energy charge in murine peritonitis. Arch Surg 1987, 122:328-31.

[64] Jorge LB, Coelho FO, Sanches TR, Malheiros D, Ezaquiel de Souza L, Dos Santos F, de Sa Lima L, Scavone C, Irigoyen M, Kuro OM, Andrade L: Klotho deficiency aggravates sepsis-related multiple organ dysfunction. Am J Physiol Renal Physiol 2019, 316:F438-F48.

[65] Li Y, Nourbakhsh N, Pham H, Tham R, Zuckerman JE, Singh P: Evolution of altered tubular metabolism and mitochondrial function in sepsis-associated acute kidney injury. Am J Physiol Renal Physiol 2020, 319:F229-F44.

[66] Yang S, Hauptman JG: The efficacy of heparin and antithrombin III in fluid-resuscitated cecal ligation and puncture. Shock 1994, 2:433-7.

[67] Kuhlmann MK, Shahmir E, Maasarani E, Akhtar S, Thevanayagam V, Vadgama JV, Kopple JD: New experimental model of acute renal failure and sepsis in rats. JPEN J Parenter Enteral Nutr 1994, 18:477-85.

[68] Pedersen PV, Warner BW, Bjornson HS, Hiyama DT, Li S, Rigel DF, Hasselgren PO, Fischer JE: Hemodynamic and metabolic alterations during experimental sepsis in young and adult rats. Surg Gynecol Obstet 1989, 168:148-56.

[69] Iskander KN, Craciun FL, Stepien DM, Duffy ER, Kim J, Moitra R, Vaickus LJ, Osuchowski MF, Remick DG: Cecal ligation and puncture-induced murine sepsis does not cause lung injury. Crit Care Med 2013, 41:159-70.

[70] Gonnert FA, Recknagel P, Seidel M, Jbeily N, Dahlke K, Bockmeyer CL, Winning J, Losche W, Claus RA, Bauer M: Characteristics of clinical sepsis reflected in a reliable and reproducible rodent sepsis model. J Surg Res 2011, 170:e123-34.

[71] Gentile LF, Nacionales DC, Lopez MC, Vanzant E, Cuenca A, Cuenca AG, Ungaro R, Szpila BE, Larson S, Joseph A, Moore FA, Leeuwenburgh C, Baker HV, Moldawer LL, Efron PA: Protective immunity and defects in the neonatal and elderly immune response to sepsis. J Immunol 2014, 192:3156-65.

[72] Gentile LF, Nacionales DC, Lopez MC, Vanzant E, Cuenca A, Szpila BE, Cuenca AG, Joseph A, Moore FA, Leeuwenburgh C, Baker HV, Moldawer LL, Efron PA: Host responses to sepsis vary in different low-lethality murine models. PLoS One 2014, 9:e94404.

[73] Wynn JL, Scumpia PO, Delano MJ, O'Malley KA, Ungaro R, Abouhamze A, Moldawer LL: Increased mortality and altered immunity in neonatal sepsis produced by generalized peritonitis. Shock 2007, 28:675-83.

[74] Brook B, Amenyogbe N, Ben-Othman R, Cai B, Harbeson D, Francis F, Liu AC, Varankovich N, Wynn J, Kollmann TR: A Controlled Mouse Model for Neonatal Polymicrobial Sepsis. J Vis Exp 2019.

[75] Starr ME, Steele AM, Saito M, Hacker BJ, Evers BM, Saito H: A new cecal slurry preparation protocol with improved long-term reproducibility for animal models of sepsis. PLoS One 2014, 9:e115705.

[76] Lee MJ, Kim K, Jo YH, Lee JH, Hwang JE: Dose-dependent mortality and organ injury in a cecal slurry peritonitis model. J Surg Res 2016, 206:427-34.

[77] Jian W, Gu L, Williams B, Feng Y, Chao W, Zou L: Toll-like Receptor 7

Contributes to Inflammation, Organ Injury, and Mortality in Murine Sepsis. Anesthesiology 2019, 131:105-18.

[78] Shaver CM, Paul MG, Putz ND, Landstreet SR, Kuck JL, Scarfe L, Skrypnyk N, Yang H, Harrison FE, de Caestecker MP, Bastarache JA, Ware LB: Cell-free hemoglobin augments acute kidney injury during experimental sepsis. Am J Physiol Renal Physiol 2019, 317:F922-F9.

Chapter 8

Animal Pain Models for Spinal Cord Stimulation

Joseph M. Williams, Courtney A. Kelley, Ricardo Vallejo, David C. Platt and David L. Cedeño

Abstract

Spinal cord stimulation (SCS) is an electrical neuromodulation technique with proven effectiveness and safety for the treatment of intractable chronic pain in humans. Despite its widespread use, the mechanism of action is not fully understood. Animal models of chronic pain, particularly rodent-based, have been adapted to study the effect of SCS on pain-like behavior, as well as on the electrophysiology and molecular biology of neural tissues. This chapter reviews animal pain models for SCS, emphasizing on findings relevant to advancing our understanding of the mechanism of action of SCS, and highlighting the contribution of the animal model to advance clinical outcomes. The models described include those in which SCS has been coupled to neuropathic pain models in rats and sheep based on peripheral nerve injuries, including the chronic constriction injury (CCI) model and the spared nerve injury model (SNI). Other neuropathic pain models described are the spinal nerve ligation (SNL) for neuropathic pain of segmental origin, as well as the chemotherapy-induced and diabetes-induced peripheral neuropathy models. We also describe the use of SCS with inflammatory pain and ischemic pain models.

Keywords: spinal cord stimulation, animal models, neuropathic pain, inflammatory pain, ischemia

1. Introduction

The field of electrical neuromodulation was developed under the hypothesis that the activation of large, myelinated nerve fibers could modulate sensory nociceptive signals carried by A-delta and C nerve fibers into the dorsal horn in the spinal cord. The gate control theory (GCT) formulated by Melzack and Wall [1], served as inspiration for the use of peripheral nerve stimulation and spinal cord stimulation (SCS) to treat pain. The simplicity of the proposed mechanism, based on the understanding of pain in 1965, granted researchers with the ability to formulate finite mathematical and complex computational models to assess the effects of different variables of the electrical signal on the neuronal conduction. The GCT's enduring value in neuromodulation for more than 50 years is due to its simplicity and utility as a working tool to postulate therapies to patients in pain. Unfortunately, as the German psychologist Wolfgang Köhler explains: "premature simplifications and systematization in science, could ossify science and prevent vital growth" [2].

The early 1990s marked the beginning of a revolution in the field of neuroscience in understanding the mechanism of pathological pain from a molecular perspective. The use of animal models has helped unravel the role of neuroinflammatory processes driven by glial cells in the development and maintenance of chronic neuropathic pain. Those advances though, were largely neglected in the field of electrical neuromodulation, which remained focused on the effects of electrical signals on neuronal conduction, ignoring the benefit of understanding how these signals could affect biological processes at the neuron-glia interaction. The differential electrophysiological characteristics of neurons and glial cells is now at the core of our quest to understand how electrical signals affect such biological processes. To begin with, the resting membrane potential of these cell populations is different, driven by the fact that the main neuronal intracellular cation is potassium, while sodium is the predominant one in glial cells [3]. Considering the critical roles that various specialized glial cell populations play in the intimate communication between neurons and glial cells, it is pertinent to briefly describe these roles. Following peripheral injury, persistent release of neurotransmitters at the synaptic cleft activates microglial and astrocyte membrane receptors generating transcriptional changes that generate the synthesis and release of pro-inflammatory and anti-inflammatory cytokines. Astrocytes are critical to maintain homeostasis at the synapse. The synaptic cleft is surrounded by astroglial perisynaptic processes in what is now known as the tripartite synapse. Perisynaptic glial processes are densely packed with numerous transporters, which provide proper homeostasis of ions and neurotransmitters in the synaptic cleft, for local metabolism support, and for release of astroglia-derived scavengers of oxygen species [4]. For example, membrane ionotropic and metabotropic glutamate receptors in the astrocyte regulate glutamate concentration. Interestingly, a single astrocyte provides processes that extend over distance to surround over 100,000 synapses. During intense neuronal firing, the release of neurotransmitters, such as glutamate and GABA, induces the elevation of calcium ion concentrations in glial cells, causing Ca^{2+}-dependent release of molecules that affects neural excitability and synaptic transmission and plasticity. Even more thought-provoking is that although astrocytes are unable to generate action potentials, they can raise intracellular calcium concentrations that spread from astrocyte to astrocyte through gap channels that allow propagation of so-called calcium waves as a way of cell-to-cell communication. The presence of Ca^{2+}mobilizations mediated by astrocytes implies that glial cells have some excitability and neuromodulator activities [5]. Finally, oligodendrocytes provide myelin to hundreds of surrounding axons and are known to affect the conduction velocity of action potentials propagating along the axons they surround when electrically stimulated [6].

An important distinction between glial cells and neurons is that glial cells depolarize following electrical stimulation, but do not generate action potentials. In 1981, Roitbak and Fanardjian [7] demonstrated in a live feline model that changes in the frequency and intensity of the applied pulsed electrical signals could lead to differential degrees of astrocytic depolarization. Another interesting clue on how electrical signals could affect glial cells was provided by Agnesi et al. [8], in an experiment with anesthetized rats that showed that changing the repolarization of an electrical stimulation signal from monophasic to a biphasic led to different degrees of glutamate release by the stimulated astrocytes.

The complexity of changes in neuron-glial biological processes triggered by pain and further modulation by electrical stimulation demands the use of experimental animal models. Testing such hypotheses in humans would require large-scale, well-controlled clinical trials because of the heterogeneity of genetics and pain etiology in the general population [9].

The notable anatomical, biological, and physiological resemblances between humans and animals, predominantly mammals, have encouraged researchers to investigate a large range of mechanisms and assess novel therapies in animal models before applying their discoveries to humans.

Scientists cross-examine organisms at multiple levels: molecules, cells, organs, and physiological functions in healthy or diseased conditions. Advance molecular technologies are required to get a complete portrayal and understanding of the mechanisms. Certain aspects of the responses can be evaluated using in vitro approaches (e.g., cell culture). On the other hand, the exploration of physiological functions and systemic interactions between organs requires a whole organism.

This chapter explores the efforts of diverse research groups to understand from a behavioral and molecular perspective, how spinal cord stimulation affects pathological pain by utilizing animal models. This research may provide strong hypotheses on what may be happening in humans and ways to continue improving therapeutic efficacy.

The following sections provide a description of existing, well-validated models for pain caused by neuropathies, inflammation, and ischemic conditions. Due to technical limitations, most of these are based on *Rattus norvegicus*, although recently models in a larger animal (*Ovis aries*) have been developed.

2. Animal models of SCS for neuropathic pain

Neuropathic pain is caused by damaged somatosensory neural circuits that have developed into a disease condition as a result of an injury that compromised nerve fibers. Chronic neuropathic pain affects hundreds of millions of people around the world and is one of the main sources of work-related disabilities, contributing to the socioeconomical burden on individuals as well as health systems [10]. SCS is largely indicated for chronic neuropathic pain conditions, thus the development of various animal models that resemble clinical conditions play a critical role in our understanding of the electrophysiological and molecular changes in the establishment and persistence of neuropathic pain.

2.1 SCS in partial nerve injury models

Prior to the development of the chronic constriction injury (CCI) model, animal models of pain often were lacking in their ability to accurately mimic human peripheral neuropathological conditions or did not reflect conditions involving injuries which spared a portion of a nerve's functioning [11]. The CCI model most commonly used was described by Bennet and Xie in 1988 [11]. The procedure typically involves exposing the common sciatic nerve under anesthesia at the level of the mid-thigh and freeing approximately 7 mm of the sciatic nerve from adhering tissue at a location proximal to the sciatic nerve's trifurcation. Once exposed, four sutures are tied loosely around the sciatic nerve approximately 1-2 mm apart from one another. These ligatures are tied loose enough to just barely constrict the diameter of the sciatic nerve (as observed under 25x-40x magnification), thus preserving partial nerve functioning [11–16]. Constriction of the sciatic nerve was observed histologically beneath all 4 ligature areas as early as one day following the CCI procedure. From days 2-21, adjacent constriction areas tended to progressively merge and were accompanied by thinning of the affected sciatic nerve area. Two to four months after the CCI procedure, thinning of the ligated area was still present, but the swellings typically observed in the area had dissipated.

Importantly, this CCI model has proven to be effective in eliciting a neuropathic pain state as measured by a variety of methods, including von Frey mechanical, chemogenic, and heat and cold thermal stimulation. CCI surgery typically resulted in increased paw sensitivity following von Frey stimulation by Day 2 post-lesion using both the up-down method of analysis [12, 15, 16] and the ascending filament method of analysis [12–14]. The CCI model is also sensitive to chemogenic pain. Following the application of a noxious substance (a 50% mustard oil solution) to the affected hind paw, CCI rats exhibited exaggerated physical responses and an increase in the amount of time they held their hind paw above the floor of the apparatus [11]. CCI rats also showed hypersensitivity to noxious heat sources, such as radiant beams of light being applied to the affected hind paw [11, 16] and increased allodynic responses to cold, such as a slightly chilled metal floor [11].

Although most applications of the CCI model with SCS have been performed in rats, an ovine model has also been effectively demonstrated [17]. In rats, application of SCS with pulsed signals at 50 Hz frequency, 0.2 ms pulse width (PW), and intensity at 66% of the motor threshold (MT) for 30 minutes [12, 14] decreased pain sensitivity following CCI, but did not return pain levels back to pre-injury control levels. Similar results were obtained when SCS was applied for 180 minutes in rats with CCI lesions using the following SCS parameters: 50 Hz frequency, 0.2 ms PW at 80% of the MT [12]. Lowering the intensity to 20-40% of the MT eliminated the beneficial effect of SCS. Electrodes in these rat studies were aimed at the T11-L1 regions of the spinal cord. In sheep, SCS parameters were set at 40 Hz frequency, 120 μs PW and 0.1 V intensity on a continuous setting for one week with electrodes placed at the L2-L3 region. SCS also attenuated pain responses following CCI in sheep, though also failed to return pain levels back to pre-lesion levels [17]. Most SCS studies following CCI typically utilized conventional (also called tonic) SCS at a stimulating frequency of 50 Hz. However, a more detailed investigation of frequency on treatment outcomes (in which frequency varied from 1 Hz to 150 Hz) found a response curve that suggested that while the GCT could account for a subset of efficacious SCS responses, it is unlikely to be the only mechanism underlying the beneficial effects of SCS [18].

In addition to demonstrating that SCS was effective in decreasing pain sensitivity, the CCI model also has proven valuable in elucidating the biological mechanisms behind the increase in pain following injury and the beneficial effect of SCS. After CCI lesions, rats exhibited an increase in the toll-like receptor 4 and nuclear factor κβ [15, 16], which subsequently could increase the release of pro-inflammatory cytokines such as IL-1β, IL-6, and TNF-α. SCS significantly reduced these CCI-induced increases, perhaps by inhibiting the activation of glial cells. Indeed, the co-administration of the microglial inhibitor minocycline was shown to decrease CCI-induced pain and prolonged the effect of SCS [12]. However, this same study also showed an increase in the microglial-reactive marker OX-42 and the astrocyte reactive marker GFAP in the lumbar region of CCI-lesioned rats following SCS treatment. This paradoxical increase may limit the effectiveness of SCS and may partially explain why SCS is not effective in all patients and why pain relief often does not return to baseline levels following SCS. Other studies utilizing SCS in CCI-lesioned rats have identified roles of the adenosine and GABAergic systems in mediating the beneficial effects of SCS. Administration of adenosine or the adenosine A1 receptor agonist R-N6-phenylisopropyladenosine (R-PIA), decreased pain in CCI rats [14]. In addition, giving sub-effective doses of R-PIA to non-responders to SCS during stimulation led to effective pain relief. Zhang et al. [18] also found that administration of bicuculline, a $GABA_A$ receptor antagonist, decreased inhibitory responses to SCS.

Although the CCI model has provided significant value in (1) serving as a valid model of neuropathic pain, (2) demonstrating that the use of SCS is effective in reducing neuropathic pain, and (3) advancing our understanding of the biological mechanisms underlying SCS, its use has perhaps been surpassed in recent years by another animal model of partial nerve injury called partial sciatic nerve ligation (PSNL). Most PSNL studies utilize the Seltzer technique [19]. The procedure typically involves exposing the sciatic nerve under anesthesia at high-thigh level. The sciatic nerve is freed from adhering tissue at a location near the trochanter just distal to the point at which the posterior biceps semitendinosus nerve branches off the common sciatic nerve. Once the sciatic nerve is properly exposed, a suture with a curved cutting mini needle is inserted into the nerve. Unlike the CCI procedure, which involves a loose ligation of the sciatic nerve, the PSNL procedure involves tightly ligating approximately 1/3 to 1/2 of the dorsal nerve thickness [19, 20]. As with the CCI procedure, the goal is to partially reduce, but not completely block sciatic nerve functioning.

Similar to the CCI model, the PSNL model also successfully induces a neuropathic pain state as measured by a variety of methods. The primary method is to assess mechanical allodynia using von Frey filaments [21–23]. Following PSNL surgery, rats show a decreased paw withdrawal response following mechanical stimulation of the affected paw, as compared to control rats, pre-surgery baseline levels, and paw withdrawal thresholds (PWT) following stimulation of the contralateral, unaffected paw [23, 24]. This increased pain sensitivity usually develops by Day 2 post-PSNL lesion [21] and is still typically observed after two weeks post-PSNL lesion [20, 24, 25]. Meuwissen et al. [26] recorded decreased PWT over 40 days following the PSNL lesion. Although the PSNL technique overall has been successful in inducing a neuropathic pain state, it should be noted that there is a wide range of pain responsiveness across studies, with some studies reporting 100% of subjects exhibiting hyperalgesia with von Frey testing of the affected hind paw [20, 24] and other studies reporting less than 40% of subjects showing hyperalgesia [27, 28]. Increased paw sensitivity to thermal stimuli has also been observed following the presentation of both heat stimuli (e.g., a radiant light beam) and cold stimuli, such as a cold spray directed at the affected paw [19, 29]. However, the degree of thermal sensitivity can vary depending upon the location of the PSNL ligature. Other studies have also confirmed hypersensitivity to pain following PSNL surgery by using a pneumatic pressure device [30] and by observing gait/posture [31]. Overall, the PSNL technique has proven successful at inducing a neuropathic pain state as assessed by numerous methodologies.

The PSNL model has also proven effective at evaluating SCS treatment for chronic neuropathic pain. Both tonic and burst SCS attenuated the pain sensitivity observed in rat PSNL neuropathic pain models [20, 24]. In rats, tonic SCS (50 Hz frequency, 0.2 ms PW, intensity at 66% of the MT) attenuated PSNL-induced hyperalgesia following 30 minutes of stimulation [23, 32, 33] and 60 minutes of stimulation [20, 22, 24]. Though tonic SCS successfully decreased pain sensitivity, SCS treatment typically did not return pain levels in rats back to pre-injury control levels. In a mouse model, SCS treatment following PSNL lesions proved particularly efficacious, with 80% of mice in one study [34] and 100% of mice in another study [25] responding positively to tonic SCS treatment. In this latter study, unlike the typical rat study, the mice returned to baseline levels of paw withdrawal following SCS treatment.

Although most rat studies investigating the effect of SCS following PSNL lesions have utilized conventional stimulation parameters and have shown a significant benefit of tonic SCS treatment, it is clear that not all PSNL rat subjects benefit from SCS treatment, leading researchers to investigate different SCS parameters in hopes of improving efficacy. Some factors that have proved to have significant impact on SCS efficacy following PSNL lesions include: (1) electrode placement, (2) stimulus intensity, (3) timing of treatment, and (4) utilizing a burst (vs tonic) stimulation pattern. Electrodes placed at the T13 level of the spinal cord typically yielded more efficacious treatment outcomes than electrodes placed at the T11 area [28, 31, 35] or L5 and L6 regions [36]. In a study that directly compared the efficacy of electrode location at T13 and T11 [21], the T13 placement yielded significantly better pain relief than placement at T11 with 63% vs 15% improvement, respectively, following 15 minutes of electrical stimulation and 48.5% vs. 18.4% improvement, respectively, following 30 minutes of electrical stimulation. Lowering the intensity to

30-50% of the MT reduced the beneficial effect of tonic SCS [24]. In terms of timing, early SCS treatment given within 24 hours of lesion led to significantly better treatment outcomes than late SCS given 16 days post-lesion [32]. Interestingly, an early round of SCS treatment followed by a subsequent late round of SCS treatment increased the efficacy of the late SCS treatment [37]. Lastly, burst stimulation typically led to similar response rates as tonic stimulation [20, 22, 26]. However, burst stimulation patterns did produce slightly different outcomes. For instance, one study [24] found that tonic SCS was most effective at 66% of the MT, while burst SCS was most effective at 50% of the MT. In addition, burst stimulation took longer following stimulus onset to achieve therapeutic benefits, but the benefits of the burst stimulation lasted longer after the stimulation was turned off [38]. Burst SCS stimulation also led to greater performance than tonic SCS on a mechanical conflict avoidance system (MCAS) task which measured the cognitive-motivational aspects of pain, rather than the more typical mechanical allodynic physical response to pain [26]. These results suggest that although equally efficacious, tonic, and burst SCS stimulation may work, at least in part, by different biological mechanisms.

Given the beneficial effect of SCS treatment following PSNL lesions, many PSNL studies have sought to investigate the biological mechanisms behind it. Many studies have utilized a paradigm in which sub-effective doses of pharmaceutical treatments are given to SCS non-responders to determine if the combination of these treatments can yield beneficial effects. Song et al. [29] showed that sub-effective doses of the muscarinic agonist oxotremorine turned SCS non-responders into SCS responders, suggesting that the cholinergic system (particularly M2 and M4 muscarinic receptors) plays an important role in SCS efficacy. A subsequent study by these same authors [39] indicated an important serotonergic role in the pain-relieving effect of SCS, particularly the 5-HT2A and 5-HT4 serotonin receptor subtypes. Similarly, blocking NMDA receptors with sub-effective doses of ketamine followed by 30 minutes of SCS also turned SCS non-responders into SCS responders, indicating that the glutamate system also plays an important role in the beneficial effects of SCS [22]. While blocking the excitatory glutamatergic system likely plays a role in successful SCS treatment, enhancing the inhibitory GABAergic system might also play a significant role in successful SCS treatment [27, 32]. SCS treatment decreased intracellular GABA levels in SCS responders but not SCS non-responders [32], while increasing extracellular GABA levels in the spinal cord [27]. Lastly, SCS stimulation in PSNL rats also led to an increase in levels of *c-fos*, suggesting immediate early gene modulation may trigger longer term changes which could explain pain relief both during and after SCS stimulation [40]. Overall, PSNL has proven to be a valuable tool in examining the biological mechanisms behind the beneficial treatment effects of SCS.

2.2 SCS in the spared nerve injury model

The Spared Nerve Injury (SNI) was developed by Decosterd and Woolf in 2000 [41] to evaluate peripheral neuropathic pain in the rat model. The SNI is considered superior to previous denervation and partial denervation models due to its specificity of the affected region, as well as its prompt and long-lasting effect. Unlike other models that were designed to test acute nociceptive pain through behavioral and electrophysiological measurements, denervation and partial denervation models induce sensations such as hypersensitivity that more accurately reflect true clinical chronic pain conditions.

The SNI procedure targets the sciatic nerve at its point of trifurcation (**Figure 1A**) in the hindlimb of the rat. Located directly under the biceps femoris muscle, the nerves are exposed and identified as the tibial, common peroneal, and

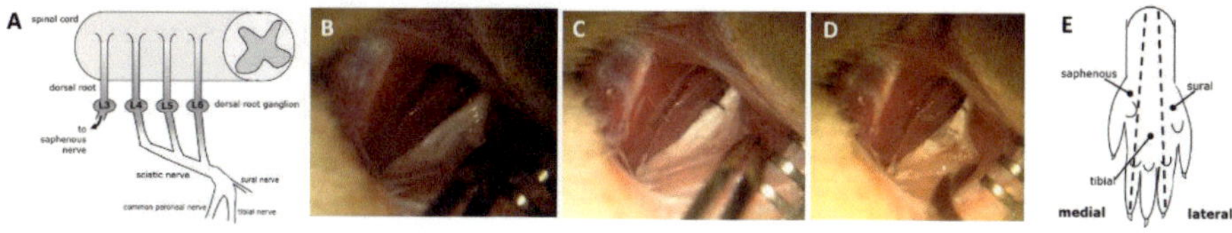

Figure 1.
(A) A scheme depicting the anatomical innervation of the sciatic nerve into the spinal cord of the rat. (B-D) Photographic sequence of the localization, ligation, and sectioning of the tibial and peroneal nerves. (E) Map of nerve coverage to plantar hind paw surfaces.

sural branches (**Figure 1B**). Distal to the point of trifurcation and in the direction of the terminal end, both the tibial and common peroneal branches are individually ligated with silk sutures (**Figure 1C**). Then, 2–4 mm of nerve is sectioned and removed to ensure a complete disruption of nerve transmission (**Figure 1D**). The incision is then closed, leaving the sural branch fully intact and undisturbed. Minor amendments, such as carefully separating the gluteus superficialis and biceps femoris muscles instead of cutting through to expose the sciatic nerve, were made in some later studies in attempt to reduce unnecessary tissue damage [42]. Hypersensitivity is rapidly established in this model, with behavioral onset occurring at just 24 hours post-induction, lasting no less than 6 months, with peak sensitivity around 2 weeks [41]. The duration of the SNI effectiveness allows for considerable flexibility when considering study design. Per the original study, non-responders are virtually nonexistent so long as the model is induced correctly.

As shown in **Figure 1E**, the hind paw of the rat is subdivided into three zones which are innervated by the sciatic and saphenous nerves. Transecting two of the three sciatic nerve branches, allows for precise and consistent behavioral testing of the lateral portion of plantar surface, corresponding to the sural nerve. This model permits mechanical and thermal allodynia, as well as thermal hyperalgesia to be evaluated [41] and has been used extensively in basic science studies investigating the use spinal cord stimulation (SCS) for the treatment of neuropathic pain.

In 2015, the SNI-SCS model was taken a step further when Tilley et al. [42] developed a model of continuous stimulation in an awake and freely moving rat, allowing stimulation to be delivered for 72 continuous hours. This method allowed for more clinically relevant testing since human patients receive continuous stimulation. A miniaturized four-electrode cylindrical lead was implanted in the epidural space of the rat and anchored into the musculature in the back (**Figure 2**). The lead exited through the incision and was secured through a custom-made harness and tubing up to a circuit board and stimulator suspended in a swivel so that the full assembly could turn and move with the rat. The rat cage lid was modified to allow free movement of the tubing. In later studies, the lead has been attached to an ethernet port secured to the rat harness with a coiled ethernet cord running to the stimulator connector suspended in the swivel [43]. Mechanical (von Frey filament) and cold thermal (acetone drop) allodynia were tested in this study. SCS was set at 50 Hz frequency, 20 μs PW, and at 70% of the MT. While there was no apparent improvement in cold allodynia following SCS, mechanical allodynia was significantly alleviated 24 and 72 hours after the start of SCS. A follow-up genomic study revealed the biological processes uniquely modulated by the SNI model and SCS in the spinal cord and dorsal root ganglion tissues (**Table 1**) [44]. The primary affected processes in both types of tissues included inflammatory response, ion channel regulation, and immune response.

Following the initial development of the SNI model, Li et al. [35] tested variations in an effort to optimize the model specifically for SCS studies. The study included the original SNI procedure, peroneal axotomy, tibial axotomy, tibial tight ligation (no sectioning), and partial tibial ligation (1/3 to 1/2 of its diameter ligated,

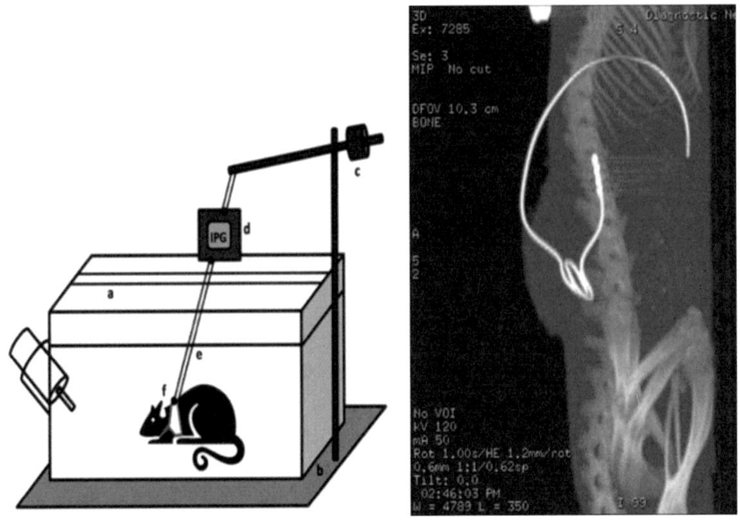

Figure 2.
Left: A diagram of the setup for continuous SCS setup reported in references [42, 44]. a: plexiglass lid, b: supporting floor, c: counterweight swivel system, d: connecting board/stimulator (IPG), e: connecting cable, f: harness with lead connector. Right: a lateral x-ray image showing a quadripolar SCS lead placed in the dorsal epidural space of a rat.

without sectioning). SCS was delivered through an implanted 2 mm disc cathode placed on the dura at the T11 level. The 4 mm anode was placed on the chest wall, subcutaneously. Stimulation parameters were set at 50 Hz frequency, 0.2 ms PW, and amplitude at 90% of the MT. SCS was delivered for a 30-minute duration. Measuring mechanical allodynia via von Frey filament testing, authors found that all variations of the model produced allodynia within one week, lasting for at least 3 weeks. All variations except the partial tibial ligation lasted 7-10 weeks. Paw posture was noted as one difference between models, where peroneal axotomy resulted in an inverted position of the paw which tended to be dragged behind the rat. The other variations presented an eversion posture, with the partial tibial ligation being less prominent. Contrary to the original study, where no non-responders were reported and the contralateral hypersensitivity rate was zero, Li et al. found only 53% of SNI operated rats developed hypersensitivity and 25% had some hypersensitivity in the contralateral paw. Response to SCS showed the SNI group with the smallest responder rate at just 8%, compared to the 40-50% responder rate of the variation groups. The researchers concluded there was an inverse relationship between degree of hypersensitivity and efficacy of SCS, agreeing with previous literature in similar models [45], and that these variations of the SNI may provide better models for use in SCS animal studies. However, it should be mentioned that some later studies report higher responder rates to the original variation of the SNI model and subsequent SCS treatment.

Most recently, Sluka and coworkers [46] evaluated tonic SCS on multiple pain models, including the SNI. Implanting an epidural lead and corresponding neurostimulator, the rats were stimulated for 15 minutes per day at 60 Hz, 0.25 ms PW, and at 90% of the MT. Two weeks after SNI induction, the effect of SCS was evaluated. They found that neuropathic pain was alleviated by tonic SCS, measured by von Frey filaments, with significantly increased withdrawal thresholds. Twenty-four hours after stimulation was turned off, behavioral testing revealed that the effect of SCS was lost. The authors attribute the analgesic effect of tonic SCS on the SNI model to the activation of large Aβ dorsal column axons (supporting the GCT), as well as the electrochemical alteration of cell membranes and the involvement of neurotransmitters, receptors, and glial cells.

	FDR *p*-value (increase/decrease)	Relevant Biological Processes Modulated by SCS in the SNI model
Spinal Cord	0.063 (↑)	Inflammatory response; Immune related
	0.097 (↓)	Ion channel regulation (Voltage gated); Generation of neurons; synaptic transmission
	0.057 (↓)	Vesicle transport; regulation of calcium ion
	0.064 (↓)	Cell growth; cell activity pathways such as MAPKK, JUN kinase
	0.011 (↑)	Ribosomal proteins, 50% unknown proteins
	0.069 (↓)	Ion transport (cation and anion); GABA signaling, neuron development
	0.011 (↓)	Transmembrane/transporter activity, mostly ion transport; proton transport
	0.011 (↓)	Cell regulation changes; neuron differentiation and development
	0.016 (↑)	Activation of immune response
Dorsal Root Ganglion	0.012 (↓)	Ion transmembrane transport
	0.012 (↓)	Mitochondrial respiratory chain; regulation of superoxide, mechano-sensory perception of pain
	0.009 (↑)	Inflammatory response: cytokine and apoptosis regulation; Immune response to stimulus
	0.009 (↑)	Innate immune response; Adaptive immune response
	0.009 (↑)	Regulation of immune response: T-cell activation and differentiation
	0.074 (↑)	Histone acetylation; regulation of neuron migration; regulation of rho GTPase activity
	0.018 (↑)	Cell adhesion; cell development, wound healing
	0.086 (↓)	Calcium ion transmembrane transport
	0.062 (↑)	Cell development; extracellular matrix organization

Table 1.
Gene ontology biological processes modulated in the ipsilateral dorsal quadrant of the spinal cord (directly under the electrode) and ipsilateral L5 dorsal root ganglion demonstrating molecular changes caused by SCS therapy with the SNI model. Reelevant processes obtained after WGCNA and gene ontology analyses performed on microarray results. Only modules with significant False Discovery Rate (FDR) p-values are shown. Data from reference [44].

Previously, this group looked at frequency-dependent outcomes of SCS, particularly regarding opioid receptors [47] and glial cell activation with SCS [48]. In the opioid receptor study [47], SNI-induced rats were administered naloxone or naltrindole (both opioid antagonists), or were made morphine tolerant. Rats then received SCS at 4 Hz, 60 Hz, or no SCS daily for 6-hour periods, lasting 4 days for each treatment. Testing for mechanical allodynia, they found naloxone prevented the analgesic effect produced by 4 Hz and 60 Hz stimulation, though a higher dose was required to block the effect of 60 Hz. Interestingly, naltrindole had no effect on 4 Hz SCS, but successfully impeded the effect of 60 Hz SCS. When testing the morphine-tolerant rats, they found that 4 Hz SCS did not have the same analgesic effect that it did in normal rats, while 60 Hz stimulation remained efficacious. This work resulted in the understanding that the frequency of SCS may determine the mechanism by which pain relief is achieved, and in this case, engaging different opioid receptors.

Glial activation, via immunohistochemical staining with known markers (GFAP, MCP-1, and OX-42), was measured in a separate study using 30-minute and 6-hour SCS durations and varying the intensity (as percent of the MT) [48]. Two weeks after the SNI was induced, mechanical hypersensitivity increased, as expected, as well as glial cell activity. The results indicated that withdrawal thresholds were positively correlated with increasing SCS duration (6 h vs 30 min) and by stimulating at higher intensities (90% vs 75% vs 50% MT). Glial cell activation was significantly decreased in both 4 and 60 Hz SCS, delivered for 6 hours at 90% MT.

Additional studies focused on the question of frequency importance in SCS, utilizing the SNI as a pain model. Song et al. investigated conventional 50 Hz (200 μs PW, 80% MT) SCS compared to high frequency (HF) SCS at lower intensity (500, 1000, and 10000 Hz; 24 μs PW, 40–50% MT) [49]. A miniaturized 4-electrode plate lead was implanted into the epidural space of the T13 vertebral level. Performing behavioral testing for mechanical hypersensitivity (von Frey filaments) and thermal hypersensitivity (ethyl chloride spray for cold, modified Hargreaves test for heat), they found no significant difference in the overall analgesic effect of conventional SCS versus SCS at higher frequencies. They did, however, found that conventional SCS had significant effect on increasing the gracile nucleus neuron discharge rate. HF SCS had no effect whatsoever. These results suggest that conventional and HF SCS have different mechanisms of action.

Building on the idea that SCS can be designed to modulate neuron-glial interactions, Vallejo et al. [50] utilized the SNI model with continuous SCS to evaluate a differential target multiplexed programming (DTMP) approach compared to high rate and low rate SCS. The DTMP approach utilizes multiple signals that are intended to target neuron and glial cells differentially. It was found that all SCS treatments resulted in significant reduction of mechanical hypersensitivity, but the DTMP approach provided more significant improvement as well as reduced thermal hypersensitivity (hot/cold plate test) after 48 hours of continuous stimulation. RNA-sequencing was performed to confirm the phenotypes. **Figure 3** provides a heatmap illustrating the significant effect of DTMP on sets of genes (modules) with similar expression patterns obtained through a Weighted Gene Co-expression Network Analysis (WGCNA) showing that the effect of DTMP SCS correlated stronger with the expression patterns of modules in naïve rats, compared to the pattern of untreated animals (No-SCS). In a follow up study, Cedeño et al. [51] demonstrated that the DTMP approach modulated neurons and glial cells (microglia, astrocytes, and oligodendrocytes) in a differential manner by using set of genes that were uniquely expressed (cell-specific transcriptomes) by each of the type of neural cell. The effect of DTMP on each of these cell-specific transcriptomes correlated strongly with the expression pattern of naïve animals, indicating a return of gene expression toward the state of naïve (healthy) animals.

2.3 SCS in the spinal nerve ligation model

The spinal nerve ligation model (SNL) is one of the most popular preclinical models of neuropathic pain due to its reproducibility and lack of autotomy. During the surgery, initially described by Kim and Chung [52], the L5 spinal nerve is ligated with a 6-0 silk suture at a point just distal to the dorsal root ganglion (DRG), and cut distally, after the removal of the paraspinal muscles at the level of the L5 spinous process down to the sacrum, and the removal of the L6 transverse process.

Since the introduction of paresthesia-free stimulation parameters in the clinical setting, questions were raised on the value of the GCT as a practical construction to generate models to optimize SCS parameters. To find answers to some of these questions, Guan and coworkers have used the SNL model [53] to understand the specific

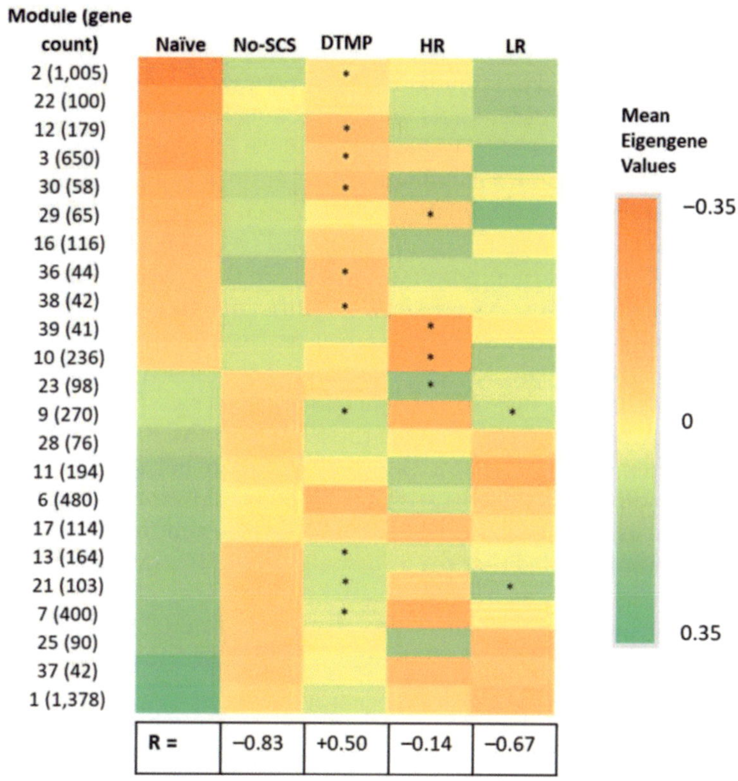

Figure 3.
Heat map of mean module eigengene values for modules with significantly different comparisons (FDR-p < 0.2) between SNI untreated animals (No-SCS) and naïve animals. A total of 23 modules out of the total 39 are affected. Asterisks (*) indicate significantly different module eigengene values when comparing the SCS treatment to untreated animals (No-SCS). R is the Pearson coefficient for the correlation between eigengene values for naïve and each of the other groups. A negative value indicates an opposite trend. DTMP: differential target multiplexed programming; LR: low rate; HR: high rate; SCS: spinal cord stimulation. Reproduced from reference [50].

effects of different components of the electrical signals in SCS treatment. Before paresthesia-free SCS, common frequencies used in clinical and animal models ranged from 50 to 60 Hz, since referred to as conventional SCS. Due to the lack of agreement regarding the optimal frequency and stimulation intensity to maximize analgesia, these authors hypothesized that kilohertz-level SCS and conventional 50Hz SCS might differently activate gate-control mechanisms and affect peripheral afferent conduction properties [53].

Using the SNL rodent model of neuropathic pain, the authors evaluated intensity-dependent (20%, 40%, and 80% MT) pain inhibition of SCS at various frequencies (50 Hz, 1 kHz, and 10 kHz) while maintaining the PW constant (24 μs). They further compared the effects of conditioning stimulation of the dorsal column, the primary structure targeted by SCS, at 50 Hz and 1 kHz on the conduction property of afferent Aα/β-fibers and inhibition of dorsal horn wide dynamic range (WDR) neuronal responses.

In their experiments, Guan and coworkers [53] advanced a custom-made quadripolar epidural SCS electrode up to the T10-12 spinal levels, via a small laminectomy at the level of T13. Mechanical hypersensitivity was assessed by determining the PWT using von Frey filaments. To further evaluate clinical conditions in the SNL model, the authors choose stimulation intensities set at either 20%, 40%, or 80% of the MT to test the effect of the described frequencies on pain-like behavior.

Stimulation was conducted for 30 mins on days 12, 13, and 14 (week 1) and days 19, 20, and 21 (week 2) post-SNL. Behavioral testing was done at time 0, 15 (within the activation of SCS), 30 (end of stimulation), and 60 min. A cross-over design was implemented to avoid the order effect while switching the different frequencies.

Interestingly, rats exposed to 10 kHz SCS at 80% MT often exhibited signs of discomfort. For comparison, a small number of animals were implanted, but not stimulated, and served as a stimulation sham. When stimulation was applied at 20% MT, the effect was marginal for all the tested frequencies. The average mean PWT across the three treatment days was increased from the pre-stimulation level in all SCS groups but was statistically significantly higher than that of sham stimulation only in the 1 kHz and 10 kHz groups. Notably, there was a trend for SCS induced inhibition to increase gradually from the first to the third treatment in all groups. When using 80% MT the mean PWT was significantly increased from the first day of stimulation in both the 1 kHz and the 10kHz SCS groups. Of notice, the mean PWT in the 1 kHz and 10 kHz were both higher than that of the 50 Hz group on the first day of stimulation. The inhibitory effect of 50 Hz stimulation increased progressively during the second and third days of stimulation. The authors concluded that the SCS analgesia in SNL rats depends on both intensity and frequency, and high-intensity kilohertz level SCS provides earlier inhibition of mechanical hypersensitivity than conventional 50 Hz SCS. These results imply that analgesia from kilohertz and 50 Hz SCS may involve different mechanisms.

In a follow-up report, Guan and coworkers [54] explored how charge delivery affects pain inhibition by different frequencies at intensities that seem to be below the sensory threshold (40% MT), and which component of stimulation runs the therapeutic actions. Epidural electrodes were implanted 5 to 7 days post-SNL, in a similar fashion described by this group previously [53]. Based on the frequency, PW, and intensity, the authors calculated the charge-per-pulse, duty time, and charge-per-second. Then, four patterns of high-dose subthreshold active recharge biphasic signals at different frequencies with similar duty times were produced by adjusting the PW (200 Hz with 1 ms PW, 500 Hz with 0.5 ms PW, 1.2 kHz with 0.2 ms PW, and 10 kHz with 0.024 ms PW). Finally, the authors included one 50 Hz with 0.2 ms PW at subthreshold and a sham (no SCS) group. Because clinical and animal data suggest that subthreshold SCS may have a slower onset, stimulation was carried for 120 mins (one session per day) from days 14 to 17 (week 1). The behavioral response was determined by measuring the PWT 30 mins pre-SCS, at 0, 30, and 60 mins during SCS, and 0, 30, and 60 mins post-SCS to evaluate carry-over effects. In those groups that showed increased tolerance to mechanical hypersensitivity, the peak effect appeared at 60 to 90 mins after initiation of SCS and faded shortly after the stimulation was completed. The onset of significant PWT increase was observed from day one in the 200 Hz and 10 kHz groups and was observed on day two in the 1.2 kHz group. Although 200 Hz SCS had the longest PW, the highest charge-per-pulse and the lowest charge-per-second, and 10 kHz had the shortest PW, the lowest charge-per-pulse, and the highest amplitude and charge-per-second, the two groups provided comparable improvements in PWT. These findings suggest that the efficacy of the inhibitory effect is not correlated to the difference in individual SCS parameters (frequency, PW) but is positively correlated with the electrical dose. Probably, the most interesting finding is that at subthreshold SCS amplitudes, mechanical hypersensitivity was not only inhibited by 10 kHz but also at lower frequencies (200 Hz). The authors concluded that using low-frequency subthreshold SCS and longer PWs, could be a more energy-efficient stimulation paradigm for inhibition of mechanical hypersensitivity when compared with 10 kHz SCS.

2.4 SCS in a chemotherapy-induced neuropathic pain model

The administration of chemotherapy agents for the treatment of cancer often results in the onset of neuropathic pain due to peripheral nerve damage. Recently, Sivanesan et al. [55] reported on the efficacy of SCS in reducing mechanical and thermal hypersensitivity in a rodent model of chemotherapy-induced peripheral neuropathy (CIPN). The chemotherapeutic paclitaxel (PTX), common in the treatment of ovarian, breast, and lung cancers, can induce painful peripheral neuropathy even at therapeutic dosages. Often this pain is severe enough to necessitate a reduced dose of PTX and persists after cessation of the drug in nearly a third of cases. Other chemotherapeutic agents, including platinum-based agents, and proteasome inhibitors like bortezomib, are also known to induce similar neuropathies [56].

Induction of the model began by acclimation of a group of adult male rats that were divided into three groups: (1) SCS + PTX, (2) PTX, or (3) naïve. Behavioral testing consisted of assessments of mechanical hypersensitivity (von Frey filaments) and thermal hypersensitivity (via dry ice application) of the hind paws.

Animals assigned to receive SCS underwent a T13 laminectomy and were implanted with a quadripolar miniaturized lead in the dorsal epidural space corresponding to the T13-L1 spinal cord. Stimulation parameters were set to conventional settings with 50 Hz frequency, 0.2 ms PW, and current intensity at 80% MT. Subsequently, animals in the PTX and SCS + PTX groups were administered 1-2 mg/kg PTX, via intraperitoneal (i.p.) injection, every other day for four days. Naïve animals received i.p. injections of the vehicle used in the PTX groups. SCS was administered daily for 6-8 hours over the course of two weeks. To substantiate whether SCS can avert the development of CIPN, PTX was administered at the same time as the stimulation. Implanted animals that did not receive SCS treatment were included as control animals.

Rats developed hypersensitivity one week after the first administration of PTX that was sustained for 25 days. Interestingly, early administration of SCS attenuated the development of mechanical hypersensitivity associated with neuropathic pain-like behavior induced by administration of PTX (**Figure 4**). SCS did not fully recover to the PWT in naïve animals, but the preemptive effect of SCS is noteworthy. Early application of SCS also prevented the development of cold hypersensitivity. It is also important to note that the analgesic effect of SCS persisted for at least 2 weeks after stopping SCS treatment.

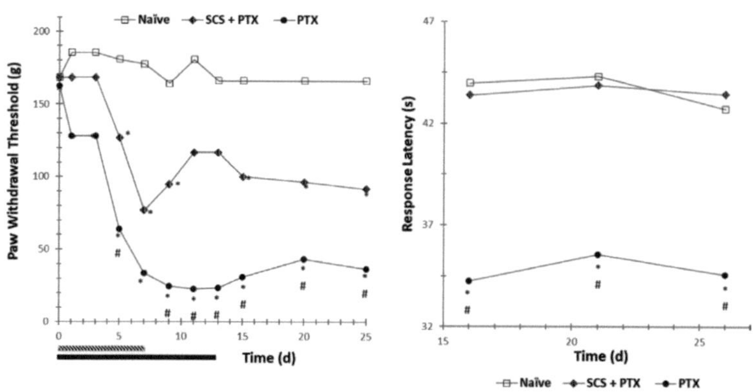

Figure 4.
*Mechanical hypersensitivity (left) and cold thermal hypersensitivity (right) of animals treated with SCS (SCS + PTX), untreated (PTX) and naïve. The patterned box indicates the time of PTX administration. The black box indicates the time of SCS administration. * indicates significant differences ($p < 0.05$) relative to naïve, # indicates significant differences ($p < 0.05$) relative to PTX + SCS. Values obtained from reference [55].*

L3-L6 spinal cord tissue was harvested 17 days after SCS was applied, and RNA in the samples was sequenced to investigate changes in gene expression and biological processes of treated, untreated, and naïve animals. It was found that some genes associated with mechanosensation, neuroimmune response, and glial activation were affected by the CIPN model. The authors hypothesized that repetitive dosing of SCS increased the expression of genes that enhance adenosine-related activity, which has been shown to enhance pain inhibition by SCS when using the CCI model [14]. The authors also observed that SCS downregulated GABA reuptake-related genes, which is consistent with a previous observation in rats after sciatic nerve injury [57]. They postulated that downregulation of genes such as *Gat3* (a GABA transporter expressed by glial cells) by SCS may increase GABAergic signaling that inhibits neurotransmission in CIPN rats. The GABAergic inhibition of excitatory neurotransmitters may involve then the suppression of calcium influx into presynaptic terminals, which is regulated by astrocytes.

2.5 SCS in a model of painful diabetic neuropathy

Originally developed in the early 1960's for studying diabetes mellitus, the streptozotocin (STZ)-based painful diabetic neuropathy model (SPDN) uses an antibiotic derived from *Streptomyces achromogenes* to selectively kill insulin secreting β-cells in the pancreas [58]. The results replicate symptoms seen in type 1 diabetes including dysregulation of blood glucose, decreased body weight, and peripheral artery disease leading to painful diabetic neuropathy.

Early investigations with this model to study the effects of SCS were conducted by Wu et al. [59] to explore the effect of SCS on blood flow in the periphery. Adult male rats were divided into two groups: (1) diabetic rats and (2) non-diabetic rats. Diabetic rats were injected with 50 mg/kg streptozotocin i.p., while the non-diabetic animals were injected with an equivalent volume of vehicle (citrate buffer). Animals were monitored weekly for weight loss and blood glucose levels. After four weeks, animals were tested for vasodilation in response to SCS provided via a spring-loaded unipolar ball electrode placed on the right or left side of the subdural face of the dorsal columns at the L2-L3 spinal segments. SCS was set to 50 Hz frequency, 0.2 ms PW, with monophasic rectangular pulses. Current was applied for 2 minutes at 30, 60, or 90% of the MT. It was found that MT in diabetic rats was significantly higher than in non-diabetic rats, and that SCS at the largest intensity attenuated SCS-induced vasodilation in diabetic rats. Furthermore, increasing SCS from 30% to 90% of MT increased blood flow in non-diabetic rats but not in diabetic rats. The study suggested that SCS-induced vasodilation improves peripheral blood flow, although this seems partially impaired in the diabetic animals.

In a later study, van Beek et al. [60] utilized the SPDN model to explore the effect of increasing the stimulation frequency on mechanical hypersensitivity induced by the model. In this study the dosage of STZ was increased to 65 mg/kg, to ensure the development of type-1 diabetes in four days instead of four weeks. Animals were implanted with a quadripolar lead via a T13 laminectomy into the dorsal epidural space of the T10-T12 spinal cord. Stimulation parameters were set to 200 μs PW, intensity at 67% MT and frequency at either 5, 50, or 500 Hz. Sham-stimulated animals were used as controls. SCS sessions were 40 minutes/day for four consecutive days. It was found that SCS at all frequencies alleviated mechanical sensitivity similarly, but stimulation at 500 Hz elicited a delayed response.

In other study, van Beek et al. [61] utilized the SPDN model to evaluate the long-term efficacy (10 weeks) of conventional SCS treatment. As before, the SPDN model was induced in male rats using an i.p. injection of 65 mg/kg STZ. Animals were monitored for weight loss and blood glucose to establish response to the model.

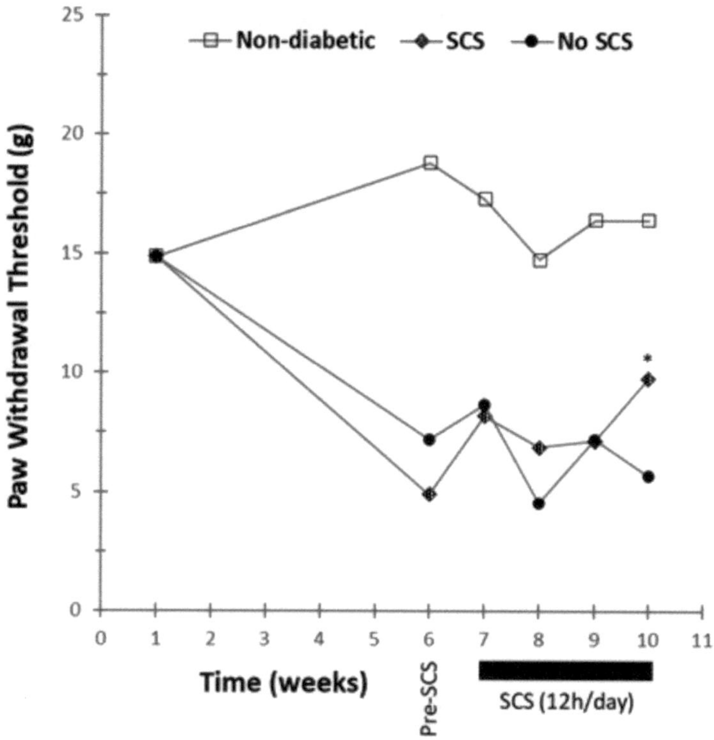

Figure 5.
*Effect of conventional SCS on mechanical hypersensitivity in a diabetic neuropathic pain model. * indicates a significant difference ($p < 0.05$) relative to No-SCS. Values obtained from reference [61].*

An internally implanted pulse generator fitted with a quadripolar lead was required due the longer duration of the study. The quadripolar lead was implanted via a L1 laminectomy into the dorsal epidural space of the L2-L5 spinal cord. Stimulation parameters were 50 Hz frequency, 210 μs PW, intensity at 67% of the MT, 12 h/day for four weeks. A group of implanted SPDN animals sham for SCS were included as a control. The results indicate that long-term conventional SCS decreases mechanical hypersensitivity even after cessation of SCS in the SPDN model (**Figure** 5).

3. Animal models of SCS for inflammatory pain

The injection of a chemical inflammatory agent in a skin dermatome has been effectively used for the study of the mechanism of acute and persistent inflammatory pain [62]. Such agents include solutions of formalin, complete Freund's adjuvant, or carrageenan (CAR). The CAR model has been adapted to study the effect of SCS in inflammatory pain in the limbs of rodents. Cui et al. [63] reported the first account of the utilization of a carrageenan-based model of chronic nociceptive pain coupled to SCS. The pain model was adapted from Woolf and Doubell [64] and consisted of the injection, under standard halothane anesthesia, of 0.15 mL solution of carrageenan lambda (in 0.9% saline to a concentration of 1%) in the mid plantar part of the hind paw. The inflammatory agent induces an edema at the site of injection and decreases the threshold for paw withdrawal or vocalization to mechanical stimuli in the affected area. Adult male Sprague-Dawley rats epidurally implanted, under anesthesia, with a monopolar cathode (2 x 3 mm^2) placed retrograde in the L1-L3 vertebral region via a laminectomy in T11. The anode was placed subcutaneously in the supravertebral region adjacent to the cathode. Rats were allowed to recover for 3 days post-surgery before any experimentation. Current-controlled SCS was applied using a pulsed signal with a width of 200 μs at a frequency of 50 Hz. The intensity was set to 67% of the MT and was on average 1.0 (± 0.3) mA. These parameters correspond to those used clinically during conventional SCS therapy. Treatment was applied for 30 minutes at 3 h, 1, 3, 5, 7 and 9 days after injection of the CAR solution. SCS was also applied to another group of animals 3 days (30 minutes/day) before injection besides the timepoints after injection. The study also included control animals that were injected with CAR but were not implanted with the SCS system, and animals that were subjected to SCS but were not injected with CAR. The extent of local inflammation was determined by measuring the circumference of the metatarsal region and mechanical sensitivity was measured by recording paw withdrawal or vocalization upon applying pressure to the affected paw. A pressure gauge measured the force (in g) that elicited the withdrawal or vocalization response.

The mean circumference of the edema at the paw was around 30 mm before injection (no edema) and increased to a maximum at around 43 mm 3 hours after injection. The edema gradually decreased back to baseline at day 7-9 post-injection. The mean paw withdrawal/vocalization threshold was 215-220 g before CAR injection and decreased to 77 g at 3 hour after CAR injection. Mechanical hypersensitivity reduced gradually and reached baseline at around day 7 post-injection. The reduction in mechanical hypersensitivity correlated well with the reduction in the edema (**Figure 6**). The application of 30 min of SCS at every time point produced a significant increase of the size of the edema until day 5 post-injection (**Figure 7**). However, mechanical sensitivity was only significantly increased by SCS at the 3h point after CAR injection. At day 3, mechanical sensitivity was reduced significantly relative to the pre-stimulation value and was similar at days 7 and 9 post-injection. Authors reported that application of SCS pre-emptively did not provide a beneficial effect. Application of SCS in the absence of the inflammatory insult did not produce significant changes in circumference size and mechanical sensitivity.

Authors concluded that this model is a representation of subacute pain between the third day post CAR injection and the 14th day, which is concomitant to the invasion of different types of inflammatory cells, while the stage previous to the

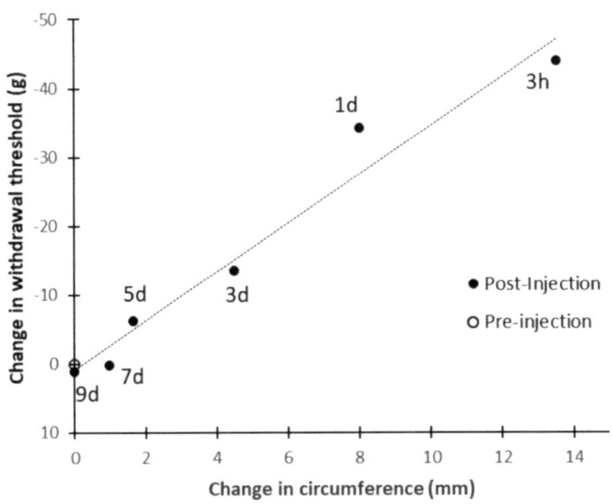

Figure 6.
Correlation between edema size resulting from CAR injection as measured by the mean circumference of the metatarsal level of the paw and the change in the threshold force (g) that elicits paw withdrawal or vocalization. Labels by every post-injection point indicates the time point. The values at days 7 (7d) and 9 (9d) post-injection are the same as the pre-injection values. Values obtained from reference [63].

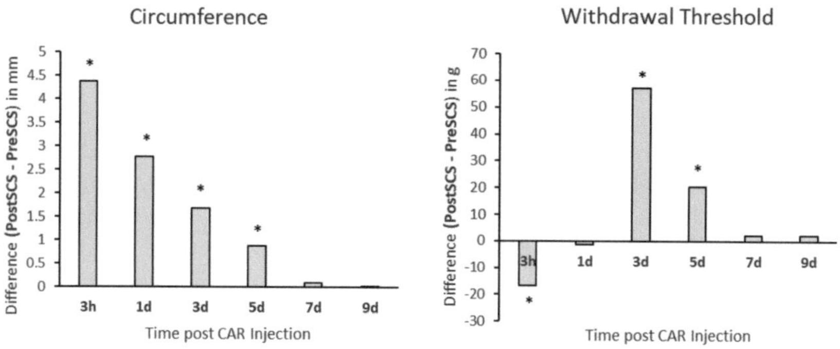

Figure 7.
*Change in the edema size (left) and mechanical hypersensitivity (right) as a result of 30 minutes/day of SCS. A positive change in withdrawal threshold is equivalent to a reduction in hypersensitivity. * indicates a significant difference ($p < 0.05$). Values obtained from reference [63].*

third day post-injection represents an acute pain phase. It was surprising to observe that the SCS signal applied in this study increased the size of the edema as well as mechanical sensitivity in the early stage of the acute phase. However, the increase in hypersensitivity was not likely causal to the edema, and rather may be due to plasticity changes in the dorsal horn as a result of the stimulating signal and the acute inflammatory process. Once the inflammatory processes have settled in during the subacute phase, authors hypothesized that SCS provides an analgesic effect due to the inhibition of neuronal hyperexcitability due to A fiber-mediated wind up.

Years later, the same group reported [49] on using the CAR-based inflammatory pain model to assess the effect of signal rate at low intensities in the acute stage of the model. This was motivated by a shift in SCS paradigm resulting from the clinical introduction of a SCS therapy that provided pain relief at intensities below the perception threshold, thus removing the need for paresthesia overlap of the painful dermatome required by conventional SCS which operates at low frequency (50 Hz), in contrast to the high frequency (10 kHz) used by the novel therapy. The authors utilized signals at 50 Hz (conventional frequency), and 10 kHz, which is referred to as high frequency SCS (HF SCS). In the same report, the authors also studied the effects on HF SCS (500 Hz, 1 kHz, and 10 kHz) on the SNI model, which was allowed to develop more chronically (2 weeks after nerve injury) before SCS intervention. In this work, authors used male adult Wistar rats, which were injected with 0.15 mL of a 1% saline solution of CAR in the hind paw as previously described [63]. Animals were implanted with a SCS system consisting of a paddle lead with four circular poles (0.9-1.0 mm diameter) spaced by 1.8-2.0 mm, which was introduced epidurally via laminectomy at the T13 vertebral level and placed anterograde to cover the T10-T12 levels. This was a variation from the previous report [63]. Animals were left to recover from surgery for 48 hours before any additional experimental intervention. Pain-like behavior was tested before injection (baseline, before stimulation and after 120 minutes of SCS at days 1, 2 and 3 after CAR injection. The test consisted of applying force progressively with clamping forceps (algometer) terminated in a blunt tip in the affected paw until the animal withdraws the paw. The algometer was equipped with a pressure gauge that reads the force exerted (in g) at the threshold of paw withdrawal. In contrast to the previous study by this group, the circumference of the metatarsal level of the paw was not measured, so the effect of SCS frequency on the edema was not determined. SCS was distributed to the four contacts in the paddle lead using adjacent bipoles (+-+-, rostral to caudal). Conventional SCS (50 Hz) used monophasic pulses 200 µs wide and current-controlled intensity set to 80% of the MT, corresponding to intensities in the 0.48 to 0.64 mA range. The HF-SCS (10 kHz) monophasic pulses were 24 μs wide with intensities set in the range 0.3-0.4 mA, which correspond to 40-50% of the MT, which were defined as subparesthetic based on observation of behavioral responses. Untreated animals served as control. Mean paw withdrawal threshold was 72 g before injection and decreased to around 19 g 1 day after CAR injection. As expected, for this model, the mean withdrawal threshold gradually increased reaching around 30 g and 56 g at days 2 and 3 post-injection, respectively (**Figure 8**).

Neither conventional SCS nor HF-SCS provided a significant improvement of acute inflammatory pain over the course of 3 days, although it is worth mentioning that, in contrast, their previous work reported a significant difference at 3 days post CAR injection. The authors did not comment on their counter results, but is plausible that the position of the lead, which was reported to be a differing factor may have influenced the outcome. A lumbar location may modulate neural circuits of the hind paw more effectively than a thoracic location used in this study. The findings for the acute inflammatory pain were similar to what was found when healthy animals were subjected to SCS and a test of acute pain (pinch force with a pointy tip in the algometer), but in contrast to the results observed in the neuropathic chronic pain model, in which 120 minutes of both conventional and HF-SCS treatments reduced mechanical hypersensitivity significantly. Thus, it can be concluded from the study that neither HF-SCS nor conventional SCS provide relief from acute inflammatory pain (as well as acute nociceptive pain), in agreement with previous clinical and well-controlled observations [65–67] and had led to the establishment of a segmental mechanism of action in which SCS works by modulating conduction of dorsal column fibers within a particular segmental circuitry that has reached

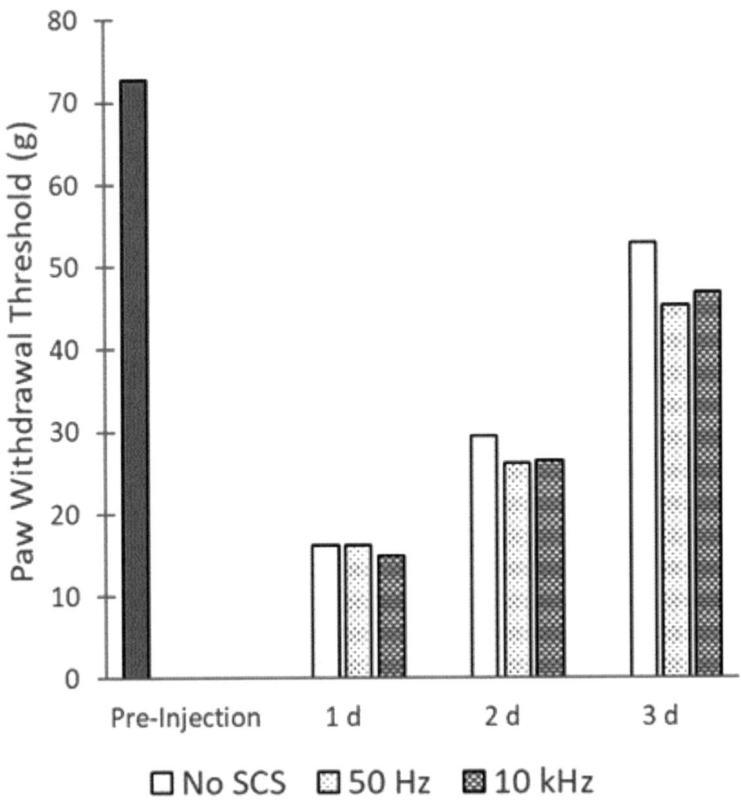

Figure 8.
Effect of SCS treatments on acute inflammatory pain. Values obtained from reference [49].

a level of central sensitization during the establishment of chronic pain due to a peripheral injury, such as in the SNI model of neuropathic pain tested.

Recently, Sato et al. [46] reported the utilization of a CAR-based model to study the effect of conventional SCS on joint inflammatory pain. This group had previously found [68] that the unilateral intraarticular anterior injection of 0.1 mL of a 3% solution of lambda carrageenan (type IV, dissolved in 0.9% saline) into the left knee joint of rats induces pain-like behavior that manifests as increased thermal (hot) and mechanical hyperalgesia in the ipsilateral hind paw and knee. The model can be used to evaluate acute or chronic onset of inflammatory pain. In their recent work, they implemented this joint inflammatory pain model to test the effect of short doses (15 min/day) of conventional SCS (60 Hz, 250 μs PW, intensity at 90% of the MT) on thermal and mechanical hyperalgesia using an acute stage of the model. The SCS system had been previously described [48, 69] and consisted of a stimulation lead epidurally introduced, under anesthesia, via laminectomy at the T13 vertebral level and positioned rostrally. The authors did not provide details on the lead design and final position of it relative to spinal levels within the epidural space. Lead wires were tunneled to an internal neurostimulator (Interstim iCon, model 3058, Medtronic Inc., Minneapolis, MN) implanted subcutaneously in the left flank. This allowed animals to roam freely in their cages while being stimulated. Animals were tested for both paw and knee withdrawal to noxious mechanical stimuli before CAR injection, and 30 min before and after SCS (15 min) on days 1, 2, 3, and 4 after injection. Paw withdrawal thresholds were obtained using von Frey filaments with bending force in the range 1-402 mN applied to the plantar surface of the paw ipsilateral to the affected joint. Measurements in the contralateral paw served as internal controls. Knee withdrawal thresholds were measured by compressing the affected extended knee with a pair of calibrated forceps (30 mm^2 tip) until the knee was withdrawn due to the applied force. Mean paw and knee withdrawal thresholds are shown in **Figure 9**.

An acute application of conventional SCS, as applied in this work, improved mean withdrawal thresholds significantly relative to the pre-SCS state, implying that conventional SCS may be used to treat acute inflammatory pain. The study did not address the effects of a chronic inflammatory state, which is achievable with this CRA model. Similar to what was reported for effects on the SNI neuropathic pain model, the effect is reversible and reproducible over the different days of treatment. It has been established that SCS modulates inflammatory processes in the stimulated area of the spinal cord that contain neural circuits associated with the painful areas. These

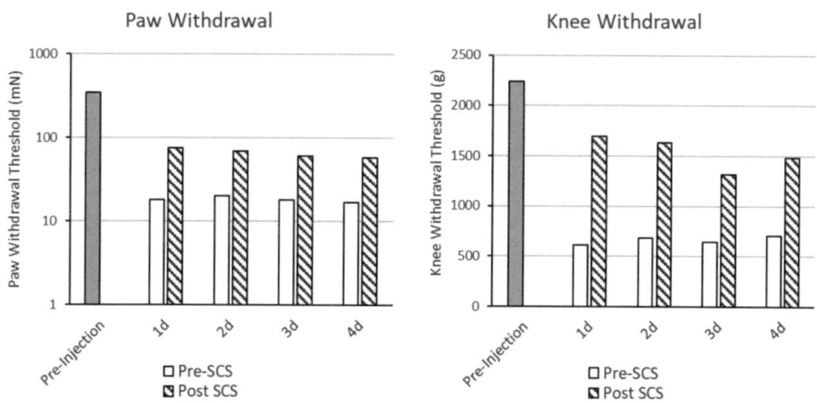

Figure 9.
Effect of SCS treatments on acute inflammatory joint pain as reflected in the ipsilateral paw and knee. All post-SCS values are significantly increased ($p < 0.05$) relative to Pre-SCS values. Pre-SCS values are significantly reduced relative to pre-injection. There is no significant difference between treatment days. Values obtained from reference [46].

neural circuits contain neurons and other abundant non-neuronal cells that are highly involved in the establishment and chronification of pain, even at early stages. It is quite interesting to note that the effect of SCS sets in as early as 1 day to alleviate hyperalgesia associated with acute knee inflammation, which was not observed by Linderoth and coworkers when inflammation was elicited in the hind paw [49, 63]. It is plausible that the circuits operating in the thoracic region for inflammation of the hind paw are not as effective for SCS, in contrast to treat inflammation of the knee joint.

4. Animal models of SCS for ischemic pain

It has been established that SCS modulates vasodilation in the lower limbs and feet dermatomes associated with vertebral segments being stimulated [70]. This has justified SCS as an alternative treatment for nociceptive pain and associated symptoms related to advanced cases of peripheral arterial occlusion disease (PAOD), which leads to ischemia and the subsequent neuropathy due to the lack of blood supply to nerve terminals. Other clinical uses of SCS related to vasodilation modulation include Rynaud's syndrome and angina pectoris. In the absence of a pain model related to PAOD, animal models that measure the modulation of blood flow and vasodilation have been used to demonstrate the mechanism of action of SCS treatment of peripheral vascular diseases. Although there is no evidence that SCS is effective on acute nociceptive pain, the modulation of vasodilation is hypothesized as the mechanism of action for relieving ischemic conditions and recover the flow of nutrients into the affected nerve terminals. Linderoth and Foreman's groups have collaborated to measure the effect of low rate SCS on blood flow changes in the skin dermatomes of the hind paws of anesthetized rats. In one experiment [71], a spring-loaded monopolar ball cathode was placed in the subdural surface of the L1-L3 dorsal columns (left or right) of anesthetized rats to assess the role of SCS in modulating the sympathetic autonomous system. SCS monophasic pulses (50 Hz, 200 μs PW, 66% of the MT) were applied for 2 minutes. Blood flow was monitored using laser-based doppler probes placed in the glabrous surfaces of the hind paws ipsilateral and contralateral to the stimulation. Another group of animals was subjected to total sympathectomy, while the other was subjected to the ganglionic transmission blocker hexamethonium. In a separate experiment [72], the effect of SCS on the sympathetic nervous system was determined by evaluating the role of ganglionic transmission (with hexamethonium blockade), alpha-adrenergic receptors (phentolamine or prazosin blockade), beta-adrenergic receptors (propanolol blockade), and adrenal catecholamine secretion (adrenal demedullation) in paralyzed anesthetized animals. The left L1-L2 vertebral region was stimulated epidurally with a monopolar ball cathode (0.9 mm diameter) that delivered pulses at 50 Hz, 200 μs PW, and 0.6 mA of intensity. Blood flow was monitored using laser Doppler probes in each hind paw. Although both studies concurred that SCS increases peripheral blood flow in the ipsilateral limb by about 200% concomitant to a reduction of flow resistance of ~50%, there were disagreements in the role of sympathetic contributions, which prompted the formulation of a second hypothesis involving the antidromic activation of the release of vasodilators, such as calcitonin gene-related peptide (CGRP) and nitric oxide. A further report [73] explored the effect of SCS pulse rate on blood flow, finding that pulsing at 500 Hz provided a significant increase of vasodilation relative to pulsing at 200 Hz and 50 Hz at similar pulse widths and intensities. The frequency effect seems to be related to increased release of CGRP, induced by activation of fibers containing the capsaicin receptor (TRPV-1). In conclusion, the reduction of nociceptive lower limb pain due to ischemia has been indirectly associated with SCS-induced vasodilation that provides an increase in blood flow and the concomitant decrease of flow resistance in the affected limb. It is plausible that vasodilation is due to the release of agents CGRP and nitric oxide from the stimulated fiber afferents and at some extent by modulation of the sympathetic nervous system.

5. Translational equivalence of animal models

Besides rodent (mostly rat) models, there have been reports of SCS effects on ovine models of neuropathic pain. As presented in section 2.1 above, Reddy et al. [17] reported on the utilization of female sheep to develop a CCI model to study the effect of tonic SCS. The advantage of using a large animal model is that it provides a way to bridge the translation of SCS parameters toward clinical application for longer exposures in anatomical environments that are more similar to that of humans. These authors found that the model provided a significant reduction of mechanical hypersensitivity upon continuous SCS for one week. A closer examination of the

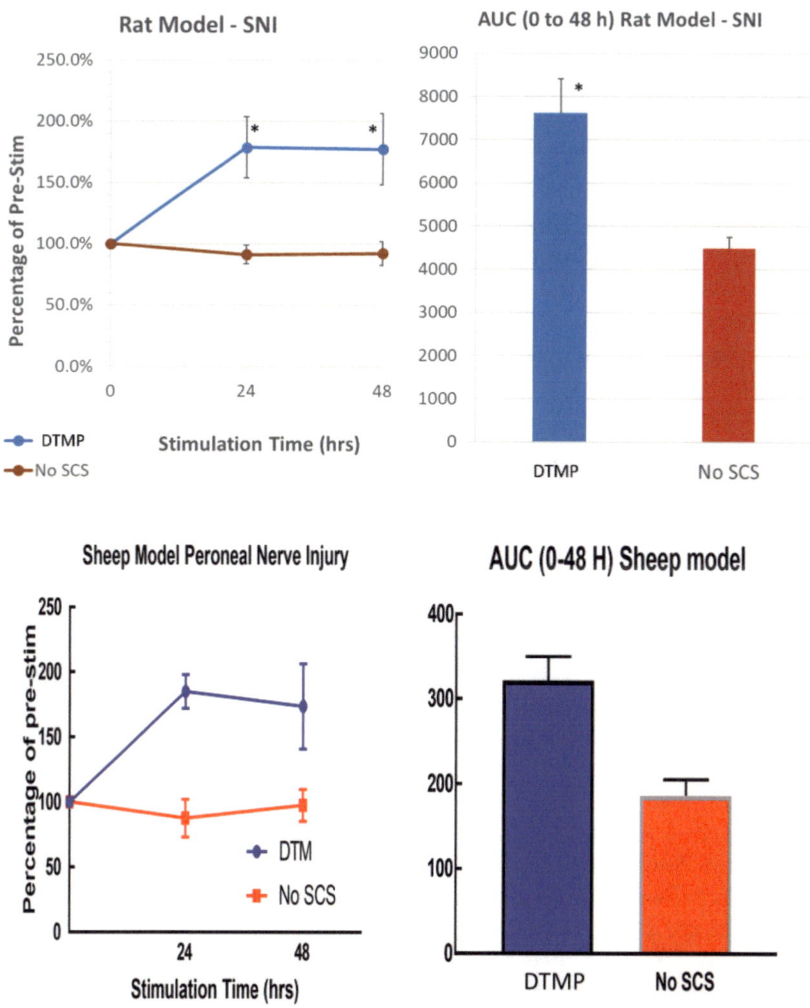

Figure 10.
*Top row: Mechanical hypersensitivity of rats subjected to SCS with a DTMP approach in comparison with untreated animals (No SCS) and corresponding areas under the curve (AUC). Bottom row: equivalent measurement obtained from sheep. * denotes significant differences ($p < 0.05$) between treated and untreated animals.*

reported data for 5 animals, reveals that one of them was a non-responder to the pain model since there was not a decrease of the limb withdrawal threshold (WT). If data from this animal is discarded, the CCI model reduced the WT to a mean 51% (± 6%) relative to the mean WT of the control measurements in the contralateral limb. The mean WT of the responders after SCS corresponded to 85% (± 13%) of the mean WT of the control. This is consistent with the findings in rodents, although a direct comparison is not possible because there are not reports on rodent CCI models with continuous SCS.

Vallejo et al. [74] reported on a comparison of the effect of SCS based on the DTMP approach on a rat and sheep models after 24 and 48 h of continuous treatment. The pain model in the rats was the SNI as previously described [42, 43], while the sheep model is the equivalent peroneal nerve injury (PNI) developed by Wilkes et al. [75] and adapted for SCS by implanting a cylindrical octapolar human-grade lead (1.3 mm diameter) in the L1-L3 epidural space. DTMP consisted of multiplexing 4 pulsed signals with frequencies in the 50 Hz to 1.2 kHz and PW of 200 µs at an intensity of 50% of the MT. Mechanical hypersensitivity was obtained before starting SCS, as well as at 24 h and 48 h of continuous SCS, using an electronic von Frey anesthesiometer. In order to compare rodent and ovine results, the WT were normalized to the pre-SCS values (**Figure 10**). Rodent data is for individual subjects (N = 13). Ovine data is from two sheep that were evaluated in a crossover experiment, in which one sheep was stimulated while the other one served as a No-SCS control. After a one-week break for washing out the effects of SCS, the animal that had not been treated was subjected to SCS while the other one was the No-SCS control. This process was repeated until obtaining a set of six measurements.

DTMP significantly relieved mechanical hypersensitivity in the rat model equivalent to 78.6% at 24h and 77.3% at 48 h in the rat model relative to the pre-SCS and No-SCS measurements. Similar effects were seen in the sheep model where the decrease in mechanical hypersensitivity was 84.8% at 24h and 73.7% at 48 h. These results demonstrate translational equivalence between two animal models of neuropathic pain for the first time.

6. Conclusion

Certain limitations exist in the development of animal models that simulate human pathological conditions of pain. For instance, the most common clinical indication for SCS has become the treatment of intractable neuropathic pain of the lower back and legs, largely associated with failed surgical spine interventions (failed back surgery syndrome, FBSS), which causes axial back pain that radiates to the limbs in a unilateral or bilateral manner. The existing rat models of neuropathic pain, which are described in this chapter, are mostly peripherally induced (nerve injury) and test the manifestation of mechanical hypersensitivity in the paws, not necessarily in the leg of the animals. An animal model that resembles FBSS has yet to be developed. Such peripheral nerve injury models, however, resemble symptoms found in other pain-related syndromes such as complex regional pain syndrome (CRPS), which are also indicated for SCS treatment in humans. Despite these limitations, the existing models have proven extremely useful to understand the effects of various modalities of SCS on pain-like behavior of the animals, and more importantly, on the mechanistic understanding of SCS via the molecular analysis of samples obtained from neural tissues (spinal cord, DRG) that cannot be obtained in clinical assessments. Such molecular evaluations have made use of pharmacological approaches that use the coadministration of neurotransmitters agonists and antagonists, opioids, receptor blockers, etc., as well as immunohistochemical analysis that target cellular markers of glial activation. Recent approaches are most robust and utilize high throughput transcriptomic and proteomic analysis in combination with many bioinformatic tools that provide an understanding of the effects of SCS on complex biological processes that involve a multitude of proteins and their encoding genes. These advancements should provide the field with tools to enhance current therapies and improvements on pain diagnostics that could ultimately lead to an integral and personalized treatment of painful conditions in humans. Animal models will continue to play a crucial role in the development of the science and technology of electrical neuromodulation for treating pain.

Acknowledgements

The authors want to acknowledge our colleagues, Dana Tilley, William Smith, Ashim Gupta, Cynthia Cass, Maggie DeMaegd, Randi Wilson, Louis Vera-Portocarrero, Melanie Goodman-Keiser, Samuel Thomas, Alejandro Vallejo, and Tina Billstrom who have provided their help in developing our own SCS animal models.

Conflict of interest

DLC and RV are consultants and scientific advisors for Medtronic Inc. They are also coinventors in patents related to differential target multiplexed (DTM) spinal cord stimulation.

Author details

Joseph M. Williams[1], Courtney A. Kelley[1,2], Ricardo Vallejo[1,2,3,4], David C. Platt[1,2] and David L. Cedeño[1,2,3]*

1 Department of Psychology, Illinois Wesleyan University, Bloomington, USA

2 Lumbrera LLC, Bloomington, USA

3 SGX Medical LLC, Bloomington, USA

4 National Spine and Pain Center, Bloomington, USA

*Address all correspondence to: dclumbrera@gmail.com

References

[1] Melzack R, Wall PD. Pain mechanisms: A new theory. *Science* 1965; 150: 971-979.

[2] Köhler W. On unnoticed sensations and errors of judgment. *Sel Pap Wolfgang Köhler* 1971; 13-39.

[3] Parpura V, Verkhratsky A. Homeostatic function of astrocytes: Ca2+ and Na+ signalling. *Transl Neurosci* 2012; 3: 334-344.

[4] Verkhratsky A, Nedergaard M, Hertz L. Why are astrocytes important? *Neurochem Res* 2015; 40: 389-401.

[5] Mayorquin LC, Rodriguez A V, Sutachan J-J, et al. Connexin-mediated functional and metabolic coupling between astrocytes and neurons. *Front Mol Neurosci* 2018; 11: 118.

[6] Fields RD. Oligodendrocytes changing the rules: action potentials in glia and oligodendrocytes controlling action potentials. *Neurosci* 2008; 14: 540-543.

[7] Roitbak AI, Fanardjian V V. Depolarization of cortical glial cells in response to electrical stimulation of the cortical surface. *Neuroscience* 1981; 6: 2529-2537.

[8] Agnesi F, Blaha CD, Lin J, et al. Local glutamate release in the rat ventral lateral thalamus evoked by high-frequency stimulation. *J Neural Eng* 2010; 7: 26009.

[9] Vallejo R, Gupta A, Cedeno DL, et al. Clinical Effectiveness and Mechanism of Action of Spinal Cord Stimulation for Treating Chronic Low Back and Lower Extremity Pain: a Systematic Review. *Curr Pain Headache Rep* 2020; 24: 1-13.

[10] Mills SEE, Nicolson KP, Smith BH. Chronic pain: a review of its epidemiology and associated factors in population-based studies. *Br J Anaesth* 2019; 123: e273–e283.

[11] Bennett GJ, Xie Y-K. A peripheral mononeuropathy in rat that produces disorders of pain sensation like those seen in man. *Pain* 1988; 33: 87-107.

[12] Shu B, He S-Q, Guan Y. Spinal Cord Stimulation Enhances Microglial Activation in the Spinal Cord of Nerve-Injured Rats. *Neurosci Bull* 2020; 36: 1441-1453.

[13] Wallin J, Cui J-G, Yakhnitsa V, et al. Gabapentin and pregabalin suppress tactile allodynia and potentiate spinal cord stimulation in a model of neuropathy. *Eur J Pain* 2002; 6: 261-272.

[14] Cui J-G, Sollevi A, Linderoth B, et al. Adenosine receptor activation suppresses tactile hypersensitivity and potentiates spinal cord stimulation in mononeuropathic rats. *Neurosci Lett* 1997; 223: 173-176.

[15] Yuan B, Liu D, Liu X. Spinal cord stimulation exerts analgesia effects in chronic constriction injury rats via suppression of the TLR4/NF-κB pathway. *Neurosci Lett* 2014; 581: 63-68.

[16] Xu L, Liu Y, Sun Y, et al. Analgesic effects of TLR4/NF-κB signaling pathway inhibition on chronic neuropathic pain in rats following chronic constriction injury of the sciatic nerve. *Biomed Pharmacother* 2018; 107: 526-533.

[17] Reddy CG, Miller JW, Abode-Iyamah KO, et al. Ovine model of neuropathic pain for assessing mechanisms of spinal cord stimulation therapy via dorsal horn recordings, von Frey filaments, and gait analysis. *J Pain Res* 2018; 11: 1147-1162.

[18] Zhang TC, Janik JJ, Peters R V, et al. Spinal sensory projection neuron

responses to spinal cord stimulation are mediated by circuits beyond gate control. *J Neurophysiol* 2015; 114: 284-300.

[19] Seltzer Z, Dubner R, Shir Y. A novel behavioral model of neuropathic pain disorders produced in rats by partial sciatic nerve injury. *Pain* 1990; 43: 205-218.

[20] Meuwissen KP V, de Vries LE, Gu JW, et al. Burst and tonic spinal cord stimulation both activate spinal GABAergic mechanisms to attenuate pain in a rat model of chronic neuropathic pain. *Pain Pract* 2020; 20: 75-87.

[21] Smits H, Van Kleef M, Joosten EA. Spinal cord stimulation of dorsal columns in a rat model of neuropathic pain: evidence for a segmental spinal mechanism of pain relief. *Pain* 2012; 153: 177-183.

[22] Meuwissen KP V, van der Toorn A, Gu JW, et al. Active Recharge Burst and Tonic Spinal Cord Stimulation Engage Different Supraspinal Mechanisms: a Functional Magnetic Resonance Imaging Study in Peripherally Injured Chronic Neuropathic Rats. *Pain Pract* 2020; 20: 510-521.

[23] Truin M, Janssen SPM, van Kleef M, et al. Successful pain relief in non-responders to spinal cord stimulation: the combined use of ketamine and spinal cord stimulation. *Eur J Pain* 2011; 15: 1049-e1-e9.

[24] Meuwissen KP V, Gu JW, Zhang TC, et al. Conventional-SCS vs. burst-SCS and the behavioral effect on mechanical hypersensitivity in a rat model of chronic neuropathic pain: effect of amplitude. *Neuromodulation* 2018; 21: 19-30.

[25] Truin M, van Kleef M, Verboeket Y, et al. The effect of Spinal Cord Stimulation in mice with chronic neuropathic pain after partial ligation of the sciatic nerve. *Pain* 2009; 145: 312-318.

[26] Meuwissen KP V, van Beek M, Joosten EAJ. Burst and tonic spinal cord stimulation in the mechanical conflict-avoidance system: Cognitive-motivational aspects. *Neuromodulation* 2020; 23: 605-612.

[27] Yakhnitsa V, Linderoth B, Meyerson BA. Spinal cord stimulation attenuates dorsal horn neuronal hyperexcitability in a rat model of mononeuropathy. *Pain* 1999; 79: 223-233.

[28] Stiller C-O, Cui J-G, O'Connor WT, et al. Release of γ-aminobutyric acid in the dorsal horn and suppression of tactile allodynia by spinal cord stimulation in mononeuropathic rats. *Neurosurgery* 1996; 39: 367-375.

[29] Song Z, Meyerson BA, Linderoth B. Muscarinic receptor activation potentiates the effect of spinal cord stimulation on pain-related behavior in rats with mononeuropathy. *Neurosci Lett* 2008; 436: 7-12.

[30] Simpson RK, Gondo M, Robertson CS, et al. Reduction in the mechanonociceptive response by intrathecal administration of glycine and related compounds. *Neurochem Res* 1996; 21: 1221-1226.

[31] Cui J-G, Meyerson BA, Sollevi A, et al. Effect of spinal cord stimulation on tactile hypersensitivity in mononeuropathic rats is potentiated by simultaneous GABAB and adenosine receptor activation. *Neurosci Lett* 1998; 247: 183-186.

[32] Truin M, van Kleef M, Linderoth B, et al. Increased efficacy of early spinal cord stimulation in an animal model of neuropathic pain. *Eur J Pain* 2011; 15: 111-117.

[33] Janssen SP, Gerard S, Raijmakers ME, et al. Decreased intracellular GABA levels contribute to spinal cord stimulation-induced analgesia in rats suffering from painful peripheral neuropathy: The role of KCC2 and GABAA receptor-mediated inhibition. *Neurochem Int* 2012; 60: 21-30.

[34] Truin M, Van Venrooij P, Duysens V, et al. Spinal cord stimulation in a mouse chronic neuropathic pain model. *Neuromodulation* 2007; 10: 358-362.

[35] Li D, Yang H, Meyerson BA, et al. Response to spinal cord stimulation in variants of the spared nerve injury pain model. *Neurosci Lett* 2006; 400: 115-120.

[36] Schechtmann G, Song Z, Ultenius C, et al. Cholinergic mechanisms involved in the pain relieving effect of spinal cord stimulation in a model of neuropathy. *Pain* 2008; 139: 136-145.

[37] Sun L, Tai L, Qiu Q, et al. Endocannabinoid activation of CB1 receptors contributes to long-lasting reversal of neuropathic pain by repetitive spinal cord stimulation. *Eur J Pain* 2017; 21: 804-814.

[38] Meuwissen KP V, Gu JW, Zhang TC, et al. Burst spinal cord stimulation in peripherally injured chronic neuropathic rats: a delayed effect. *Pain Pract* 2018; 18: 988-996.

[39] Song Z, Meyerson BA, Linderoth B. Spinal 5-HT receptors that contribute to the pain-relieving effects of spinal cord stimulation in a rat model of neuropathy. *Pain* 2011; 152: 1666-1673.

[40] Smits H, Kleef M V, Honig W, et al. Spinal cord stimulation induces c-Fos expression in the dorsal horn in rats with neuropathic pain after partial sciatic nerve injury. *Neurosci Lett* 2009; 450: 70-73.

[41] Decosterd I, Woolf CJ. Spared nerve injury: An animal model of persistent peripheral neuropathic pain. *Pain* 2000; 87: 149-158.

[42] Tilley DM, Vallejo R, Kelley CA, et al. A continuous spinal cord stimulation model attenuates pain-related behavior in vivo following induction of a peripheral nerve injury. *Neuromodulation* 2015; 18: 171-176.

[43] Vallejo R, Gupta A, Kelley CA, et al. Effects of Phase Polarity and Charge Balance Spinal Cord Stimulation on Behavior and Gene Expression in a Rat Model of Neuropathic Pain. *Neuromodulation* 2020; 23: 26-35.

[44] Vallejo R, Tilley DM, Cedeño DL, et al. Genomics of the Effect of Spinal Cord Stimulation on an Animal Model of Neuropathic Pain. *Neuromodulation* 2016; 19: 576-586.

[45] Smits H, Ultenius C, Deumens R, et al. Effect of spinal cord stimulation in an animal model of neuropathic pain relates to degree of tactile "allodynia". *Neuroscience* 2006; 143: 541-546.

[46] Sato KL, Sanada LS, Da Silva MD, et al. Transcutaneous electrical nerve stimulation, acupuncture, and spinal cord stimulation on neuropathic, inflammatory and, non-inflammatory pain in rat models. *Korean J Pain* 2020; 33: 121.

[47] Sato KL, King EW, Johanek LM, et al. Spinal cord stimulation reduces hypersensitivity through activation of opioid receptors in a frequency-dependent manner. *Eur J pain* 2013; 17: 551-561.

[48] Sato KL, Johanek LM, Sanada LS, et al. Spinal cord stimulation reduces mechanical hyperalgesia and glial cell activation in animals with neuropathic pain. *Anesth Analg* 2014; 118: 464-472.

[49] Song Z, Viisanen H, Meyerson BA, et al. Efficacy of kilohertz-frequency and conventional spinal cord stimulation in rat models of different pain conditions. *Neuromodulation* 2014; 17: 226-235.

[50] Vallejo R, Kelley CA, Gupta A, et al. Modulation of neuroglial interactions using differential target multiplexed spinal cord stimulation in an animal model of neuropathic pain. *Mol Pain* 2020; 16: 1744806920918057.

[51] Cedeño DL, Smith WJ, Kelley CA, et al. Spinal cord stimulation using differential target multiplexed programming modulates neural cell-specific transcriptomes in an animal model of neuropathic pain. *Mol Pain* 2020; 16: 1744806920964360.

[52] Ho Kim S, Mo Chung J. An experimental model for peripheral neuropathy produced by segmental spinal nerve ligation in the rat. *Pain* 1992; 50: 355-363.

[53] Shechter R, Yang F, Xu Q, et al. Conventional and kilohertz-frequency spinal cord stimulation produces intensity-and frequency-dependent inhibition of mechanical hypersensitivity in a rat model of neuropathic pain. *Anesthesiol* 2013; 119: 422-432.

[54] Chen Z, Huang Q, Yang F, et al. The impact of electrical charge delivery on inhibition of mechanical hypersensitivity in nerve-injured rats by sub-sensory threshold spinal cord stimulation. *Neuromodulation* 2019; 22: 163-171.

[55] Sivanesan E, Stephens KE, Huang Q, et al. Spinal cord stimulation prevents paclitaxel-induced mechanical and cold hypersensitivity and modulates spinal gene expression in rats. *Pain Reports* 2019; 4: e7854.

[56] Hopkins HL, Duggett NA, Flatters SJL. Chemotherapy-induced painful neuropathy: pain-like behaviours in rodent models and their response to commonly-used analgesics. *Curr Opin Support Palliat Care* 2016; 10: 119-128.

[57] Stephens KE, Chen Z, Sivanesan E, et al. RNA-seq of spinal cord from nerve-injured rats after spinal cord stimulation. *Mol Pain* 2018; 14: 1744806918817429.

[58] Furman BL. Streptozotocin-induced diabetic models in mice and rats. *Curr Protoc Pharmacol* 2015; 70: 5-47.

[59] Wu M, Thorkilsen MM, Qin C, et al. Effects of spinal cord stimulation on peripheral blood circulation in rats with streptozotocin-induced diabetes. *Neuromodulation* 2007; 10: 216-223.

[60] Van Beek M, Van Kleef M, Linderoth B, et al. Spinal cord stimulation in experimental chronic painful diabetic polyneuropathy: delayed effect of high-frequency stimulation. *Eur J Pain* 2017; 21: 795-803.

[61] van Beek M, Hermes D, Honig WM, et al. Long-term spinal cord stimulation alleviates mechanical hypersensitivity and increases peripheral cutaneous blood perfusion in experimental painful diabetic polyneuropathy. *Neuromodulation* 2018; 21: 472-479.

[62] Ren K, Dubner R. Inflammatory models of pain and hyperalgesia. *ILAR J* 1999; 40: 111-118.

[63] Cui J-G, Meyerson BA, Linderoth B. Opposite effects of spinal cord stimulation in different phases of carrageenan-induced hyperalgesia. *Eur J Pain* 1999; 3: 365-374.

[64] Woolf CJ, Doubell TP. The pathophysiology of chronic pain—increased sensitivity to low threshold Aβ-fibre inputs. *Curr Opin Neurobiol* 1994; 4: 525-534.

[65] Lindblom U, Meyerson BA. Influence on touch, vibration and cutaneous pain of dorsal column stimulation in man. *Pain* 1975; 1: 257-270.

[66] Lindblom U, Meyerson BA. On the effect of electrical stimulation of the dorsal column system on sensory thresholds in patients with chronic pain. In: *Progress in brain research*. Elsevier, 1976, pp. 237-241.

[67] Linderoth B, Meyerson BA. Spinal Cord Stimulation Exploration of the Physiological Basis of a Widely Used Therapy. *Anesthesiol* 2010; 113: 1265-1267.

[68] Radhakrishnan R, Moore SA, Sluka KA. Unilateral carrageenan injection into muscle or joint induces chronic bilateral hyperalgesia in rats. *Pain* 2003; 104: 567-577.

[69] Sato KL, Johanek LM, Sanada LS, et al. Spinal cord stimulation (scs) improves decreased physical activity induced by nerve injury. *Behav Neurosci* 2014; 128: 625-632.

[70] Foreman RD, Linderoth B. Neural mechanisms of spinal cord stimulation. In: *International review of neurobiology*. Elsevier, 2012, pp. 87-119.

[71] Linderoth B, Gunasekera L, Meyerson BA. Effects of sympathectomy on skin and muscle microcirculation during dorsal column stimulation: animal studies. *Neurosurgery* 1991; 29: 874-879.

[72] Croom JE, Foreman RD, Chandler MJ, et al. Reevaluation of the role of the sympathetic nervous system in cutaneous vasodilation during dorsal spinal cord stimulation: are multiple mechanisms active? *Neuromodulation* 1998; 1: 91-101.

[73] Wu M, Linderoth B, Foreman RD. Putative mechanisms behind effects of spinal cord stimulation on vascular diseases: a review of experimental studies. *Auton Neurosci* 2008; 138: 9-23.

[74] Vallejo R, Vera-Portocarrero L, Kelley C, et al. Translational comparison of rodent and sheep models of continuous differential target multiplexed spinal cord stimulation. In: *14th International Neuromodulation Society Congress*. Sydney, Australia, 2019.

[75] Wilkes D, Li G, Angeles CF, et al. A large animal neuropathic pain model in sheep: a strategy for improving the predictability of preclinical models for therapeutic development. *J Pain Res* 2012; 5: 415-424.

Section 4

Preclinical Models of Eye Diseases

Chapter 9

An Overview of Glaucoma: Bidirectional Translation between Humans and Pre-Clinical Animal Models

Sophie Pilkinton, T.J. Hollingsworth, Brian Jerkins and Monica M. Jablonski

Abstract

Glaucoma is a multifactorial, polygenetic disease with a shared outcome of loss of retinal ganglion cells and their axons, which ultimately results in blindness. The most common risk factor of this disease is elevated intraocular pressure (IOP), although many glaucoma patients have IOPs within the normal physiological range. Throughout disease progression, glial cells in the optic nerve head respond to glaucomatous changes, resulting in glial scar formation as a reaction to injury. This chapter overviews glaucoma as it affects humans and the quest to generate animal models of glaucoma so that we can better understand the pathophysiology of this disease and develop targeted therapies to slow or reverse glaucomatous damage. This chapter then reviews treatment modalities of glaucoma. Revealed herein is the lack of non-IOP-related modalities in the treatment of glaucoma. This finding supports the use of animal models in understanding the development of glaucoma pathophysiology and treatments.

Keywords: animal models, rodents, preclinical models, glaucoma, IOP, IOP-lowering, optic nerve degeneration, retinal ganglion cells

1. Introduction

Glaucoma is a heterogenous disease with numerous contributing factors including environment, genetics, and epigenetics. It is the primary cause of irreversible blindness in the world and the number of patients diagnosed is only projected to increase in the coming years. The use of preclinical animal models has exponentially progressed our understanding of the underlying pathophysiology of the disease, as well as providing a platform for generating and testing successful therapeutics. This chapter delves into the fundamentals of glaucoma including the pathologies, types, and symptoms with a subsequent description of the numerous preclinical animal models of the disease and what has been garnered from their study. We will then discuss treatments of glaucoma that are either FDA-approved or in development and conclude by summarizing how pre-clinical studies have advanced the development of new glaucoma therapeutics.

IntechOpen

1.1 Basics of glaucoma

The eye is an elaborate structure suited to performing its unique function: collecting photons of light and converting that to an electrical signal allowing for vision. Because light needs to enter the eye without impedance, the cornea and lens lack vasculature. However, a source of nutrients and waste efflux is necessary for tissue survival. This necessity is answered by way of the aqueous humor, a water-based filtrate of the blood produced by the ciliary body of the eye. As it flows from the ciliary body through the pupil, the aqueous humor carries and bathes the tissues with sugars, vitamins, and other necessary supplies for cellular survival while carrying the excreted cellular metabolic waste products back to the blood stream for removal. The exit path for the aqueous humor is through the trabecular meshwork, Schlemm's canal and supplementary outflow structures (**Figure 1A**). Any imbalance between aqueous humor production and its elimination can have an impact on intraocular pressure (IOP). As they exit the eye, the axons of retinal ganglion cells (RGCs) converge and they become the nerve fibers of the optic nerve (**Figure 1B**) [1]. RGC axon degeneration can be induced by both elevated IOP-related changes and IOP-independent factors.

Glaucoma, defined as pathological damage to the optic nerve (ON), results in visual field defects due to death of the retinal ganglion cells (RGCs) and damage to their axons. Glaucoma is the leading cause of irreversible blindness globally. Trends predict that by 2040, as many as 111.8 million people worldwide will have this disease [2]. Of the approximately 80 million current cases, 11 million are estimated to result in complete blindness [3]. Glaucoma's primary risk factor is elevated intraocular pressure (IOP), although some forms of this disease do not include this endophenotype.

This disease is classified into the conventional categories of primary open-angle glaucoma (POAG) and primary angle-closure glaucoma (PACG), as well as primary congenital glaucoma, normotensive glaucoma (NTG), and pigmentary dispersion glaucoma. Other rare types exist, such as exfoliation glaucoma and traumatic glaucoma. The most important modifiable risk factor for onset and progression of glaucoma is elevated IOP, although normotensive glaucoma patients suffer from vision loss in spite of their IOP being in the normal physiological range, highlighting the complexity of this disease. In other subtypes of

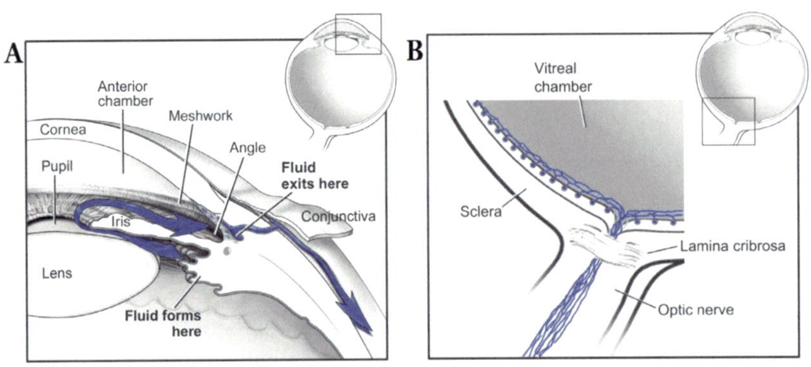

Figure 1.
Aqueous humor dynamics and retinal ganglion cells: two areas of glaucoma-related research. (A) The aqueous humor is produced by the ciliary body and exits through the trabecular meshwork and other outflow structures leaving the eye and entering the blood stream (flow shown in blue). (B) The axons of the retinal ganglion cells (blue) form the optic nerve and run through the lamina cribosa as they exit the eye. In glaucoma, retinal ganglion cells and their axons can be damaged due to IOP-related or IOP-independent mechanisms. Figures modified from Li, et al. 2012. Courtesy: National Eye Institute, National Institutes of Health.

this disease, glaucoma can also result from a variety of IOP-related mechanisms due to structural alterations that inhibit outflow of aqueous humor. These include trabecular meshwork obstruction by foreign material, trabecular endothelial cell loss, loss of phagocytic activity of the trabecular meshwork, loss of giant vacuoles from the endothelium of Schlemm's canal and reduced pore size or density in the wall of Schlemm's canal [4].

1.2 Pathophysiology of glaucoma

In the early stages of glaucoma, glial cells in the optic nerve head respond to glaucomatous change. IOP-related mechanisms of damage generally include obstruction of the trabecular meshwork, morphological changes in astrocytes such as enlargement of cell body and processes, as well as upregulation of cytoskeletal and extracellular matrix proteins. Studies have demonstrated that remodeling of astrocytes and increased deposition of extracellular matrix can occur in some forms of experimental glaucoma. Moreover, even a short period of IOP elevation can cause hypertrophy, process retraction, and simplification of the shape of astrocytes in the optic nerve without changes in gene expression. In addition, the accompanying extracellular matrix deposition is believed to be an early defense mechanism to repair or prevent damage to the blood retina barrier [5]. In later stages of glaucoma, glial scar formation can occur as a reaction to injury as a method of protection and healing. Glial cells recruit immune cells, increasing extracellular matrix deposition and inflammatory factors that prevent axonal regeneration [6].

Interestingly, different compartments of RGCs and the optic nerve die by different cellular mechanisms. Specifically, if the RGC axon is cut, the axon distal to the lesion degenerates via Wallerian degeneration, while the axon proximal to the lesion is removed by a process called dying back. Lastly, the cell body of the axon dies via apoptosis [7, 8]. All of which occur among glial scar formation. This process of RGC axon loss can be observed *in situ* during a dilated pupil fundus examination. This area of the posterior globe is termed the optic disc with its center termed the optic cup. Damage from glaucoma causes destruction of the nerve fibers around the rim of this structure and increases the size of the "cup"; an increase in the cup-to-disc ratio is one of the clinical phenotypes that is used to clinically monitor disease progression.

1.3 Classification of glaucoma and early diagnosis in humans

POAG is the most common form of glaucoma and is associated with increased IOP [9]. In broad contrast, PACG has a functional trabecular meshwork with obstructed access, while the trabecular meshwork in POAG is pathological, but open and unobstructed. The initiatory event of PACG is thought to be a blockage between the pupillary portion of the iris and the anterior lens surface, which is correlated with mid-dilation of the pupil [10]. Primary congenital glaucoma, often associated with autosomal recessive disease heritability, results from an abnormal development of the anterior segment and angle of the anterior chamber [11]. NTG is a disease that is nearly identical to POAG but lacks the increased IOP. Pigmentary glaucoma is characterized by accumulation of pigment in the trabecular meshwork and corneal endothelium [12].

Because IOP is the only known modifiable risk factor, it is the target of the majority of current treatment modalities. Increased age has also demonstrated increased risk of ocular hypertension resulting in elevation of IOP and onset of POAG [9]. Damage can also ensue from non-IOP-related mechanisms such as reduced ocular perfusion pressure, excitotoxicity from excessive glutamate, autoimmune-mediated nerve damage, loss of neurotrophic factors, failure of cellular repair mechanisms, and abnormal autoregulation of retinal and choroidal vasculature [4]. African-Caribbean descent, near-sightedness, decreased thickness of the central cornea, first-degree family history, low ocular perfusion pressure, and diabetes are other associated risk factors [13].

The clinical diagnosis of glaucoma relies on recognition of signs of optic nerve damage via slit lamp biomicroscopy and examination of the optic nerve head, followed by measurement of IOP, assessment of the angle via gonioscope and measurement of visual fields. The only directly observable pathology of the optic nerve is in the intrascleral portion which can be observed as an increased cup-to-disc ratio [14]. Glaucoma can progress over decades if it is not appropriately treated. Because it is not painful unless IOP becomes extremely elevated, the early stages of glaucoma often progress undetected. It manifests clinically in advanced stages, where it first affects the peripheral vision of the affected eye. Unfortunately, the other eye, if unaffected, often compensates for changes in the visual field, making most patients unaware of the development and slow loss of vision. Early characteristics might be identified as difficulty reading in dim light. Due to its asymptomatic and silent onset, assessment of family history and frequent clinical assessment is vital. Additionally, assessment of secondary causes of IOP elevation can be beneficial in devising a treatment strategy that can include medical, laser, and surgical modalities [5].

2. Pre-clinical models of glaucoma

While progress has been made in understanding the genetic pathophysiology of glaucoma in humans using genome-wide association studies (GWAS), pre-clinical animal models provide an extremely valuable resource for identifying and understanding cellular mechanisms of action underlying specific mutations, genetic interactions, and ultimately, a knowledge of the disease pathogenesis to better treat the condition. They have been used to observe and modify the interplay of genetic and environmental factors in complex diseases such as glaucoma. They have also been used to develop and evaluate novel therapeutics. This cycle of observation of a disease phenotype and therapeutics response in humans, followed by replication and in-depth examination in pre-clinical models, with subsequent verification in humans, is a bidirectional translation model that is essential to continual forward progression of disease and treatment studies (**Figure 2**). Although there is great value to the models that have been created, there remain unmet needs.

There are many factors to consider when selecting an animal species population for modeling disease. One is the reproduction of the experimental procedure in both the pre-clinical models and humans [15]. For example, in performing an electroretinogram (ERG), a measurement of the electrical activity of the retina in response to light stimulus, employing the use of anesthetics can affect neurotransmission and affect test results [16]. This can become a confounding issue in smaller animals which must be anesthetized. Other factors to consider include the animal's body temperature and age. If body temperature decreases enough, metabolic processes that affect the chemical reactions necessary for an ERG will be decreased, suppressing the amplitude of the ERG, mainly in mice, rats, and rabbits due to their body weight to surface area ratio [17]. Age should also be considered as it influences amplitudes as well. This has been observed in rabbits with younger rabbits exhibiting smaller amplitudes and older rabbits displaying larger amplitudes [18]. Obtaining IOP values can also be difficult and the method

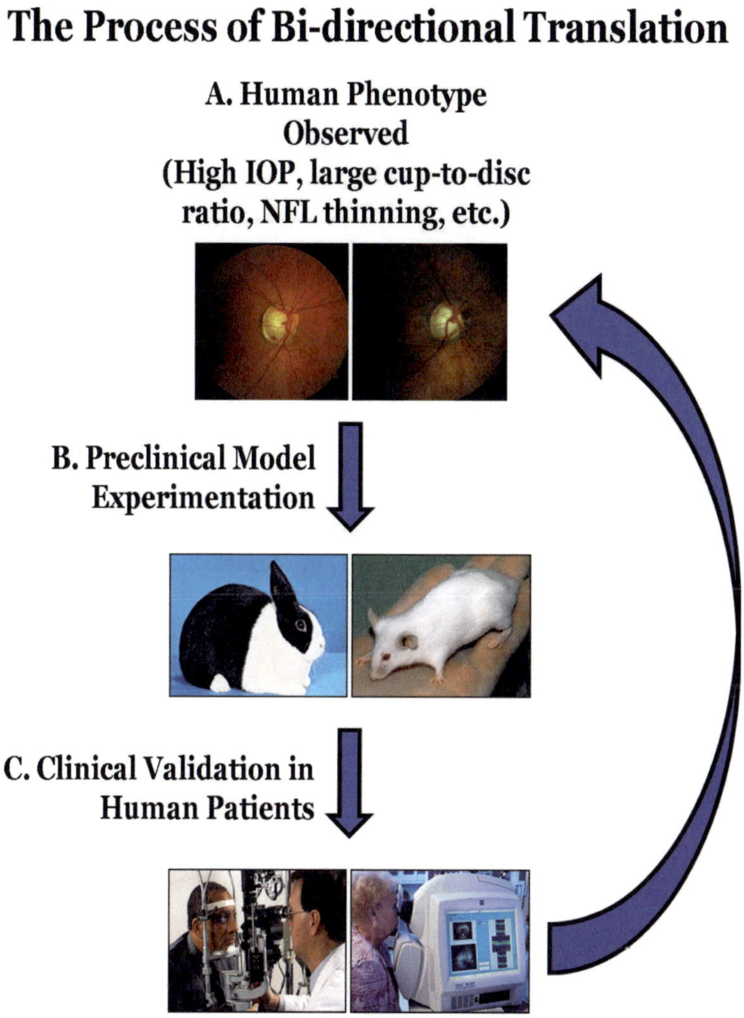

Figure 2.
The progression of bi-directional translation. (A) A disease phenotype is observed in human patients. (B) The observed phenotype is then modeled in a preclinical animal model with as much fidelity to the human condition as possible. (C) After rigorous testing in animal models, the outcomes of those tests (pharmaceutical, or other therapeutic) are then taken back to the human patients and tested for safety and efficacy. If needed, the process repeats. This cycle gives a better comprehension of the disease and how to treat it most effectively.

varies per animal model. In addition, different animal models are susceptible to variations from blood pressure, pulse, respiration, anxiety, as well as sedation and measurement complications [15].

2.1 Naturally occurring models of primary open angle glaucoma (POAG)

2.1.1 Introduction to naturally occurring animal models of POAG

Many genetic loci containing spontaneous polymorphisms have been identified in both human POAG patients and in animals. A few causative genes have been identified such as *MYOC*, *OPTN*, and *WDR36* [11]. Recent studies also postulate RGC number is a risk factor with lower numbers found with gene polymorphisms in *SIX6* (homeobox protein) and *ATOH7* (atonal basic helix–loop–helix transcription factor 7), both of which are associated with worse outcomes [19–22].

2.1.2 POAG in monkeys

Low and high tension POAG was first described in monkeys in 1993. It was found to be maternally inherited, and greater than 40% of the models showed elevated IOP. They displayed loss of RGCs, degeneration of the optic nerve, and damage to the retinal peripheral field. Though while these models are a closer mimic to the human condition, they have strong drawbacks including excessive expense, care, and more complicated handling procedures [15, 23–25].

2.1.3 POAG in dogs

An autosomal recessive POAG has been studied in beagles. Elevation of IOP was seen at 1–2 years of age due to a reduction in aqueous humor outflow. The disease was biphasic: early in the disease the iridiocorneal angle was open, followed by closure with lens subluxation and displacement from the anterior vitreous patellar fossa. The model was used in a genome wide single nucleotide polymorphism array study in which the metallopeptidase *Adamts10*, a candidate gene for POAG, was identified. One noteworthy anatomical difference between dogs and humans is that dogs have an intrascleral plexus rather than a Schlemm's canal, which may result in minor discrepancies between the two models [11, 15, 26, 27].

2.1.4 POAG in mini-pigs

Mini-pig models have also been used as their retina shows likeness to the human retina with holangiotic retinal vasculature, cone photoreceptors in the external retina, a similar scleral thickness, and three types of RGCs [28, 29]. This model can reproduce IOP elevation and can be used to study ocular regeneration with stem cells. Another benefit of this model is its suitability for OCT, corneal topography imaging, and ERG analyses [30].

2.1.5 POAG in birds

Avian models of POAG via light induction technique have been described. They have shown response to antiglaucoma drugs also, which could be beneficial in drug trials targeting IOP [11].

2.1.6 POAG in rodents

Rodent models are valued for their ease of handling and lower management costs. They also have a relatively comparable genome to humans. Drawbacks of mouse models include the lack of a collagenous lamina cribrosa, although it is replaced by one composed of astrocytes. Because the lamina cribrosa is a major location of the pathology that causes optic nerve damage, species differences must be taken into account [11].

Presently, studies have shown that the mutated human myocilin gene, *MYOC Tyr437His* mutation, causes autosomal dominant severe glaucoma with juvenile onset. Mice with a mutation in this same gene develop elevated IOP and 20% RGC loss at 18 months, as well as axonal degeneration in the optic nerve and detachment of the endothelial cells of the trabecular meshwork [31]. A *Col1a1* (alpha-1 subunit of collagen type 1) mutation abrogates matrix metalloproteinase-related cleavage, necessary for turnover of trabecular meshwork, which leads to aggregation and thus increased IOP and RGC death at 24 weeks. This finding infers a correlation between IOP regulation and the turnover of fibrillar collagen in the trabecular meshwork [32].

2.2 Naturally occurring models of PACG

Spontaneous mutations in *B10-Sh3pxd2b*^{nee}, a rare mutation seen in Frank-ter Haar Syndrome, results in glaucoma alongside skeletal and cardiovascular abnormalities. The formation of podosomes, which degrade the extracellular matrix, is impaired, causing the proliferation of the trabecular meshwork and development of iridiocorneal adhesions due to outflow blockage and high IOP resulting in RGC loss by 3–4 months in mice harboring the mutation [5]. Spontaneous mutations in another gene, the serine protease *Prss56*, mimic angle-closure glaucoma as the ocular axial length is reduced, the lens is large, and thus the angle is narrow [33].

2.3 Primary congenital glaucoma

Congenital glaucoma types include autosomal recessive mutations in *CYP1B1* (cytochrome P450 family 1 subfamily B polypeptide 1) and *LTBP2* (Latent-transforming growth factor beta-binding protein), and autosomal dominant mutations in *MYOC* (myocilin), *OPTN* (optineurin), and *WDR36* (WD repeat-containing protein 36) [5]. Another study adds that the transcription factors FOXC1 (Forkhead box C1), FOXC2 (Forkhead box C2), PITX2 (Paired Like Homeodomain 2), LMX1B (LIM homeobox transcription factor 1 beta), and PAX6 (Paired box protein) contribute to congenital glaucoma [34].

2.3.1 Congenital PACG in rabbits, rats, and cats

Naturally occurring congenital glaucoma was first observed in rabbits in 1886 [11]. It was also documented in albino New Zealand white rabbits in the 1960s that presented with anomalies in the anterior chamber [35–37]. In rats, spontaneous congenital glaucoma was seen in 1926 in an inbred family of Wistar-Albino-Glaxo rats [38]. This population presents with enlargement of the globe, elevated IOP, decreased number of RGCs, and degeneration of the optic nerve head. It has also been used in other studies [11]. Feline glaucoma has also been observed with buphthalmia and similar phenotypes to human primary congenital glaucoma, though its occurrence is rare [39].

2.3.2 Congenital PACG in dogs

Evangelho *et al.* document that the anatomy of dogs suits the development of angle closure because they have reduced ocular axial length, an enlarged lens, and a narrow angle [15]. Congenital PACG has been observed in dogs, but it is very rare, and has not been used widely for studies of this subtype of glaucoma [11, 40].

2.3.3 Congenital PACG in turkeys

In turkeys, secondary angle closure glaucoma has been observed, presenting with buphthalmia, low-grade aqueous cells and flare associated with posterior synechiae formation, resulting in pupillary block and iris bombe [41]. It provides a functional model for angle closure glaucoma, but it is also rare.

2.4 Pigmentary dispersion glaucoma

Pigmentary dispersion glaucoma, first described in the DBA/2 J mouse in 1978 presents with a continual increase of IOP until approximately 9 months coupled with early onset iris depigmentation. It is caused by spontaneous mutations in tyrosinase-related protein 1 (*Tyrp1*^{b}) and glycosylated protein nmb (*Gpnmb*^{R150X}) [15, 42]. Co-existing mutations in these two genes, leads to pigment dispersion, iris atrophy, anterior synechiae, and increased IOP, as well as loss of RGCs and optic nerve atrophy that is progressive, even after the IOP returns to lower IOP levels in older DBA/2 J mice [43–45]. Similar to humans, it progresses in severity with increasing age. Although pigmentary dispersion glaucoma can affect humans, it is not linked to mutations in either *Tyrp1* or *Gpnmb*.

2.5 Normotensive glaucoma

Normotensive glaucoma presents with the same characteristics as POAG, but it lacks an elevated IOP above the normal physiological range. Speculation concerning the mechanism includes lack of blood flow to the optic nerve, vascular spasm, and multiple mutations [11]. Recently, some investigators have used the marmoset, a small primate, as an experimental glaucoma model. Its advantages include a high reproduction rate and a short time to sexual maturation (12–18 months), as well as their ease of management and breeding [46]. The transgenic marmoset was reported in 2009 as well. Moreover, in 2019 it was documented that aged marmosets showed glaucomatous retinal and brain degeneration as well as thinning of the lamina cribrosa [46]. They did not have accompanying mutations in glaucoma-associated genes nor elevation of IOP, which suggest a normotensive glaucoma phenotype. It was noted that there was increased oxidative stress and reduced brain-derived neurotrophic factor levels, which is neuroprotective for RGCs and also reduced in human glaucoma patients [46].

3. Experimentally induced models of glaucoma

To aid in the study of glaucoma-associated optic nerve damage, models have been created by directly damaging RGC axons or indirectly through elevation of IOP. The optic nerve can be crushed with self-closing fine forceps to cause temporally synchronous injury to the RGC axons. This experimental model is useful to study the effects of RGC damage, but does not replicate the spontaneous, continuous development seen in acute or chronic glaucoma. Kimura *et al*. advocate for experimentally inducible models due to the fact that wild-type animals can be used and the experimental condition can be meticulously monitored, as well as the progression of disease [46].

3.1 POAG models

IOP can be elevated through direct or indirect blockage of the trabecular meshwork via injection of hypertonic saline into episcleral veins, cauterization of the episcleral veins, or photocoagulation with an argon laser, which all block outflow and induce an elevation of IOP [20].

3.1.1 Laser photocoagulation

Laser photocoagulation has been used as an experimental model in non-human primates. This technique damages the trabecular meshwork, which blocks outflow of aqueous humor and elevates IOP [47]. It requires three lasers in a 7-day interval to increase IOP by 60%. This method is expensive and can cause anterior peripheral synechiae, hyphema, and corneal edema. In animals subjected to this procedure, it caused loss of RGCs and thinning of the nerve fiber layer, both phenotypes associated with glaucomatous damage in humans [17, 48]. An argon laser with the slit lamp can also be used, but only for certain strains of rodents because it can cause pigment affinity and variation in elevation of IOP [49, 50]. If laser photocoagulation is combined with temporary narrowing of the iridiocorneal angle via paracentesis, this results in a sudden, 3-week increase in IOP that is not reflective of glaucoma progression in humans, although more acute changes can be evaluated. It can also cause ischemia and opacity of the central cornea [51]. To create a more chronic elevation of IOP condition, 50 microliters of hypertonic saline solution can be injected into the collecting veins of a rat eye to cause sclerotic damage to the trabecular meshwork and optic nerve. This is accomplished with specialized microneedles and a complex procedure both difficult to execute and to teach. A moderate increase in IOP is seen 7–10 days after the procedure and is recommended for use in studies exploring neuroprotection [52]. In addition, a nylon suture can be used to occlude the vein and cause an increase in IOP [15, 53].

3.1.2 Glaucoma induced by modifying the trabecular meshwork

Topical application or injection of steroids as IOP modulators has also been studied in a variety of animals as a mechanism to elevate IOP and mimic POAG [20]. Its mechanism of action is not fully delineated but is believed to function by stabilization of the lysosomal membrane and the accumulation of glycosaminoglycans polymerized in the trabecular meshwork, which creates resistance to outflow of aqueous humor. Outflow resistance is further increased by elevated expression of fibronectin, elastin, and laminin, which also hinder outflow [15]. Glaucoma induced via this mechanism has been studied in a New Zealand rabbit breed [54], which demonstrated that the angle of the anterior chamber is an important regulatory mechanism of outflow of aqueous humor. It has been used to further understand the composition of the trabecular meshwork, as well as identifying its components such as glycosaminoglycans, hyaluronic acid, keratan sulfate, heparan sulfate, and sulfate-chondroitin [55, 56].

Based on the increased presence of hyaluronic acid in the trabecular meshwork induced by steroids, it was demonstrated that a single application of 1% hyaluronic acid in rat models induced an elevation of IOP for up to 8 days, proving a useful acute model [15]. Though not well understood, this injection causes an accumulation of glycosaminoglycans in the trabecular meshwork, which obstructs outflow. This model is noteworthy for its low cost, ease of execution, and sustainability as it induces a more chronic hypertensive state and could be used for pharmacological studies [15, 57, 58]. As a candidate for animal models, rats have similar benefits to mice. There is a comparable elevation of IOP and corresponding optic nerve changes as seen in humans [11]. As such, a second steroidal approach involves topical dexamethasone used in rats to elevate IOP and study the regulation of myocilin, previously identified as a causative gene of POAG in humans. Though the model demonstrated IOP elevation, mRNA levels of myocilin in the trabecular meshwork and in proximity to Schlemm's canal were not different from the control [59].

3.1.3 Reperfusion ischemia

An additional model to mimic open angle glaucoma is via induction of reperfusion ischemia by paracentesis in the anterior chamber. In this method, the cannulation of the anterior chamber with a microneedle allows precise control of the IOP and suppression of blood flow through the retinal and uveal vasculature. This causes IOP-induced damage to the RGCs [15, 47].

3.2 PACG models

Microspheres have been injected to block the trabecular meshwork and emulate PACG. The microspheres do not block the pupil, which allows observation of the fundus, which makes this a suitable model. However, fluctuations in IOP can limit the efficacy as well as location of the microspheres. Yet, elevation of nitric oxide in the aqueous humor was detected in neovascular and angle closure subtypes, thought to be due to the inflammatory mechanism [15, 60]. Bouhenni *et al.* also writes that there are various rat, mice, and rabbit models of PACG to study the effects of elevated IOP on RGCs and the optic nerve. These models have been created with techniques such as hypertonic saline injection into the episcleral veins, cauterization or ligation of the episcleral veins, or laser photocoagulation as discussed prior [11].

4. Genetically modified models

Genetically modified models allow for a careful examination of the influence of typically a single gene mutation on the onset of elevated IOP, RGC damage, and the progression of glaucoma. They allow for manipulation of loci that contribute to this multifactorial mechanism but require a longer timeframe of study than mechanically induced models [15]. An ideal model should be easily reproducible, economical, and closely emulate human pathology [15]. Of all the species, the mouse is a very common model due to its low cost, ease of breeding and the vast genetic resources that are available. Examples of rodent glaucoma models include but are not limited to the following: intraocular injection of RGC toxins; crush or transection of the ON; manual elevation of IOP using microneedle injection into the anterior chamber; laser photocoagulation of the trabecular meshwork or episcleral veins; transgenic mice with specific mutations (reviewed in [11, 61]); and bead injection into the anterior chamber. While all of these methods have merit, none of them completely mimics the array of human disease presentation, and therefore additional models of glaucoma are still an unmet need of the vision research community.

4.1 POAG models

Transgenic models have been developed such as the *bug eye* mutant, the *lrp2* (lipoprotein receptor-related protein 2) mutant, and the *wdr36* mutant in zebrafish. The *bug eye* shows RGC death and high IOP and was used to identify *lrp2* as the gene responsible for the endophenotypes of elevated IOP, large eyes, decreased retinal neurons, activation of RGC stress genes, and optic nerve pathology [62–64]. Kimura *et al.* also reports a $P2Y_6$ (pyrimidinergic receptor) knockout (KO) mouse that presents with age-dependent optic nerve and RGC degeneration and impaired visual function due to excess production of aqueous humor [46].

4.2 PACG models

Vav2/*Vav3* (guanine nucleotide exchange factors) KO mice mimic human spontaneous development of glaucoma, but there is poor understanding of the pathophysiology. These models develop buphthalmia and the iridiocorneal angle changes before 6 months of age and ultimately chronic angle closure glaucoma occurs [65]. They have additionally been identified as candidate genes for a sub-group of open-angle glaucoma in the Japanese [20]. Bouhenni *et al.* find three notable features of this model: first, elevated IOP occurs naturally in this model; second, the incidence of this phenotype is high and occurs at a reasonably young age; third, human hypotensive glaucoma treatments have shown IOP-lowering effects in this model [11]. This makes this model useful for targeting molecular mechanisms in developing understanding of the pathophysiology.

4.3 Primary congenital glaucoma models

Knockout of *Foxc1* and *Foxc2*, genes involved in embryonic and ocular development, in mice causes death during the embryonic or neonatal periods [66]. Heterozygous *Foxc1*$^{+/-}$ mice have defects in ocular drainage structures, but do not see elevation of IOP. Moreover, *Cyp1b1* KO animals develop ocular defects comparable to human congenital glaucoma, presenting with rudimentary Schlemm's canal, abnormalities in the trabecular meshwork, adhesion of the iris to the trabecular meshwork and peripheral cornea [15]. Another model was described in an albino quail population with a similar phenotype, but due to small size, limited availability, and difficult clinical translation, it is rarely used [11].

4.4 Normotensive glaucoma models

Genetically modified mice with normal IOP have been used to further study normotensive glaucoma. Specifically, mice lacking the glutamate transporter genes, *Glast* or *Eaac1* (Excitatory amino acid transporter 3), develop RGC damage and optic nerve degeneration without the IOP elevation. *Glast* is expressed in Müller glia in the retina and aids in the removal of glutamate, sparing RGCs from the neuroexcitotoxicity due to its accumulation [46]. *Eaac1* is expressed in neurons and assists with the uptake of both cysteine and glutamate [46]. This evidence supports a protective role of these genes in preventing RGC damage.

A deficiency in apoptosis signal-regulating kinase 1 (*Ask1*) also known as mitogen-activated protein kinase 5 (Map3k5) had no neurotoxic effects or effects on IOP. It was also demonstrated that the activation of p38 MAPK and the production of inducible nitric oxide synthase was suppressed in glial cells and RGCs, implying that ASK1 activation could be involved in normotensive glaucoma [67]. Additionally, this model was used to study the neuroprotective effects of *N*-acetylcysteine, which was demonstrated to be protective in the *Eaac1* KO mice. Kimura *et al*. also added that *Glast* or *Eaac1* mutations produce an early onset phenotype, which increases the utility of this model, particularly in studying efficacy of treatments [46]. This is contrasted with the other models of normotensive glaucoma, which are comprised of overexpression of mutated optineurin E50K and tank-binding protein 1, the mutated genes associated with human normotensive glaucoma [46]. These models have a later onset, which makes them less suitable experimentally. In addition, using marmosets mentioned prior, a model is in the works targeting the *Glast* gene, which is speculated to produce a functional model with early onset glaucoma [46].

4.5 Immune response models

In the Wallerian degeneration slow (W1dS) mouse, transfection with a fusion gene of *Nmnat1* and *Ube4b* protect RGC axons by maintaining mitochondrial function. An influx of calcium was documented prior to RGC axon degeneration [68, 69]. This finding was significant, as it proves there are specific molecular mechanisms that modulate axon degeneration. Struebing *et. al* review other molecular mechanisms of RGC degeneration. For example, knocking out *Bax* promotes survival of

RGC bodies, but does not rescue axons. The JNK (c-Jun, N-terminal kinase) pathway is involved in both axonal and soma degradation as deficiency in both *Jnk2* and *Jnk3* results in protection from RGC death after optic nerve crush. Lastly, knocking out *Dlk* (dual leucine zipper kinase) causes cell death in soma but does not affect degeneration of axons [20, 70–72].

Within an investigation of an autoimmune response as a plausible mechanism of RGC damage, it was determined that serum samples of glaucoma patients have increased levels of heat shock protein 27 (HSP27) and heat shock protein 60 (HSP60). Immunization of these proteins in the Lewis rat population resulted in RGC degeneration and axonal loss 1–4 months later, supporting a role of these proteins in glaucoma [11, 73].

4.6 The BXD murine family of recombinant inbred lines of mice

Because most human glaucoma cases are not due to polymorphisms in single genes, it is not surprising that pre-clinical models that examine the effects of mutations in one gene at a time do not fully recapitulate all endophenotypes of human disease. In contrast, a polygenetic approach may advance the field of glaucoma. One approach to this is the involvement of the BXD murine family. BXD mice are a family of recombinant inbred strains that were derived by mating C57/Bl6 (B6) and DBA/2 J (D2) mice and inbreeding the F2 progeny for >20 generations, allowing for natural recombination of genes throughout the entire genome.

Each fully inbred BXD strain is genetically distinct and fixed at each locus of the genome. This family of mice is an outstanding resource as data on >1000 phenotypes and nearly 100 expression data sets (gene, protein, and metabolites) have been collected and are available on GeneNetwork (www.genenetwork.org), an open access resource for the scientific community. Moreover, all BXD and their parent strains have been fully sequenced. There are ~5.2 million single nucleotide polymorphisms, >400,000 insertions/deletions and multiple copy number variants between the progenitors which segregate among the BXD strains. Multiple data sets of the eye, retina, optic nerve phenotypes and expression data are also available on GeneNetwork to facilitate systems genetics analyses at multiple levels from gene to metabolome [74].

The BXD family has become a valuable resource for modeling human disease, including glaucoma. B6 has no glaucoma-associated pathologies with fairly constant IOP until >13 months of age. The optic nerve has little damage throughout the life of B6. In contrast, D2 parents develop pigmentary dispersion glaucoma and have an elevated IOP that reaches its maximum at ~9 months with a subsequent IOP reduction. ON damage increases throughout the lifetime of D2 mice. The influence of pigmentary dispersion on glaucoma can be studied among the afflicted progeny or be eliminated by excluding those strains that harbor mutations in *Tyrp1* and *Gpnmb* from the study plan. By quantifying specific endophenotypes across the BXD family along with gene expression and polymorphism profiles, new and informative insights regarding novel modulating genes can be revealed. Specific to this pre-clinical murine family, several BXD strains spontaneously develop elevated IOP and/or optic nerve damage due to the particular set of polymorphisms in the genome of each individual strain, similar to the human condition. Importantly, the phenotype of each BXD strain is highly reproducible because each strain is fully inbred with a fixed genome and the supply of mice from each strain is essentially unlimited.

As a testament to the power of the BXD family and the genetic/genomic information gathered from these mice, approximately 20 disease-associated strains have already been cloned from the BXD family [74]. One example of the power of using BXD mice in the virtuous cycle of bi-directional translation is the identification of the novel IOP-modulating gene, *Cacna2d1*, which has demonstrated potent IOP-lowering effects with therapeutic blocking of the function of its gene product with pregabalin in a dose-dependent and haplotype-specific manner [74].

In other studies, by examining the immune network and the response of the optic nerve to RGC damage, and comparing the two, it was determined that an innate immune network was activated by the optic nerve crush [75]. The importance of the complement cascade or innate immune network as mentioned above, has been demonstrated by knocking out *C1qa* in D2 mice. Both pigmentary dispersion glaucoma and elevated IOP are noted, however, the loss of axons in the optic nerve is lessened, which points to the role of *C1qa* in the degeneration of axons in the optic nerve [76]. A gene network of regulatory mechanisms in the retina that are activated by injury was mapped, and it was determined there are common regulatory mechanisms. In addition, there was a significant quantitative trait locus (QTL) found on chromosome 16 from 80 to 95 Mb that correlates with the expression of *C4b* in the normal retina [77]. In this region, two *cis*-acting QTLs were identified as potential modulatory genes of the innate immunity network, although the modulating gene has not yet been identified [20]. These data suggest possible shared disease mechanisms with age-related macular degeneration (AMD), in which complement proteins are found in the drusen deposits that characterize AMD [45, 78–80].

5. Therapeutics for glaucoma

5.1 Current FDA-approved therapeutics

At baseline, the goal of current glaucoma treatments is to decrease IOP, which is presently the only identified modifiable risk factor. There are a variety of medications that modify IOP by either decreasing production or increasing the outflow of aqueous humor. Factors such as patient compliance, costs, drug penetration, variations in drug metabolism and bioavailability, and even other factors such as systemic diseases, diet, alcohol, etc., all play a role in medical management. Additionally, glaucoma patients require long-term treatment to keep pressures low. Years of treatment can exacerbate ocular surface disease and cause chronic conjunctival inflammation, which may threaten the efficacy of future surgical procedures (such as trabeculectomy). IOP fluctuation can worsen disease progression, seen in the advanced glaucoma interventional study [81].

5.1.1 Modulation of aqueous production

Drugs that decrease the production of aqueous, such as beta blockers and carbonic anhydrase inhibitors, have been the mainstay in glaucoma treatment for years. However, these drugs can have systemic adverse side effects such as bradycardia, impotence, exacerbation of asthma, and also may demonstrate tachyphylaxis over time. The beta blockers, such as timolol, modulate aqueous inflow. The beta-1 receptor increases production of aqueous, and the beta blockers inhibit the production of cyclic AMP by this receptor which reduces aqueous production [13]. Carbonic anhydrase inhibitors, such as brinzolamide, decrease the production of aqueous via suppression of aqueous ducts [13], but can produce a renal metabolic acidosis as they inhibit acid secretion in the proximal tubule of the kidney as well [13]. Other drugs, such as brimonidine, modulate the production of aqueous via the alpha-2 receptor. Adverse effects to this drug can include a delayed hypersensitivity reaction and, due to their ability to cross the blood–brain barrier, they are contraindicated in children under two [13].

5.1.2 Modulation of aqueous humor outflow

Parasympathomimetic drugs, such as pilocarpine, have been used to decrease outflow. They cause contraction of the longitudinal ciliary muscles, which increases aqueous humor outflow. However, due to its three-to-four times daily dosing paradigm, myopic shift, and risk of retinal detachment, along with decreased patient compliance, it is no longer a first-line treatment [13]. Presently, prostaglandin analogs, such as latanoprost (Xalatan), have become the mainstay first-line treatment. They function by increasing outflow via modulation of uveoscleral pores, opening them as a secondary outflow mechanism that decreases outflow resistance. Most recently, Rho kinase inhibitors, such as Rhopressa, inhibit actin/myosin contraction of these muscles and improve trabecular meshwork outflow by decreasing the episcleral venous pressure. In the acute setting, hyperosmotic agents such as glycerol and mannitol can be used to lower the IOP, given intravenously, increasing the tonicity of the plasma and drawing aqueous out of the eye [13].

5.1.3 Sustained-release devices

To combat challenges of drug delivery, different models of sustained release implants have been developed. One intracameral implant called Durysta is an FDA-approved device that delivers bimatoprost into the anterior chamber over a period of four months [82]. Unfortunately, complications of Durysta use include chronic inflammation and corneal endothelial cell loss.

Other sustained-release implants in development include intracanalicular devices, subconjunctival injections, and collagen shields [83]. Examples include latanoprost micro-dose delivery with Optejet (Microprost, Eyenovia), latanoprost delivery via an intracanalicular insert (OTX-TIC, Ocular Therapeutix), and latanoprost or travoprost delivery via a punctal plug (L-evolute and T-evolute, Mati Therapeutics). The latter includes two travoprost delivery platforms, ENV515 (Envisia Therapeutics) and iDose (Glaukos) [83–85]. iDose is a titanium implant that releases a unique formulation of travoprost into the anterior chamber [84]. It releases micro-amounts of the drug over a year and eliminates the barrier of the cornea. It is composed of three parts that titrates travoprost release [84, 86]. It was reported in a randomized, double-blind phase II trial, iDose achieved a 30% reduction in IOP at 12 months, lowering the average number of glaucoma medications per patient compared to the control group of 0.5% timolol, demonstrating non-inferiority with minimal adverse effects [84]. At each stage of development of these FDA-approved therapeutics, multiple pre-clinical models were used to demonstrate safety and efficacy, making their inclusion in the drug pipeline invaluable.

5.2 Therapeutics in development

Treatments that mitigate risk factors other than IOP are an identified gap in treatment modalities [46]. These are especially needed for populations that do not respond to current IOP-lowering medications, when a lowered IOP is insufficient to halt visual field loss, and in normotensive glaucoma cases. A particular need exists for the identification of neuroprotective molecules that act directly on the optic nerve and RGC axons. Although several therapies are being evaluated in multiple laboratories across the world, there remains no FDA-approved neuroprotective option for glaucoma patients. In line with this treatment strategy, Kimura *et al.* disclosed treatment trials exploring the delivery of ciliary neurotrophic factor into the eye via modified human cells that secrete it. They postulate this mechanism has potential for neuroprotective effects in the treatment of normotensive glaucoma [46]. In addition, on the progressive end of molecular modifying, it may be possible to use stem cell therapy with CRISPR-Cas 9 technology to neutralize mutations causing glaucoma phenotypes. This capability is currently being explored [15], but will take thoughtful risk/benefit analysis.

Approaching treatment from a different angle, a unique tool to modulate IOP is being explored. The Mercury Multi-Pressure Dial (Equinox) is a pair of pressurized goggles that create a pressure vacuum around the eye, which decreases pressure from gravity and increases ocular blood flow [87]. They operate on the principal that glaucoma is likely a dual-pressure disease due to the balance between IOP and intracranial pressure (ICP) [87]. Thus, the inventors of this device postulate that glaucoma is a result of high IOP and low ICP. By applying a moderate negative pressure in the front of the eye with their goggles, the pressure inside the eye is reduced and the ICP is restored to a physiological level [87]. Moreover, it serves as a point to demonstrate that one direction glaucoma treatment might be headed is 24/7 modulation of pressure where sensors monitor pressure on-the-go, allowing physicians access to IOP data without requiring an office visit and creating a practical opportunity for a telemedicine consultation.

Experimental models of glaucoma are crucial to understanding the mechanism of disease and designing novel treatments. Assessing their axonal degeneration in optic nerve cross sections has proven beneficial in this pursuit. Specifically, the BXD genetic reference panel will be used to detect and study spontaneous models of glaucoma. This will be invaluable to the scientific community, especially in an effort to develop novel treatment options. While the development of these novel modalities takes time, animal models can be used to explore the benefit of existing drugs, a method known as drug repositioning or repurposing [67]. Neuroprotection is one particular facet of interest, and it is postulated available drug modalities for diseases of the central nervous system such as Alzheimer's or Parkinson's might also exhibit neuroprotection in glaucoma patients [88]. Examples of these trials include memantine, valproic acid, edaravone, and niacin (vitamin B3). Unfortunately, memantine was ruled ineffective in 2018 [89]. Valproic acid was demonstrated to be neuroprotective in rodent models of normotensive glaucoma, and one study from India showed improvement of advanced glaucoma cases [90, 91]. Edaravone was also shown to decrease RGC death in mouse models of normotensive glaucoma [92]. Lastly, oral niacin was demonstrated to be protective in mouse models [93]. There is also interest in the potential of dairy products being neuroprotective due to their levels of spermidine, which is a compound that has demonstrated neuroprotection in mouse models [67]. Additionally, using rodent models, Chintalapudi *et al.* have demonstrated IOP-lowering effects of pregabalin, which inhibits calcium channels containing the CACNA2D1 subunit. It is mainly used for neuropathic pain but was developed initially as an antiepileptic [74, 94]. Animal models have clearly demonstrated their necessity in testing for current and future pharmacological treatments.

6. Bidirectional translation from humans to pre-clinical models and back again

The virtuous cycle of bidirectional translation works through the observation of disease phenotypes and processes in human patients, followed by replication and examination of the specific observation in normal and pathological pre-clinical models to discover novel modulators of complex disease mechanisms, and ultimately test those outcomes back in human patients. This process should be repeated until a safe and effective treatment paradigm is obtained or the disease process of better understood. This strategy clearly supports the hypothesis that breakthroughs in human and experimental models fuel a sustainable model of human observation, pre-clinical model experimentation, and verification in humans. As direct support for this strategy, as discussed above, with the known observation that elevated IOP is the chief modifiable risk factor for POAG, Chintalapudi *et al.* used strains from the BXD family of mice and identified a novel gene modulator of IOP—calcium voltage-gated channel auxiliary subunit alpha2delta 1 (*Cacna2d1*)— that was confirmed in human GWAS investigations [74]. These findings were the platform that allowed for the discovery of pregabalin, an inhibitor of CACNA2D1, as a new IOP-lowering drug with a novel mechanism of action [74]. This, as well as the variety of molecular models discussed above, demonstrates the efficacy of bidirectional translation in driving the diagnosis, treatment, and prevention of complex diseases [95].

The collective generation of large datasets like GWAS have facilitated the identification of gene modulators of complex traits and disease mechanisms. Those tools alone, however, do not account for the complex interplay between inherited and environmental factors. Human limitations are clear; animal models are equipped with the biological resources to support the detailed analyses of disease progression. Pre-clinical models reveal instrumental pathophysiology, which when translated to humans, fuels the evolution of molecular, cellular, developmental, and physiological research [95]. However, glaucoma is a multifaceted disease, which one animal model alone cannot flawlessly emulate. Different animal models display unique features of the pathophysiology of the disease and each help further understanding of glaucoma progression as a whole.

7. Conclusion

In conclusion, the future of glaucoma treatment is in understanding disease mechanisms of glaucoma viewed with an interventional mindset. Increasingly, the safety and efficacy of drug delivery allows better control of IOP. Medical management shortly seeks to improve sustainability through products like Durysta and iDose. Innovation of medical management is in progress with formulations of *N*-acetylcysteine or ciliary neurotrophic factor, as mentioned. It is speculated that glaucoma is headed in a direction of earlier detection, earlier intervention, and chronic modulation, potentially even with tools to adequately assess pressure from home (even 24/7), and to address it with telehealth resources. Technology may permit detection of resistance sites, which allows specification of procedures specific to the individual patient. Largely, it is evident that there is a gap in the treatment of glaucoma with non-IOP-related modalities. This supports the need for animal models in developing further understanding of the pathophysiology of glaucoma, but also in studying the efficacy of present treatment mechanisms (such as IOP-lowering) as well as novel ones (*N*-acetylcysteine, ciliary neurotrophic factor, molecular mapping with animal models, CRISPR-CAS9).

Something to consider with the current information-driven culture, are mechanisms to objectively quantify the degree of pathophysiology present in these animal models, particularly when they are used to examine the efficacy of treatment modalities. Currently, a particular BXD strain which spontaneously develops glaucoma is being used to observe optic nerve pathology (including axonal degeneration and glial scarring) and objectively quantify glaucomatous degeneration. This, as well as the potential of an automated system to carry out this task, has the ability to revolutionize this field. A deep neural network is being developed to reliably assess the progression of axonal degeneration in glaucoma. It provides an opportunity to automate this process to better understand the mechanism of glaucoma—etiologically and clinically—and to assess the efficacy of treatment trials. By using a uniform stratification of disease progression, large volume studies can be conducted with greater precision, efficiency, and less bias. This will allow for exponential growth in the understanding and treatment of glaucoma as the knowledge of pathophysiology is enhanced. It showcases the use of artificial intelligence to autonomously convert subjective data to an objective form of precise stratification.

To summarize, this chapter makes one thing clear. The "virtuous cycle" of bidirectional translation is essential to further understanding of the pathophysiology of glaucoma. It is the common tool necessary to further observe disease advancement, design more molecular models, identify disease modulators, and discover new therapeutics. Moreover, this chapter reveals that pre-clinical models illuminate this path forward.

Acknowledgements

We would like to acknowledge the following funding sources: a Challenge Award from Research to Prevent Blindness (New York, NY) to the Department of Ophthalmology at the Hamilton Eye Institute; and a grant from BrightFocus National Glaucoma Research to MMJ (Clarksburg, MD).

Conflict of interest

The authors have no conflicts of interest.

Author details

Sophie Pilkinton, T.J. Hollingsworth, Brian Jerkins and Monica M. Jablonski*
Hamilton Eye Institute, University of Tennessee Health Science Center, Memphis, TN, United States

*Address all correspondence to: mjablonski@uthsc.edu

References

[1] Li H, M.M., Jablonski MM., *Relevance of miRNAs to Eye Disease.* miRNAs and Human Diseases, 2012: p. 179-196.

[2] Tham, Y.-C., et al., *Global Prevalence of Glaucoma and Projections of Glaucoma Burden through 2040: A Systematic Review and Meta-Analysis.* Ophthalmology, 2014. **121**(11): p. 2081-2090.

[3] Kingman, S., *Glaucoma is second leading cause of blindness globally.* Bulletin of the World Health Organization, 2004. **82**: p. 887-8.

[4] Anthony Khawaja MA(Cantab), M.B., MRCOphth *Primary Open-Angle Glaucoma - Eyewiki*. 2019 [cited 2021 February 13, 2021]; Available from: https://eyewiki.aao.org/Primary_Open-Angle_Glaucoma.

[5] Soto, I. and G. Howell, *The Complex Role of Neuroinflammation in Glaucoma.* Cold Spring Harbor Perspectives in Medicine, 2014. **4**.

[6] Wang, H., et al., *Portrait of glial scar in neurological diseases.* International Journal of Immunopathology and Pharmacology, 2018. **31**: p. 205873841880140.

[7] Libby, R.T., et al., *Inherited glaucoma in DBA/2J mice: Pertinent disease features for studying the neurodegeneration.* Visual Neuroscience, 2005. **22**(5): p. 637-648.

[8] Nickells, R.W. and D.J. Zack, *Apoptosis in ocular disease: a molecular overview.* Ophthalmic Genetics, 1996. **17**(4): p. 145-165.

[9] Gordon, M.O., et al., *The Ocular Hypertension Treatment Study: Baseline Factors That Predict the Onset of Primary Open-Angle Glaucoma.* Archives of Ophthalmology, 2002. **120**(6): p. 714-720.

[10] Shields, B.M., *Primary Angle-Closure Glaucoma*, in *The Glaucoma Textbook*. 1992, Williams and Wilkins: Baltimore, MD. p. 198-199.

[11] Bouhenni, R.A., et al., *Animal models of glaucoma.* Journal of biomedicine & biotechnology, 2012. **2012**: p. 692609-692609.

[12] Pradeep Ramulu, M.D. *Pigmentary Glaucoma and Pigment Dispersion Syndrome - EyeWiki*. 2020 [cited 2021 February 14, 2021]; Available from: https://eyewiki.aao.org/Pigmentary_glaucoma_and_Pigment_Dispersion_Syndrome#:~:text=Pigmentary%20glaucoma%20is%20a%20type,corneal%20endothelium%20(Krukenberg%20spindle).

[13] Prum, B.E., Jr., et al., *Primary Open-Angle Glaucoma Preferred Practice Pattern® Guidelines.* Ophthalmology, 2016. **123**(1): p. P41-P111.

[14] Cohen, L. and L. Pasquale, *Clinical Characteristics and Current Treatment of Glaucoma.* Cold Spring Harbor perspectives in medicine, 2014. **4**.

[15] Evangelho, K., C.A. Mastronardi, and A. de-la-Torre, *Experimental Models of Glaucoma: A Powerful Translational Tool for the Future Development of New Therapies for Glaucoma in Humans—A Review of the Literature.* Medicina, 2019. **55**(6): p. 280.

[16] McCulloch, D.L., et al., *ISCEV Standard for full-field clinical electroretinography (2015 update).* Documenta Ophthalmologica, 2015. **130**(1): p. 1-12.

[17] Mizota, A. and E. Adachi-Usami, *Effect of Body Temperature on Electroretinogram of Mice.* Investigative Ophthalmology & Visual Science, 2002. **43**(12): p. 3754-3757.

[18] Wang, W.H., et al., *Noninvasive measurement of rodent intraocular pressure with a rebound tonometer.* Invest Ophthalmol Vis Sci, 2005. **46**(12): p. 4617-21.

[19] Ulmer Carnes, M., et al., *Discovery and Functional Annotation of SIX6 Variants in Primary Open-Angle Glaucoma.* PLOS Genetics, 2014. **10**(5): p. e1004372.

[20] Struebing, F.L. and E.E. Geisert, *Chapter Twenty-One - What Animal Models Can Tell Us About Glaucoma*, in *Progress in Molecular Biology and Translational Science*, J.F. Hejtmancik and J.M. Nickerson, Editors. 2015, Academic Press. p. 365-380.

[21] Macgregor, S., et al., *Genome-wide association identifies ATOH7 as a major gene determining human optic disc size.* Human Molecular Genetics, 2010. **19**(13): p. 2716-2724.

[22] Prasov, L., et al., *Math5(Atoh7) gene dosage limits retinal ganglion cell genesis.* NeuroReport, 2012. **23**(10).

[23] Chen, L., Y. Zhao, and H. Zhang, *Comparative Anatomy of the Trabecular Meshwork, the Optic Nerve Head and the Inner Retina in Rodent and Primate Models Used for Glaucoma Research.* Vision, 2017. **1**(1): p. 4.

[24] Yan, Z., et al., *Analysis of a method for establishing a model with more stable chronic glaucoma in rhesus monkeys.* Exp Eye Res, 2015. **131**: p. 56-62.

[25] Ollivier, F.J., et al., *Time-specific intraocular pressure curves in Rhesus macaques (Macaca mulatta) with laser-induced ocular hypertension.* Veterinary Ophthalmology, 2004. **7**(1): p. 23-27.

[26] Vecino, E. and S. C, *Glaucoma Animal Models*. 2011, InTech.

[27] Palko, J.R., et al., *Influence of Age on Ocular Biomechanical Properties in a Canine Glaucoma Model with ADAMTS10 Mutation.* PLoS One, 2016. **11**(6): p. e0156466.

[28] Ruiz-Ederra, J., et al., *Comparative study of the three neurofilament subunits within pig and human retinal ganglion cells.* Molecular vision, 2004. **10**: p. 83-92.

[29] Middleton, S., *Porcine ophthalmology.* Vet Clin North Am Food Anim Pract, 2010. **26**(3): p. 557-72.

[30] Vecino, E., et al., *Retrobulbar Optic Nerve Section In Pig: Optical Coherence Tomography (oct) And Multifocal Electroretinography (mferg) Study.* Investigative Ophthalmology & Visual Science, 2011. **52**(14): p. 4683-4683.

[31] Zhou, Y., O. Grinchuk, and S.I. Tomarev, *Transgenic mice expressing the Tyr437His mutant of human myocilin protein develop glaucoma.* Invest Ophthalmol Vis Sci, 2008. **49**(5): p. 1932-9.

[32] Mabuchi, F., et al., *Optic nerve damage in mice with a targeted type I collagen mutation.* Invest Ophthalmol Vis Sci, 2004. **45**(6): p. 1841-5.

[33] Nair, K.S., et al., *Alteration of the serine protease PRSS56 causes angle-closure glaucoma in mice and posterior microphthalmia in humans and mice.* Nat Genet, 2011. **43**(6): p. 579-84.

[34] Johnson, T. and S. Tomarev, *Animal Models of Glaucoma*. 2016. p. 31-50.

[35] Kolker, A.E., et al., *THE DEVELOPMENT OF GLAUCOMA IN RABBITS.* Invest Ophthalmol, 1963. **2**: p. 316-21.

[36] Hanna, B.L., P.B. Sawin, and L.B. Sheppard, *Recessive buphthalmos in the rabbit.* Genetics, 1962. **47**(5): p. 519-29.

[37] Fox, R.R., et al., *Buphthalmia in the rabbit. Pleiotropic effects of the (bu) gene*

and a possible explanation of mode of gene action. J Hered, 1969. **60**(4): p. 206-12.

[38] Addison, W.H.F. and H.W. How, *Congenital hypertrophy of the eye in an albino rat.* The Anatomical Record, 1926. **32**(4): p. 271-277.

[39] McLellan, G.J., et al., *Congenital Glaucoma in the Siamese Cat – A Novel Spontaneous Animal Model for Glaucoma Research.* Investigative Ophthalmology & Visual Science, 2005. **46**(13): p. 134-134.

[40] Gelatt, K.N., et al., *Clinical manifestations of inherited glaucoma in the beagle.* Invest Ophthalmol Vis Sci, 1977. **16**(12): p. 1135-42.

[41] de Kater, A.W., et al., *The Slate turkey: a model for secondary angle closure glaucoma.* Invest Ophthalmol Vis Sci, 1986. **27**(12): p. 1751-4.

[42] Howell , G.R., et al., *Axons of retinal ganglion cells are insulted in the optic nerve early in DBA/2J glaucoma.* Journal of Cell Biology, 2007. **179**(7): p. 1523-1537.

[43] John, S.W., et al., *Essential iris atrophy, pigment dispersion, and glaucoma in DBA/2J mice.* Invest Ophthalmol Vis Sci, 1998. **39**(6): p. 951-62.

[44] Chang, B., et al., *Interacting loci cause severe iris atrophy and glaucoma in DBA/2J mice.* Nat Genet, 1999. **21**(4): p. 405-9.

[45] Anderson, M.G., et al., *Mutations in genes encoding melanosomal proteins cause pigmentary glaucoma in DBA/2J mice.* Nature Genetics, 2002. **30**(1): p. 81-85.

[46] Kimura, A., T. Noro, and T. Harada, *Role of animal models in glaucoma research.* Neural Regeneration Research, 2020. **15**(7): p. 1257.

[47] Johnson, T.V. and S.I. Tomarev, *Rodent models of glaucoma.* Brain Res Bull, 2010. **81**(2-3): p. 349-58.

[48] Mittag, T.W., et al., *Retinal damage after 3 to 4 months of elevated intraocular pressure in a rat glaucoma model.* Invest Ophthalmol Vis Sci, 2000. **41**(11): p. 3451-9.

[49] WoldeMussie, E., et al., *Neuroprotection of retinal ganglion cells by brimonidine in rats with laser-induced chronic ocular hypertension.* Invest Ophthalmol Vis Sci, 2001. **42**(12): p. 2849-55.

[50] Ueda, J., et al., *Experimental glaucoma model in the rat induced by laser trabecular photocoagulation after an intracameral injection of India ink.* Jpn J Ophthalmol, 1998. **42**(5): p. 337-44.

[51] Biermann, J., et al., *Evaluation of intraocular pressure elevation in a modified laser-induced glaucoma rat model.* Experimental eye research, 2012. **104C**: p. 7-14.

[52] Morrison, J.C., et al., *A rat model of chronic pressure-induced optic nerve damage.* Exp Eye Res, 1997. **64**(1): p. 85-96.

[53] Sharif, N.A., *iDrugs and iDevices Discovery Research: Preclinical Assays, Techniques, and Animal Model Studies for Ocular Hypotensives and Neuroprotectants.* J Ocul Pharmacol Ther, 2018. **34**(1-2): p. 7-39.

[54] Werner, L., J. Chew, and N. Mamalis, *Experimental evaluation of ophthalmic devices and solutions using rabbit models.* Vet Ophthalmol, 2006. **9**(5): p. 281-91.

[55] Knepper, P.A., et al., *Intraocular pressure and glycosaminoglycan distribution in the rabbit eye: Effect of age and dexamethasone.* Experimental Eye Research, 1978. **27**(5): p. 567-575.

[56] Acott, T.S., et al., *Trabecular meshwork glycosaminoglycans in human and cynomolgus monkey eye.* Invest Ophthalmol Vis Sci, 1985. **26**(10): p. 1320-9.

[57] Moreno, M.C., et al., *A new experimental model of glaucoma in rats through intracameral injections of hyaluronic acid.* Exp Eye Res, 2005. **81**(1): p. 71-80.

[58] Benozzi, J., et al., *Effect of brimonidine on rabbit trabecular meshwork hyaluronidase activity.* Invest Ophthalmol Vis Sci, 2000. **41**(8): p. 2268-72.

[59] Sawaguchi, K., et al., *Myocilin gene expression in the trabecular meshwork of rats in a steroid-induced ocular hypertension model.* Ophthalmic Res, 2005. **37**(5): p. 235-42.

[60] Au - Ito, Y.A., et al., *A Magnetic Microbead Occlusion Model to Induce Ocular Hypertension-Dependent Glaucoma in Mice.* JoVE, 2016(109): p. e53731.

[61] McKinnon, S.J., C.L. Schlamp, and R.W. Nickells, *Mouse models of retinal ganglion cell death and glaucoma.* Experimental Eye Research, 2009. **88**(4): p. 816-824.

[62] John, S.W., et al., *Characterization of the Zebrafish bug eye Mutation, Exploring a Genetic Model for Pressure-induced Retinal Cell Death.* Investigative Ophthalmology & Visual Science, 2003. **44**(13): p. 1125-1125.

[63] Veth, K.N., et al., *Mutations in zebrafish lrp2 result in adult-onset ocular pathogenesis that models myopia and other risk factors for glaucoma.* PLoS Genet, 2011. **7**(2): p. e1001310.

[64] Skarie, J.M. and B.A. Link, *The primary open-angle glaucoma gene WDR36 functions in ribosomal RNA processing and interacts with the p53 stress-response pathway.* Hum Mol Genet, 2008. **17**(16): p. 2474-85.

[65] Fujikawa, K., et al., *VAV2 and VAV3 as Candidate Disease Genes for Spontaneous Glaucoma in Mice and Humans.* PLOS ONE, 2010. **5**(2): p. e9050.

[66] Seo, S., et al., *Foxc1 and Foxc2 in the Neural Crest Are Required for Ocular Anterior Segment Development.* Investigative Ophthalmology & Visual Science, 2017. **58**(3): p. 1368-1377.

[67] Harada, C., et al., *Recent advances in genetically modified animal models of glaucoma and their roles in drug repositioning.* British Journal of Ophthalmology, 2019. **103**(2): p. 161-166.

[68] Barrientos, S.A., et al., *Axonal Degeneration Is Mediated by the Mitochondrial Permeability Transition Pore.* The Journal of Neuroscience, 2011. **31**(3): p. 966-978.

[69] Sunio, A. and G.D. Bittner, *Cyclosporin A Retards the Wallerian Degeneration of Peripheral Mammalian Axons.* Experimental Neurology, 1997. **146**(1): p. 46-56.

[70] Libby, R.T., et al., *Susceptibility to Neurodegeneration in a Glaucoma Is Modified by Bax Gene Dosage.* PLOS Genetics, 2005. **1**(1): p. e4.

[71] Fernandes, K.A., et al., *JUN regulates early transcriptional responses to axonal injury in retinal ganglion cells.* Experimental Eye Research, 2013. **112**: p. 106-117.

[72] Fernandes, K.A., et al., *DLK-dependent signaling is important for somal but not axonal degeneration of retinal ganglion cells following axonal injury.* Neurobiology of Disease, 2014. **69**: p. 108-116.

[73] Wax, M.B., et al., *Induced autoimmunity to heat shock proteins elicits glaucomatous loss of retinal ganglion cell neurons via activated T-cell-derived fas-ligand.* J Neurosci, 2008. **28**(46): p. 12085-96.

[74] Chintalapudi, S., et al., *Systems genetics identifies a role for Cacna2d1 regulation in elevated intraocular pressure and glaucoma susceptibility.* Nature Communications, 2017. **8**.

[75] Templeton, J.P., et al., *Innate Immune Network in the Retina Activated by Optic Nerve Crush.* Investigative Ophthalmology & Visual Science, 2013. **54**(4): p. 2599-2606.

[76] Howell, G.R., et al., *Molecular clustering identifies complement and endothelin induction as early events in a mouse model of glaucoma.* The Journal of Clinical Investigation, 2011. **121**(4): p. 1429-1444.

[77] Templeton, J.P., et al., *A crystallin gene network in the mouse retina.* Experimental Eye Research, 2013. **116**: p. 129-140.

[78] Crabb, J.W., et al., *Drusen proteome analysis: An approach to the etiology of age-related macular degeneration.* Proceedings of the National Academy of Sciences, 2002. **99**(23): p. 14682-14687.

[79] Johnson, P.T., et al., *Individuals homozygous for the age-related macular degeneration risk-conferring variant of complement factor H have elevated levels of CRP in the choroid.* Proceedings of the National Academy of Sciences, 2006. **103**(46): p. 17456-17461.

[80] Zhou, J., et al., *Complement activation by photooxidation products of A2E, a lipofuscin constituent of the retinal pigment epithelium.* Proceedings of the National Academy of Sciences, 2006. **103**(44): p. 16182-16187.

[81] *The Advanced Glaucoma Intervention Study (AGIS): 7. The relationship between control of intraocular pressure and visual field deterioration.The AGIS Investigators.* Am J Ophthalmol, 2000. **130**(4): p. 429-40.

[82] Medeiros, F.A., et al., *Phase 3, Randomized, 20-Month Study of Bimatoprost Implant in Open-Angle Glaucoma and Ocular Hypertension (ARTEMIS 1).* Ophthalmology, 2020. **127**(12): p. 1627-1641.

[83] Shouchane-Blum, K., N. Geffen, and A. Zahavi, *Sustained drug delivery platforms – A new era for glaucoma treatment.* Clinical and Experimental Vision and Eye Research, 2019. **2**: p. 22-29.

[84] Dick, H.B., T. Schultz, and R.D. Gerste, *Miniaturization in Glaucoma Monitoring and Treatment: A Review of New Technologies That Require a Minimal Surgical Approach.* Ophthalmology and therapy, 2019. **8**(1): p. 19-30.

[85] Singh, R.B., et al., *Promising therapeutic drug delivery systems for glaucoma: a comprehensive review.* Therapeutic advances in ophthalmology, 2020. **12**: p. 2515841420905740-2515841420905740.

[86] Sarwat Salim Md, F., *Glaucoma Drainage Devices - EyeWiki.* 2020.

[87] Thompson, V., et al., *Short-Term Safety Evaluation of a Multi-Pressure Dial: A Prospective, Open-label, Non-randomized Study.* Ophthalmology and Therapy, 2019. **8**: p. 1-9.

[88] Cheung, W., L. Guo, and M.F. Cordeiro, *Neuroprotection in Glaucoma: Drug-Based Approaches.* Optometry and vision science : official publication of the American Academy of Optometry, 2008. **85**: p. 406-16.

[89] Weinreb, R., et al., *Oral Memantine for the Treatment of Glaucoma.* Ophthalmology, 2018. **125**.

[90] Kimura, A., et al., *Valproic acid prevents retinal degeneration in a murine model of normal tension glaucoma.* Neuroscience letters, 2014. **588**.

[91] Mahalingam, K., et al., *Therapeutic potential of valproic acid in advanced glaucoma: A pilot study.* Indian Journal of Ophthalmology, 2018. **66**: p. 1104.

[92] Akaiwa, K., et al., *Edaravone suppresses retinal ganglion cell death in a mouse model of normal tension glaucoma.* Cell Death & Disease, 2017. **8**(7): p. e2934-e2934.

[93] Williams, P., et al., *Vitamin B 3 modulates mitochondrial vulnerability and prevents glaucoma in aged mice.* Science, 2017. **355**: p. 756-760.

[94] Toth, C., *Pregabalin: latest safety evidence and clinical implications for the management of neuropathic pain.* Therapeutic advances in drug safety, 2014. **5**(1): p. 38-56.

[95] Nadeau, J.H. and J. Auwerx, *The virtuous cycle of human genetics and mouse models in drug discovery.* Nature Reviews Drug Discovery, 2019. **18**(4): p. 255-272.

Chapter 10

An Overview of Age-Related Macular Degeneration: Clinical, Pre-Clinical Animal Models and Bidirectional Translation

Jonathan Rho, Paul Percelay, Sophie Pilkinton, T.J. Hollingsworth, Ilyse Kornblau and Monica M. Jablonski

Abstract

Age-related macular degeneration (AMD) is a multifactorial disease that results from a complex and unknown interplay among environmental, genetic, and epidemiologic factors. Risk factors include aging, family history, obesity, hypercholesterolemia, and hypertension, along with cigarette smoking, which is the most influential modifiable risk factor. Single nucleotide polymorphisms (SNPs) in numerous genes such as complement factor H (*CFH*) pose some of the known genetic risks. The pathophysiology in AMD is incompletely understood, but is known to involve oxidative stress, inflammation, dysregulated antioxidants, lipid metabolism, and angiogenesis. Animal models have been integral in expanding our knowledge of AMD pathology. AMD is classified as non-exudative or exudative. Because there is no perfect animal model that recapitulates all aspects of the human disease, rodents, rabbits, and non-human primates offer different advantages and disadvantages to serve as models for various aspects of the disease. Scientific advances have also allowed for the creation of polygenic pre-clinical models that may better represent the complexity of AMD, which will likely expand our knowledge of disease mechanisms and serve as platforms for testing new therapeutics. There have been, and there continues to be, many drugs in the pipeline to treat both exudative and non-exudative AMD. However, Food and Drug Administration (FDA)-approved therapies for exudative AMD that mainly target angiogenic growth factors are the only therapeutics currently being used in the clinics. There remains no FDA-approved therapy for the non-exudative form of this disease. This chapter contains a basic overview and classification of AMD and multiple animal models of AMD are highlighted. We include an overview of both current FDA-approved treatments and those in development. Lastly, we conclude with a summary of the important role of pre-clinical studies in the development of therapeutics for this highly prevalent disease.

Keywords: age-related macular degeneration, pre-clinical models, animal models, rodents, non-human primates, geographic atrophy, neovascularization, anti-VEGF complement, retina

IntechOpen

1. Introduction

Age-related macular degeneration (AMD) is a multifactorial disease that results from interplay among genetic, environmental, and epidemiologic factors. It is the leading cause of irreversible blindness in people over 60 years of age, with numbers projected to increase over time. Animal models have been integral for understanding pathophysiology of and to develop treatments for AMD. This chapter reviews the basics of AMD including pathophysiology and classification. We then highlight specific examples of animal models and the insight they provide. We discuss both current FDA-approved treatments and those in development. Lastly, we conclude with a summary of the important role of pre-clinical studies in the development of therapeutics for AMD.

1.1 Basics of AMD

The retina plays an integral role in vision by converting light to an electrical stimulus, which is ultimately processed as an image in the occipital lobe of the visual cortex. The macula, located in the posterior pole of the retina, contains the highest concentration of cone photoreceptors across the retina and is responsible for central, high-resolution, and color vision [1]. AMD is a multifactorial disease of the elderly that progressively affects vision through pathological changes to the retinal pigment epithelium (RPE) and loss of photoreceptors in the macula [2]. AMD is classified as non-exudative or exudative. Non-exudative AMD is defined by the presence of drusen — aggregates of lipid, protein, and immune complexes — underneath the RPE with subsequent thickening of Bruch's membrane [3, 4]. AMD is responsible for about 8.7% of blindness and remains as a leading cause of blindness in people over 60 years of age in the developed world [5, 6]. The disease burden will increase as the population ages with longer life expectancies. The global estimate of AMD cases was 196 million in 2020 and is expected to be 288 million by 2040 [6].

Although age is the most impactful risk factor, others include obesity, hypercholesterolemia, hypertension, lighter iris colors, lack of exercise, cigarette smoking, Western diet, elevated C-reactive protein, and family history [7–10]. Cigarette smoking is the most influential modifiable risk factor [11].

In addition to the above risk factors, genetics plays an important role in this multifactorial disease. The International Age-Related Macular Degeneration Genomics Consortium conducted a genome-wide association study of 43,566 subjects that revealed 52 genetic variants of AMD shared between 34 loci. Some of these include genes encoding for collagen type IV (*COL4A3*), matrix metalloproteinases (*MMP9, MMP19*), ATP binding cassette (*ABCA1*) involved in cholesterol transport, paired immunoglobin like type 2 receptor beta (*PILRB*) involved in immune regulation, vascular endothelial growth factor A (*VEGFA*) involved in angiogenesis, and various components of the complement cascade including complement factor H (*CFH*), complement factor I (*CFI*), and complement factors 3 and 9 (*C3, C9*) [12]. Among the 34 AMD loci, burden testing of rare (frequency < 0.1%) variants identified 4 protein-altering genes — *CFH, CFI*, tissue inhibitor of metalloproteinases 3 (*TIMP3*), and solute carrier family 16 member 8 (*SLC16A8*) — that contribute to AMD pathology [12]. For example, a knockout mutation in *SLC16A8* resulted in defective lactate transport with consequent acidification along with dysfunction of the retina and photoreceptors [12]. Discovering susceptible AMD loci helps expand knowledge of factors underlying the pathophysiology of this multifactorial disease, along with plausible therapeutic targets.

1.2 Pathophysiology of AMD in humans

Although incompletely understood, AMD is a complex disease that results from a mix of genetic predisposition, environmental factors, and age. There are many models that attempt to explain the pathophysiology of AMD, the underlying disease mechanisms of which are multifaceted and not mutually exclusive. These can be categorized as oxidative stress, inflammation, dysregulated antioxidants, lipid metabolism, and angiogenesis [13]. This chapter highlights the multifactorial etiology of RPE damage and dysfunction, a key event in AMD pathogenesis and briefly touches on other aspects of AMD pathophysiology [3].

A properly functioning RPE is important for retinal homeostasis because of the multiple roles it plays including: transportation of nutrients from the choroidal vasculature; absorption of stray photons of light; phagocytosis of photoreceptor outer segments; metabolism of fatty acids; formation of the blood-retinal barrier; regulation of subretinal water transport; and regeneration of visual pigments during the visual transduction cascade [14]. Some retinal changes that are characteristic of AMD include dysfunction of the RPE, sub-RPE deposition of lipids and proteins, neovascularization of the choroid or retina, and disciform scar formation [13]. Most people develop asymptomatic extracellular lipid deposition underneath the RPE. However, as these lesions enlarge they can cause dysfunction of the RPE [15]. Although an exact stepwise development of disease is not clear, early AMD is defined by the appearance of drusen under the RPE with thickening of Bruch's membrane (BrM). Consequently, this impairs the ability of the RPE to efflux fluids across BrM and to deliver nutrients such as glucose, vitamin A (all-*trans* retinal), and docosahexenoic acid (DHA), causing stress on the RPE and photoreceptors [15]. The impaired transport across BrM may exacerbate formation of drusen, thus causing a vicious cycle of pathology.

Moreover, the RPE is susceptible to oxidative stress from high oxygen utilization, prolonged exposure to visible light, lipid oxidation by photoreceptors and drusen, and cigarette smoking [4, 13]. During phototransduction, visual pigments called opsins use the chromophore 11-*cis* retinal to absorb photons of light. Upon absorption, the 11-*cis* configuration becomes all-*trans*, the initiating step for phototransduction. To convert the all-*trans* back to 11-*cis*, it must proceed through the retinoid cycle whereby the RPE re-isomerizes the molecule back to its 11-*cis* conformation. A byproduct of this cycle is A2E, which accumulates in lipofuscin — particularly in the macula — and reacts with oxygen to form free radicals. This may partly explain why the macula is preferentially affected in AMD [15]. Lipofuscin also accumulates in aging eyes which may exacerbate oxidative stress by forming free radicals and inhibiting the RPE's function of degrading organelles [4, 13]. In short, there are many etiologies of oxidative stress and the literature supports that it is an important part of AMD pathophysiology [13].

Identification of SNPs in several complement factor components sheds light on its role in AMD pathogenesis. The complement system is beneficial for its role in innate immunity and encouraging phagocytosis and removal of unwanted cellular material; however, dysregulation of this system can cause damage and inflammation in surrounding tissue [4]. Similarly, inflammation is a cascade of events that is beneficial in the short term in response to foreign and damaged material, yet chronic inflammation can be harmful and may contribute to the development of AMD [16]. There are many genetic variants of complement genes associated with AMD and one example is the Y402H polymorphism in the *CFH* gene. CFH normally regulates the alternate complement pathway by interfering with C3b and factor B interaction and inhibiting the formation of C3 convertase [17]. However, the

Y402H polymorphism prevents CFH from binding to BrM or to malondialdehyde, a byproduct of lipid peroxidation, ultimately causing unregulated complement activation and chronic inflammation [4, 13, 17].

Antioxidants scavenge reactive oxygen species (ROS) thereby attenuating oxidative stress. Nuclear factor erythyroid 2-related factor 2 (NRF2) is a transcription factor that upregulates antioxidants when signaled by oxidative stress. Studies of *Nrf2*$^{-/-}$ mice showed retinal damage and changes such as thickened BrM, sub-RPE deposits, and complement activation. Thus, antioxidants may protect against AMD, and in contrast, the loss of antioxidants, as shown in the *Nrf2*$^{-/-}$ mice, may exacerbate AMD progression [13].

In humans, the inner and outer retina are supplied by the retinal artery and choroidal circulation, respectively. The choroidal circulation is located beneath BrM, which acts as a physical barrier. Drusen accumulation may disrupt this barrier and when conditions favor angiogenesis, permeable blood vessels lacking endothelial tight junctions and pericytes can develop between the retina and choroidal blood vessels. These vessels can grow into the central retina, a process called choroidal neovascularization (CNV) as seen in exudative AMD [15, 18, 19]. Neovascularization may also originate from the retina in a process called retinal angiomatous proliferation (RAP) [17]. Vascular endothelial growth factor (VEGF) plays a major role in angiogenesis. There is sufficient evidence that points to the role of VEGF in exudative AMD pathogenesis, given the higher VEGF levels in AMD patients and the successful decrease in neovascularization with anti-VEGF agents [13]. Pigment epithelium-derived growth factor (PEDF) is an antiangiogenic molecule whose expression is reduced in eyes with AMD. This imbalance between angiogenic VEGF and antiangiogenic PEDF suggests that homeostasis of vascular factors is disrupted in exudative AMD [15]. In summary, AMD is a multifaceted disease with genetic and environmental risk factors that likely progresses due to a combination of oxidative stress and inflammation, combined with dysregulated antioxidants, lipid metabolism, and increased angiogenesis.

1.3 Classification of AMD

Disease classification can elucidate pathophysiological processes, prognosis, and guide in clinical decision-making. Drusen, the hallmark lesion of AMD, is visible by fundoscopy and can be classified by their size and border characteristics [15]. Specifically, drusen can be small (< 63 mm), intermediate (63–124 mm), or large (>124 mm). They can also be stratified as hard (well demarcated), soft (poorly demarcated), or confluent (contiguous) [20, 21]. Higher number and larger size of drusen portends greater likelihood of progression in AMD. Moreover, compared to hard drusen, soft drusen tend to be located in the macula and increase risk of progression [21].

AMD is categorized as non-exudative or exudative. There are many ways to stratify AMD, but this chapter uses the classification of the Age-Related Eye Disease Study (AREDS) as follows: no AMD (no or few small drusen), early AMD (multiple small drusen, few intermediate drusen, or mild RPE abnormalities), intermediate AMD (numerous intermediate drusen, at least one large drusen, or geographic atrophy without center foveal involvement), and advanced AMD (geographic atrophy with center foveal involvement or neovascular maculopathy) [22].

Each stage has defining characteristics. The advanced non-exudative form of AMD is known as geographic atrophy (GA) and is defined by slow progressive atrophy of the photoreceptors, RPE, and the choriocapillaris that form sharply demarcated lesions [23]. Advanced exudative AMD represents 10–15% of all AMD and is characterized by growth of choroidal blood vessels through BrM and into the retina, consequently causing intraretinal or subretinal leakage, hemorrhage, and RPE detachment. These changes can cause acute vision loss [15, 18, 24]. Follow-up data from the AREDS found that progression to advanced AMD is associated with the following retinal risk factors: increased baseline drusen severity, the presence of a large drusen within 1 disc diameter of the fovea, the presence of bilateral medium drusen, the presence of advanced AMD in the fellow eye, and the simultaneous presence of AMD RPE abnormalities and large drusen [25].

2. Preclinical models of AMD

Animal models have been generated by multiple laboratories by reconstructing specific features of AMD. These models have become integral for providing insight into the pathophysiology of this disease, as well as to develop proof-of-principle studies to support the advancement of new therapies [26]. In general, an optimal animal model is inexpensive and mimics the features of the human disease in a timely manner to allow for efficient studies [17]. In studies focused on AMD, these changes include a thickened BrM, sub-RPE deposits, RPE atrophy and hyperplasia, accumulation of immune cells or complement, photoreceptor atrophy, CNV, and fibrosis [17]. However, when trying to recapitulate AMD, animal models can be challenging because AMD is a complex disease with multiple polymorphisms able to be influenced by environmental and epidemiologic factors [15]. Furthermore, there are inherent differences in the eyes of animals and humans, such that no single model perfectly captures all features of AMD. Although space limits inclusion of all animal models, this review highlights the weaknesses and strengths of specific animal models and how they have been useful for understanding aspects of AMD development, progression, and treatment.

2.1 Introduction to rodent models

Rodents have been the "go-to" model for retinal disease for decades. There are many advantages to the rodent model. Economically, rodents are small animals that require little space and resources, are easy to breed and handle, have short gestation times while producing many offspring, and have short life spans. Diseases can also progress relatively quickly allowing for efficient studies [17, 27]. Mouse, rat, and human genomes have been sequenced, and each were found to have around 30,000 genes, 95% of which are shared among all three species. Further, advances in molecular genetic techniques allow for ease of genetic manipulation [27]. Anatomically, mice have key retinal structures — RPE, BrM, and choriocapillaris — that are affected in human AMD [15]. The economic, genetic, and anatomic benefits of rodents make them invaluable animal models for studying human disease and testing treatments. Clinicians and scientists alike have been working to recapitulate the human AMD phenotype in mice by taking what is known about the human condition and applying it to mice. This may come in the form of genetic manipulation to induce SNPs in known AMD-associated genes or applying risk factors for AMD to mice such as exposure to cigarette smoke or inducing obesity. Several of these manipulations will be discussed below.

It is important to highlight that there are some structural differences in the retinas of humans and rodents. Unlike humans, rodents do not have a macula, defined anatomically as having at least two layers of ganglion cells with a mixture of rod and cone cells [26]. Rodents also lack an area of the retina with high density of cones similar to the fovea. Moreover, interpretation of findings from early murine AMD models was confounded by a spontaneous point mutation in Crumbs homolog 1

(*Crb1*) that segregated in a sub-strain of the C57B/6 J mouse from the Jackson Laboratories. The *Crb1* mutation affects photoreceptor health and development, but is not relevant in human AMD pathogenesis [28]. This mutation is now screened for prior to use of mouse strains originated from the C57B/6 J mouse strain. Although rodents are not the perfect animal model, they have shed light on many aspects of AMD, of which numerous examples are highlighted in this review.

2.2 Rodent models of oxidative stress

The retina is susceptible to oxidative stress due to its high metabolic demand, lipid oxidation by photoreceptors, and the presence of molecules that form ROS mentioned in section 1.2. Below we present several mouse models that mimic AMD pathology induced by the lack of antioxidants or the addition of oxidative stress.

2.2.1 Superoxide dismutase knockout (Sod$^{-/-}$) mice

There are two isoforms of SOD, the primary antioxidant enzyme in the retina that catalyzes the breakdown of potentially harmful ROS [28]. After 7 months of age, knockout mice lacking SOD1 (*Sod1*$^{-/-}$) develop sub-RPE deposits that share similar composition to drusen found in human AMD. Other pathology in these mice include thickened BrM, RPE atrophy, and CNV in about 10% of mice [17]. This model, however, is also a model of amyotrophic lateral sclerosis resulting in extra-retinal phenotypes which can complicate the use of this mouse strain [29]. Similarly, mouse models transduced with an adenovirus-mediated ribozyme delivery system to inactivate SOD2 showed signs of oxidative damage like *Sod1*$^{-/-}$ models, with the caveat that SOD2 null mice did not show signs of CNV. Therefore, SOD2 depletion is not a good model for exudative AMD but may be useful for studying non-exudative AMD [17, 28].

2.2.2 Mice immunized with carboxyethylpyrrole (CEP)-adducted proteins

Oxidized DHA forms CEP-adducted proteins that are present in drusen at higher concentrations in AMD eyes compared to eyes without AMD. In studies performed to test the effects of adding oxidative stress, two groups of mice — 3-month-old mice given a strong inoculation (short-term) and 1-year-old mice given a weaker inoculation (long-term) — were immunized with CEP-adducted proteins. The short-term group developed complement deposition in BrM, sub-RPE deposits, RPE lysis, and the presence of macrophages. The long-term group developed a thickening of BrM [17]. However, neither group developed CNV, making this a potential model for non-exudative AMD. A benefit of this model is that there is no genetic manipulation of the mice, so this model can be combined with other genetically modified models, a condition that may be beneficial for a multifaceted disease such as AMD [17].

2.2.3 Nuclear factor erythroid 2-related factor 2 knockout (Nrf2$^{-/-}$) mice

NRF2 is a transcription factor that encodes for detoxifying and antioxidant enzymes such as SOD. *Nrf2*$^{-/-}$ mice developed hard drusen-like deposits at 8–11 months of age and larger soft drusen-like deposits at 11–18 months of age similar to changes in early AMD. At 11–17 months of age, 18% of the mice developed CNV. Other changes include RPE atrophy and hyperpigmentation with increased autofluorescence, thickened BrM and choriocapillaris endothelium, photoreceptor atrophy, and increased levels of complement and vitronectin by 12 months of age. This model is a promising model for both non-exudative and exudative AMD because it has characteristics of both conditions [26].

2.2.4 Ceruloplasmin/hephaestin double knockout (DKO) mice

Iron can be a source of oxidative stress and its transport is mediated by ceruloplasmin, transferrin, and hephaestin [15, 17]. Humans lacking ceruloplasmin can develop AMD in middle age. Ceruloplasmin/hephaestin DKO mice by 6–9 months of age developed focal RPE hypertrophy, increased lipofuscin, photoreceptor atrophy, and subretinal deposits and neovascularization [15, 17]. Retinal changes peak by about 12 months of age, showing signs of oxidative damage and complement deposition [15]. Studying the retinal changes in older mice of this DKO strain is limited, however, due to a movement-related premature death caused by the DKO of ceruloplasmin/hephaestin [17]. Hadziahmetovic *et al.* showed that oral iron chelator deferiprone given to ceruloplasmin/hephaestin DKO mice decreases iron levels and can mitigate retinal degeneration [30]. These findings suggest that iron may play a role in AMD pathology.

2.2.5 Cigarette smoke/hydroquinone exposure in mice

Cigarette smoke contains many toxins and oxidants, the most abundant of which is hydroquinone (HQ). C57BL/6 J mice at 16 months of age were fed a high-fat diet (HFD) for 4.5 months causing the mice to develop sub-RPE deposits when exposed to oxidative stress. The mice were then divided into two groups to examine the additive effects of cigarette smoke and HQ on a HFD. The mice were exposed to a combination of HFD with blue light (positive control), cigarette smoke, or oral HQ. Espinosa-Heidmann *et al.* found that mice fed a HFD yet had no oxidative stress exposure showed normal retinal morphology, while mice exposed to oxidative stress through blue light, cigarette smoke, or oral HQ demonstrated retinal changes similar to early AMD, such as sub-RPE deposits and BrM thickening [31]. Furthermore, mice treated with HQ in their drinking water were found to have more proangiogenic VEGF compared to anti-angiogenic PEDF. The imbalance of angiogenic factors from HQ may contribute to CNV [17]. These findings may partly explain why cigarette smoking is an influential risk factor in AMD.

2.3 Rodents models of inflammation

Inflammation is associated with AMD onset and progression with complement being a major component. Inflammatory components found in drusen further support inflammation taking a role in AMD pathogenesis [15]. Below are a few example models of inflammation and the complement pathway.

2.3.1 Complement factor H knockout ($Cfh^{-/-}$) mice

CFH is a regulatory protein that prevents C3b from binding to complement factor B and ultimately prevents the formation of C3 convertase. Loss of regulation of this pathway causes deposition of C3 in the kidneys and ultimately membranoproliferative glomerulonephritis (MPGN) Type II. These patients also develop drusen similar to those in AMD [17]. $Cfh^{-/-}$ mice also developed MPGN and retinal changes such as increased retinal autofluorescence, complement deposition, and disorganization of photoreceptor outer segments (POS). However, these mice also showed thinning of BrM, which is atypical of AMD, possibly from increased phagocytic activity mediated by complement [17].

2.3.2 Transgenic CFH Y402H mice

The CFH Y402H polymorphism causes chronic inflammation by disrupting the binding of CFH to C-reactive protein and heparan sulfate [26]. At one year of age, transgenic mice with this polymorphism were found to have more drusen-like deposits compared to wild-type or *Cfh*$^{-/-}$ mice [17]. The CFH Y402H mice also exhibited thickening of BrM and increased accumulation of immune cells and complement in the subretinal space and basement membrane, respectively. Unlike *Cfh*$^{-/-}$ mice, CFH Y402H mice did not show photoreceptor atrophy possibly because the mice studied were younger by one year of age or from retaining partial functionality of CFH [17].

2.3.3 Transgenic mice overexpressing C3

Implied by the regulation of C3b through CFH, C3 plays an important activating role in complement pathways. Transgenic mice transduced using adenovirus expressing C3 have higher levels of C3 and a pathology similar to AMD including loss of photoreceptor outer segments and RPE, along with the accumulation of complement. Another finding in these mice was the migration and proliferation of endothelial cells in the retina which may correspond to RAP documented in patients with exudative AMD. However, this model is limited because these mice also exhibit retinal detachments, which are not seen in AMD. It is possible that the injected adenovirus may contribute to some of the unexpected retinal changes [17].

2.3.4 Cluster of differentiation 46 (*Cd46*$^{-/-}$) mice

Like CFH regulating C3b, CD46 is a regulatory cofactor that aids in inactivating C3b and C4b. *Cd46*$^{-/-}$ mice at 12 months of age exhibit increased complement in the RPE with hypertrophic and vacuolated RPE. These findings along with increased autofluorescence, lipofuscin, and autophagosomes of the RPE suggest degeneration of this retinal layer. Other findings in these mice include sub-RPE deposits with thickening of BrM, decreased choriocapillary lumen and fenestrations, and decreased number of nuclei in the outer nuclear layer of the retina. In this model there were low levels of VEGF and no signs of neovascularization, positioning this mouse as a model to the study of non-exudative AMD [26].

2.3.5 Inflammasome mice

Inflammasomes are multiprotein complexes that respond to pathogen-associated molecular patterns or other cellular stresses. Inflammasome activation leads to secretion of proinflammatory substances such as caspase-1, interleukin-1β (IL-1β), and interleukin-18 (IL-18). The NOD-, LRR- and pyrin domain-containing protein 3 (NLRP3) inflammasome has been implicated in many inflammatory conditions such as gout, autoimmune diseases, atherosclerosis, and AMD [32]. Eyes with GA have lower levels of Double-Stranded RNA-Specific Endoribonuclease (DICER1), a micro-RNA, which leads to increased levels of Arthrobacter luteus (Alu) RNA. Alu RNA activates the NLRP3 inflammasome leading to increased levels of myeloid differentiation primary response 88 (MYD88) and IL-18 and ultimately causing RPE atrophy [26]. However, in *Myd88*$^{-/-}$ mice and *Il18r1*$^{-/-}$ mice, Alu RNA did not cause RPE degeneration [33]. These findings suggest that inflammasome activation may have a role in AMD pathogenesis and present potential targets for future therapies.

2.4 Polygenic rodent models

As discussed, AMD is a multifactorial disease resulting from a mixture of multiple genetic and environmental factors. Because monogenic animal models do not represent the complexity of human AMD, combining multiple SNPs with nongenetic factors to create a polygenic animal model may prove beneficial for studying AMD pathogenesis as well as providing platforms on which to test new therapeutics that are being developed in laboratories across the world. Mice make excellent candidates for polygenic models of AMD due to the relative ease of manipulating their genomes and simplicity of affecting their environment [17, 34].

2.4.1 Peroxisome proliferator-activated receptor gamma coactivator – 1 alpha (Pgc1α)/Nrf2 DKO mice

As stated previously, NRF2 is a transcription factor that regulates the expression of detoxifying and antioxidant enzymes. PGC-1α regulates angiogenesis and oxidative stress, among other functions. Single $Nrf2^{-/-}$ mice present signs of AMD, such as degenerated RPE and photoreceptor outer segment atrophy. When fed a HFD, $Nrf\ 2^{-/-}$ mice exhibited exacerbated signs of AMD such as RPE hyper/hypopigmentation. On a similar HFD, $Pgc\text{-}1\alpha^{+/-}$ mice also develop increased lipofuscin accumulation, another indication of AMD [26].

PGC-1α/Nrf2 DKO mice exhibit AMD signs and dysfunctional photoreceptors by 12 months of age. Autophagy and oxidative damage were greater in the DKO compared to single knockout mice [26]. This polygenic model may better represent the multifactorial nature of AMD. Environmental factors such as cigarette smoke or HFD exposure have not yet been tested in this model, which may be useful for future studies.

2.4.2 Systems genetics and the BXD family of mice

In recent years, the use of systems genetics to uncover genes underlying the pathological mechanisms of retinal diseases has become an invaluable tool in the study of multiple human diseases. Specifically, applying this approach to the BXD family of mice has elucidated novel genes associated with ocular hypertension and optic nerve necrosis in glaucoma [35, 36]. As a brief background, the BXD family of mice were generated by breeding the standard C57B/6 J mouse with the DBA/2 J strain from the Jackson Labs. Offspring were then inbred for 20 or more generations to allow for a homologous recombination-induced variety of genetic backgrounds [37]. Currently, studies are underway to use the BXD family of mice to generate a more accurate model of AMD in the mouse. This is being done by delving into the genomes of each strain of BXD mouse to find different combinations of haplotypes in AMD-associated genes which contain SNPs similar to those found in humans, or that result in an altered protein function as observed in humans. Currently, multiple strains have shown promise for not just AMD, but other retinal diseases as well.

2.5 Rabbit models

Although rodents are the most studied, the larger eye size of rabbits make them advantageous for certain pharmacological and pathological studies. While rabbits are more expensive than rodents, they are less expensive than non-human primates (NHP). Rabbits are also relatively easy to handle and breed. Furthermore, the size of the rabbits allow for easy administration of subretinal injections and vectors for gene therapy [38]. Rabbits possess a visual streak where rods and cones are dense, but they do not have a macula which, like mice, can present a caveat for direct translation to human AMD [38, 39].

Promoting a wet AMD phenotype using conventional methods of inducing CNV in rodents and primates, such as laser-induced damage of BrM and injection of proangiogenic factors, have not worked for rabbit models; however, Qui *et al.* created an exudative AMD model in rabbits by injecting Matrigel, a membrane matrix mixture that includes growth factors like basic fibroblast growth factor and endothelial growth factor. Growth factors from the Matrigel are slowly released for up to 9 weeks, with subsequent production of CNV lesions and BrM disruption that are reminiscent of AMD. This shows promise of a way to test new therapies for exudative AMD on an inexpensive and reproducible model with similar pathological features of AMD [39].

2.6 Non-human primate models

Although primates and humans have the most similar anatomy, primates are disadvantageous as models because they are difficult to genetically manipulate, expensive, and their disease course is relatively long [17]. Furthermore, they are difficult to handle and breed [38]. Historically, there were limitations to exudative AMD models, however new techniques have generated some exudative AMD models, discussed below.

Because AMD affects the cone dense macula, a major limitation of animal models such as rodents, canines, and felines is the lack of a macula [40]. NHPs are the only pre-clinical animals that have a macula and a similar organization of photoreceptors within the macula like humans [17, 41]. Another advantage of NHP models is their shared similarity in organization of the visual pathway. The macula only receives nutrients and removes waste from the choroidal circulation. Furthermore, since the macula is responsible for high acuity central vision, copious amounts of light are focused on the macula subjecting it to high levels of ROS. These details may explain why the macula is affected in AMD in both humans and NHP [17].

Genetic risk factors are also suspected in NHPs with AMD. Polymorphisms in age-related maculopathy susceptibility 2 (*ARMS2*) and high-temperature requirement factor A1 (*HTRA1*) were linked to significantly higher rates of drusen formation in both humans and rhesus monkeys. These findings suggest shared genetic risk factors and can further infer that humans and rhesus monkeys have commonality in pathophysiology [17].

Another shared risk factor between humans and NHPs is diet. Rhesus monkeys with a diet without lutein or zeaxanthin formed drusen earlier than monkeys fed a standard diet. In another study, monkeys without carotenoids and omega-3 fatty acids developed some RPE atrophy [17]. In fact, the AREDS2 study found that human subjects in the bottom quartile of nutrition benefited the most from vitamin supplementation [42].

2.6.1 Primate models for early onset drusen

Some NHP species such as rhesus macaque monkeys spontaneously develop drusen and early to intermediate AMD. The amount of drusen increased with age [43]. Drusen analyzed in these monkeys were found by immunohistochemical analysis to have similar location and composition as human drusen, sharing compounds such as apolipoprotein E, amyloid P component, complement components, immunoglobulins, vitronectin, membrane cofactor protein, annexins, and crystallins [17, 28].

Interestingly, a group of cynomolgus macaques and Japanese macaques were found to have early-onset drusen in the macula and periphery at around 1–2 years of age. The drusen in these groups of monkeys were also similar in composition to human drusen. This syndrome exhibited a dominant inheritance which along with early onset drusen may serve as a useful animal model for future studies [17].

2.6.2 Primate models for neovascularization

NHP models do not spontaneously develop advanced forms of AMD. Laser induced NHP models of exudative AMD only provide vascular leakage for about 2–3 weeks. However, Patel *et al*. created a NHP model for chronic neovascularization by intravitreal (IVT) injection of DL-alpha-aminoadipic acid, a selective glial cytotoxin, in African green monkeys. In this model, neovascularization progressed for 8–10 weeks after injection and maintained leakage for over 90 weeks. Importantly, anti-VEGF injections decreased leakage at 2–4 weeks, then neovascularization resumed at 4–8 weeks, and repeat anti-VEGF injections at 90 weeks decreased neovascular lesions. These findings are important because this may serve as a good model for testing short and extended-release therapeutics for exudative AMD in model eyes that resemble human eyes [19].

3. FDA-approved treatments for AMD

3.1 Vitamin supplementation for AMD

Lifestyle modifications are thought to delay progression of AMD. The American Academy of Ophthalmology recommends smoking cessation, an antioxidant-rich diet with healthy unsaturated fats or omega-3 supplements, management of other medical conditions, routine exercise, and regular eye examinations for all AMD patients [44]. Additionally, antioxidant vitamins and minerals have been demonstrated to slow progression to advanced AMD according to the AREDS [45]. The original formulation consisted of: 500 mg vitamin C, 400 international units (IU) vitamin E, 15 mg beta carotene, 80 mg of zinc (zinc oxide), and 2 mg of copper (cupric oxide) [45]. Copper was added to the formulation as zinc supplementation can cause copper-deficiency anemia. Smoking cessation is specifically recommended because the high dose of beta-carotene supplementation is subject to a small increased risk of lung cancer [46]. The subsequent AREDS 2 investigation evaluated adding lutein + zeaxanthin and DHA + eicosapentaenoic acid [EPA], or lutein + zeaxanthin + DHA + EPA to the original AREDS preparation. It also explored removal of beta carotene and decreased the original dose of zinc. It adapted the formula to include: 10 mg of lutein and 2 mg of zeaxanthin, 350 mg DHA and 650 mg EPA, no beta-carotene, and 25 mg zinc [47]. They found that lutein + zeaxanthin or DHA/EPA did not further halt the progression of AMD; however, removal of beta-carotene from the lutein + zeaxanthin formulation proved to be protective against AMD and better for patients due to the decreased risk of lung cancer in patients using the beta carotene poor formulation. Additionally, the decreased quantity of zinc was deemed less protective than the higher doses administered in AREDS. In short, AREDS 2 concluded administration of 500 mg vitamin C, 400 IU vitamin E, 10 mg of lutein and 2 mg of zeaxanthin, 80 mg of zinc (zinc oxide), and 2 mg of copper (cupric oxide), without beta carotene was beneficial in decreasing the progression to advanced AMD in patients with intermediate and advanced AMD in at least once eye [47].

3.2 Past therapeutics for AMD

Past therapies for AMD include photodynamic therapy, photocoagulation, low vision rehabilitation, and radiation therapy [44, 46]. First introduced in the 1990's, photodynamic therapy (PDT) involved injecting verteporfin (Visudyne) into an arm vein. The injected medication collects in pathologic neovascular membranes in the central macula. The verteporfin is light activated by using a 690 nm laser over the affected area, causing the formation of ROS. Unfortunately, new models of the PDT laser are no longer available for sale in the United States, although a single model is available in Europe. PDT has become obsolete for AMD treatment with the rise of anti-VEGF therapeutics, although it is still used for other retinal conditions [46]. A second method, photocoagulation treatment, uses a laser to accomplish the same goal. This may also require retreatment; however, the laser can produce scarring, which can cause blind spots. For this reason, it is no longer used to treat pathology within the macula. Moreover, increased damage to the macula lowers the success rate of treatment.

Studies in the 1980s examined the use of photocoagulative therapies in minimizing the progression of disease due to CNV lesions. These assessed laser therapy of the extrafoveal, juxtafoveal, and subfoveal neovascular membranes [46]. It was determined that laser therapy of extrafoveal or juxtafoveal sites was more effective than subfoveal sites. Subfoveal photocoagulation was associated with increased risk of vision loss [46]. However, with increased anti-VEGF therapies, the use of photocoagulation is also declining [46]. A third treatment is low vision rehabilitation, which is used as supplemental therapy to accommodate the central vision changes that may ensue from AMD. This can include implementation of reading glasses, magnifiers, additional lighting, among others [44]. New advances in wearable technology use individualized deficit mapping and artificial intelligence to assist users in navigating their environment and common activities of daily living. The fourth form, radiotherapy, has been used to inhibit neovascularization, but the effectiveness of this method is unclear [46].

3.3 Current therapeutics for AMD

Although there is no current treatment to delay the onset of non-exudative AMD, once the disease progresses to the exudative form, there are treatments to delay its progression, preserve remaining vision, and sometimes recover lost vision [44]. Most of these therapies target the neovascularization and associated fluid leakage and hemorrhage. These drugs inhibit VEGF, the main proangiogenic factor that contributes to neovascularization. Current treatments include bevacizumab (Avastin, Genetech), ranibizumab (Lucentis, Genentech), aflibercept (Eylea, Regeneron Pharmaceuticals), and brolucizumab (Beovu, Novartis).

Pegaptanib (Macugen, Pfizer) was the first anti-VEGF therapy approved by the FDA in 2004 and is an oligonucleic aptamer specifically targeting VEGF-165. Ranibizumab is a monoclonal antibody fragment to all VEGF-A that was approved by the FDA in 2006 based on the results of the phase III MARINA and ANCHOR trials [48, 49]. Aflibercept is a receptor-antibody fusion protein of VEGF receptors 1 and 2 fused to the Fc portion of IgG1 that blocks VEGF-A and B. Aflibercept was approved by the FDA in 2011 based on the VIEW-1 and 2 phase III trials [18, 46]. Brolucizumab is a single-chain antibody fragment approved by the FDA in October 2019 based on the phase III HAWK and HARRIER trials [46, 50]. Ranibizumab, aflibercept, and brolucizumab were created specifically for the treatment of exudative AMD, while bevacizumab was approved for colon cancer and is used off-label.

Bevacizumab is considerably less expensive at an average of $50 per treatment versus $1,800 or $2,000 for the other three available treatments and has been shown to be equally efficacious in the Comparison of Age-Related Macular Degeneration Treatments Trials (CATT) studies [51].

In any of the treatment trials that are evaluating the efficacy of the anti-VEGF family of therapies, patients are monitored for exudation and treatment response using optical coherence tomography after intravitreal injection [45]. Frequency of injections varies, but most patients require multiple doses and repeat treatments. Brolucizumab is groundbreaking as it is the first anti-VEFG therapy that has demonstrated similar efficacy from a single injection, 4 times a year [46]. Unfortunately, adoption of Brolucizumab has been limited by intraocular inflammation, vasculitis, and vascular occlusion causing visual decline that was seen in 4.6% of trial participants [52]. Potential adverse effects of anti-VEGF therapies include conjunctival hemorrhage, vitreous hemorrhage, increased intraocular pressure, cataract progression, and, rarely, retinal detachment, infection, and intraocular inflammation [44].

4. Potential therapeutics for AMD

There are many studies that have evaluated potential therapies for non-exudative and exudative AMD. Along with vitamin supplementation, there are three main classes of therapies being investigated: antibody, gene, and cell-based therapies.

Aside from the successful anti-VEGF therapies, antibodies targeting the complement pathway show some promise. Because activation of the alternative complement pathway contributes to AMD pathology, antibodies targeting components of this pathway, such as C3 and C5, may attenuate inflammation and damage to the retina by reducing complement mediated cell lysis [53, 54].

Gene therapy involves introducing genetic material, typically a viral vector, into tissues of interest to replace the blueprint of a protein product. The most used viral vectors are adeno-associated viral vectors due to their lower immunogenicity and extended duration of gene expression [54].

Another way to treat AMD is through cellular therapy which works by replacing a protein product, like gene therapy; however, instead of replacing the genetic code, the cells that produce the protein of interest are replaced or supplemented. Cellular therapy allows for the replacement of dead or diseased tissue with healthy tissue. For AMD, this typically involves replacement of the RPE. Replacement of neural retinal tissue is challenging as it relies on the re-establishment of neural connections. In contrast, the RPE does not have neural connections, but serves to maintain healthy photoreceptors by providing nutrients and removing waste products. For these reasons, the RPE is currently the primary target of cell-based therapy for AMD [54]. Another promising cellular therapy for exudative AMD is replacement of the choroidal endothelial layer as this may prevent neovascularization [55]. However, there are many challenges associated with the delivery of cell-based therapy such as immune rejection, high rates of tumor formation, and differentiation into unintended cell types. Previous studies have shown the dangers of using stem cell therapy in the treatment of AMD citing complications like IVT fibrosis and tractional retinal detachment [56]. Furthermore, the timing of RPE transplant is critical to its success. It must be performed early enough so that the underlying retinal cells can still be salvaged; however, performing the therapy too early runs the risk of complications from prepathological intervention [54].

4.1 Failed therapeutics for non-exudative AMD

Lampalizumab, a fragment antigen binding portion of a humanized monoclonal antibody that selectively binds and inhibits complement factor D [57], showed success early on as it passed both Phase I and II clinical trials. Unfortunately, it failed to show superior effects to sham treatment in treating non-exudative AMD with GA in Phase III trials [58]. Eculizumab is another antibody, which targets complement component C5. It was investigated in the COMPLETE trial to assess the progression of GA in patients with non-exudative AMD. While it demonstrated safety, it did not prove to be efficacious in slowing the rate of GA progression [59]. Much like eculizumab, LFG316, another C5 inhibitor, failed to progress past Phase II when it did not show success in stunting the growth of GA [60].

A study evaluating the safety of transplanting subretinal RPE cells derived from human umbilical tissue showed complications associated with the method of delivery. This study reported high rates of retinal perforations and detachments [61].

A unique technique of delivering cell therapy to a tissue of interest is through encapsulated cell technology (ECT). A study utilizing this technology with the NT-501 ECT implant showed promising results. A capsule containing a mass of RPE cells engineered to produce and release ciliary neurotrophic factor (CNTF) was implanted into the eye. CNTF can diffuse across the capsule and act on retinal cells to induce differentiation and promote survival of retinal cells. The exact mechanism of CNTF remains to be elucidated [62]. Studies proved this method is safe, but visual acuity (VA) did not show significant improvement. There was, however, significant improvement in the thickness of the macular region, which has been shown to be associated with increased stabilization of VA regardless of baseline best corrected visual acuity (BCVA) [63, 64]. Despite a lack of significant improvement in VA in AMD patients, this technology has since been repurposed for use in macular telangiectasia type 2 and is effective at improving BCVA and slowing progression of retinal degeneration [65].

4.2 Therapeutics in development

4.2.1 Non-exudative AMD therapies in development

There is hope that an IVT formulation of Zimura, a C5 inhibiting RNA aptamer, will show more promising results than eculizumab and LFG316 [66]. A C3 inhibitor called APL-2 passed Phase II clinical trials in the FILLY study when it demonstrated the ability to impede progression of GA [67]. Two Phase III trials of this drug are underway with the Oaks and Derby trials (Apellis). These are multicenter, randomized, double blind, sham-controlled studies that are estimated to complete around December 2022 [68].

There are studies evaluating the utility of combination antibody therapy. This concept involves inhibition of two separate pathogenic mechanisms contributing to disease progression to elicit compounding effects. A Phase I trial evaluating the combination of LFG316 and CLG561, an inhibitor of complement regulator properdin, is underway for GA [69].

Bone marrow stem cells (BMSCs) have shown safety and efficacy in patients affected by non-exudative AMD. The Stem Cell Ophthalmology Treatment Study (SCOTS) trial showed improvement in BCVA and demonstrated both safety and tolerability [70]. The trial consisted of 32 eyes affected by non-exudative AMD that were treated with autologous BMSC transplant by a variety of methods. Over a one-year period, 63% of eyes showed improvement in VA while 34% maintained a stable VA. There were no complications, and as these were autologous transplants, no immunosuppression was required.

Current gene therapy in development for non-exudative AMD works to target the complement pathway. Gene supplementation of CD59 inhibits formation of the membrane attack complex (MAC) and is being investigated with the drug AAVCAGsCD59 [71]. By preventing formation of the MAC, inhibition of complement-mediated cell lysis reduces retinal cell death, thus slowing progression of GA. Results from the recently finished Phase 1 clinical trials for AAVCAGsCD59 are being evaluated. Another promising drug, GT005, holds genetic information coding for complement factor I. It will be delivered using a recombinant, non-replicating adeno-associated viral vector. Phase I/IIa clinical trials are underway [72].

4.2.2 Exudative AMD therapies in development

The use of a port delivery system involves implanting a device into the eye that slowly releases drug over an extended period. With this device in place, the patient can have fewer office appointments and less injections. The Phase 2 Ladder study has already shown promise with this type of drug administration [73]. Bifunctional antibodies, antibodies that can bind two or more targets, are being investigated for use in exudative AMD. By targeting both the VEGF and the complement pathway it is hypothesized that patients may require fewer injections and/or show improved outcomes, similarly to the non-exudative AMD combined therapy. IBI302 is an antibody with domains for both VEGF and complement. It is undergoing dose escalation Phase I clinical trials [74]. Another drug being developed for exudative AMD is abicipar pegols, a designed ankyrin repeat protein that is part of the designed ankyrin repeat proteins (DARPin) class that inhibits all isoforms of VEGF-A. While it showed similar efficacy to ranibizumab, the FDA currently denied its approval because of reports of associated intraocular inflammation [75].

A Phase I clinical trial involving only two patients with severe exudative AMD and no control group showed successful implantation of fully differentiated human ESC-derived RPE cells that were grown on a synthetic basement membrane. VA at 12 months showed improvement in 29 and 21 letters. The patch of RPE cells appeared intact and healthy when visualized through biomicroscopy and optical coherence tomography (OCT) [76].

There are documented cases of successful autologous and allogenic transplants of induced pluripotent stem cells. However, the cost of these studies and unexpected genetic changes have been discouraging [78, 79]. Further endeavors in cell-based treatment of AMD are aimed at generating a layer of multipotent stem cells from RPE cells. Proliferation and differentiation of these stem cells may restore function to diseased retina [77].

Exudative AMD gene therapy mainly targets the VEGF pathway, but other areas of intervention include PEDF, angiostatin, and endostatin. Phase II clinical trials of rAAV.sFLT-1, which codes for a soluble, full length version of the VEGFR-1 protein, are currently underway [78]. A Phase I clinical trial evaluating safety and tolerability is currently underway for a recombinant, replication-deficient adeno-associated virus (AAV.7 m8-aflibercept) IVT injection gene therapy carrying an aflibercept coding sequence [79]. A Phase I clinical trial demonstrated safety for using an adeno-associated virus vector carrying genetic information for human PEDF (AdPEDF.11) [80]. Endostatin and angiostatin, are proteins that inhibits angiogenesis. A combination drug of endostatin and angiostatin (RetinoStat) demonstrated safety and tolerability [81]. There are many promising therapies in different stages of clinical trials for the treatment of AMD.

5. Bidirectional translation from humans to pre-clinical models and back again

In summary, the "virtuous cycle" of bidirectional translation allows the examination of the outcome of experimental modulation in normal and pathological phenotypic animal models to discover novel regulators with the potential to evade, delay, or overturn human disease [82]. This cycle demonstrates that breakthroughs in human and experimental models facilitate a recurring sequence of human observation, pre-clinical model experimentation, followed by verification in humans (**Figure 1**). Animal models are fundamental to this discipline, as they advance the progression of understanding of the genetic framework that produces the pathological condition of interest and is a potentially vital target for novel therapeutics. It is proven that this series of bidirectional translation efficiently drives the investigation of diagnosis, treatment, and prevention of congenital, progressive, and adult conditions alike [82].

At baseline, this methodology is possible due to advanced genetic and molecular technologies, as well as the Human Genome Project, which propelled the identification of complex traits and pathways causing disease. Those resources alone, however, do not account for the complex interplay between inherited and environmental factors. Animal models provide a degree of experimental control, not possible in humans, to explore just that [82]. Both phenotype-based (forward

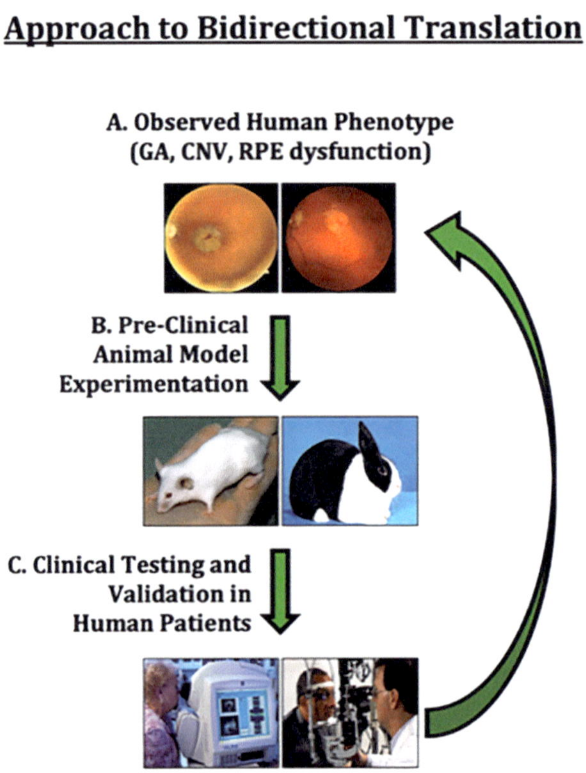

Figure 1.
Model of the "virtuous cycle" of bidirectional translation. (A) Bidirectional translation begins with the discovery of a human disease phenotype. (B) After observing a phenotype, animal models are generated to mimic the human condition as accurately as possible. This allows for a deeper understanding of the pathophysiology as well as a model on which to test therapeutics. (C) With the knowledge gained from animal models, treatments are carried back into human patients to test clinically the efficacy and tolerability of the therapeutics. The cycle then repeats allowing for a better understanding of both the disease itself and how to treat it more efficaciously.

genetics) and gene-based (reverse genetics) approaches permit linkage of genes and phenotypes in experimental animal models. Traditionally, genetic variants are accepted to relate in an additive fashion with functions that are stationary. Yet, there are many complexities in understanding these relationships, specifically in multigenic traits, with factors such as modifier genes, gene–gene interactions, gene–environment and gene-age interactions, and unconventional genetic complexities [82]. This is precisely where the beauty of animal models shines. They are the solution, the medium capable of exploring these intricacies. Puzzle pieces necessary to address gene–gene interactions, modifier genes, gene–environment interactions, and gene-age interactions can be tried and tested in pre-clinical models.

Although animal models cannot entirely replicate the human biological environment, they can reveal information that has been used to formulate hypotheses about the human manifestation of disease. This step has led to the discovery of genetic regulators and therapeutic modulators of disease, as part of the virtuous cycle of bidirectional translation. For example, the studies performed in mice undergoing oxidative stress (*Sod1*$^{-/-}$ and *Nrf2*$^{-/-}$ models) and the discovery that waste material from drusen contribute to RPE atrophy led to the development of treatments for lowering ROS and oxidative damage. Other studies demonstrated that loss of RPE cells and their functionality leads to an AMD-like phenotype, which then inspired the idea of RPE cell therapy [76]. Similarly, animal models (*Cfh*$^{-/-}$ mice) revealed the role of complement in AMD pathophysiology, which inspired the development of novel non-exudative AMD therapies that target complement such as Zimura and APL-2 [66, 67]. Finally, studies in which VEGF inhibition in animals led to the successful therapeutics (bevacizumab, ranibizumab, aflibercept, and brolucizumab) that are currently used to treat exudative AMD in humans [44]. In summary, observed phenotypes can be linked to specific genotypes (and vice versa) that can be corroborated between humans and pre-clinical models. This bidirectional translation and the virtual cycle using a cross-species approach has accelerated the discovery of novel disease-associated genes and the development of targeted therapies.

Nadeau and Auwerx recapitulate that the virtuous cycle pairs the trajectory of observations in humans with the potential of experimental animal models and confirmation in human cases. Human limitations are apparent, while animal models house the biological tools to foster disease onset and progression. They expose pathophysiology that illuminates related disease mechanisms in humans and are deemed vital for the prosperity of molecular, cellular, developmental, and physiological experimentation.

6. Conclusion

AMD is a complex, multifaceted disease that is becoming more prevalent in the aging population. Animal models provide insight into our current understanding of disease pathophysiology including an interplay of oxidative stress, inflammation, dysregulated antioxidants, lipid metabolism, and angiogenesis juxtaposed with genetic and environmental risk factors, the greatest of which are aging and cigarette smoking. Mice are the most used animal models and have provided information such as the roles of antioxidants and inflammation in AMD pathophysiology. Mice also provide excellent polygenic models which may better represent the complex pathology of AMD. Although other animal models, such as rabbits, have been helpful, NHP eyes are the most like human eyes making them an invaluable resource; however cost and ethical issues limit their widespread use.

After disease progresses to exudative AMD, there are several FDA-approved treatments such as bevacizumab, ranibizumab, aflibercept, and most recently brolucizumab that block members of the VEGF family of proteins. Through the AREDS 2 study, vitamin supplementation consisting of 500 mg vitamin C, 400 IU vitamin E, 10 mg of lutein and 2 mg of zeaxanthin, 80 mg of zinc (zinc oxide), and 2 mg of copper (cupric oxide) can slow the progression to advanced AMD. Although treatment options are currently limited, there are studies in various clinical phases evaluating potential therapies for both non-exudative and exudative AMD. Three main classes under investigation are antibodies, genes, and cell-based therapies. The virtuous cycle of bidirectional translation, along with the use of improved animal models, enhances our understanding of AMD pathophysiology and opens the doors to innovative treatment options.

Acknowledgements

We would like to acknowledge the following funding sources: a Challenge Award from Research to Prevent Blindness (New York, NY) to the Department of Ophthalmology at the Hamilton Eye Institute; and a Catalyst Award for Innovative Research Approaches for Age-Related Macular Degeneration to MMJ from Research to Prevent Blindness (New York, NY) and the International Retinal Research Foundation (Birmingham, AL).

Conflicts of interest

The authors declare no conflict of interest.

Author details

Jonathan Rho, Paul Percelay, Sophie Pilkinton, T.J. Hollingsworth, Ilyse Kornblau and Monica M. Jablonski*
Hamilton Eye Institute, University of Tennessee Health Science Center, Memphis, TN, United States

*Address all correspondence to: mjablonski@uthsc.edu

References

[1] Loskutova, E., et al., *Macular pigment and its contribution to vision.* Nutrients, 2013. **5**(6): p. 1962-1969.

[2] Nivison-Smith, L., et al., *Age-related macular degeneration: linking clinical presentation to pathology.* Optom Vis Sci, 2014. **91**(8): p. 832-848.

[3] Ambati, J. and B.J. Fowler, *Mechanisms of age-related macular degeneration.* Neuron, 2012. **75**(1): p. 26-39.

[4] Bowes Rickman, C., et al., *Dry age-related macular degeneration: mechanisms, therapeutic targets, and imaging.* Investigative ophthalmology & visual science, 2013. **54**(14): p. ORSF68-ORSF80.

[5] Geerlings, M.J., E.K. de Jong, and A.I. den Hollander, *The complement system in age-related macular degeneration: A review of rare genetic variants and implications for personalized treatment.* Molecular immunology, 2017. **84**: p. 65-76.

[6] Wong, W.L., et al., *Global prevalence of age-related macular degeneration and disease burden projection for 2020 and 2040: a systematic review and meta-analysis.* Lancet Glob Health, 2014. **2**(2): p. e106–e116.

[7] Lambert, N.G., et al., *Risk factors and biomarkers of age-related macular degeneration.* Progress in retinal and eye research, 2016. **54**: p. 64-102.

[8] Seddon, J.M., et al., *Association between C-reactive protein and age-related macular degeneration.* Jama, 2004. **291**(6): p. 704-710.

[9] Shahid, H., et al., *Age-related macular degeneration: the importance of family history as a risk factor.* Br J Ophthalmol, 2012. **96**(3): p. 427-431.

[10] Chapman, N.A., R.J. Jacobs, and A.J. Braakhuis, *Role of diet and food intake in age-related macular degeneration: a systematic review.* Clin Exp Ophthalmol, 2019. **47**(1): p. 106-127.

[11] Velilla, S., et al., *Smoking and age-related macular degeneration: review and update.* Journal of ophthalmology, 2013. **2013**: p. 895147-895147.

[12] Fritsche, L.G., et al., *A large genome-wide association study of age-related macular degeneration highlights contributions of rare and common variants.* Nature genetics, 2016. **48**(2): p. 134-143.

[13] Abokyi, S., et al., *Central Role of Oxidative Stress in Age-Related Macular Degeneration: Evidence from a Review of the Molecular Mechanisms and Animal Models.* Oxidative medicine and cellular longevity, 2020. **2020**: p. 7901270-7901270.

[14] McCannel, C.A., O. European Board of, and O. American Academy of, *Retina and vitreous*. 2018.

[15] Zeiss, C.J., *REVIEW PAPER: Animals as Models of Age-Related Macular Degeneration: An Imperfect Measure of the Truth.* Veterinary Pathology, 2010. **47**(3): p. 396-413.

[16] Kauppinen, A., et al., *Inflammation and its role in age-related macular degeneration.* Cellular and molecular life sciences : CMLS, 2016. **73**(9): p. 1765-1786.

[17] Pennesi, M.E., M. Neuringer, and R.J. Courtney, *Animal models of age related macular degeneration.* Molecular aspects of medicine, 2012. **33**(4): p. 487-509.

[18] Hernández-Zimbrón, L.F., et al., *Age-Related Macular Degeneration: New Paradigms for Treatment and*

Management of AMD. Oxidative medicine and cellular longevity, 2018. **2018**: p. 8374647-8374647.

[19] Patel, C., et al., *Primate model of chronic retinal neovascularization and vascular leakage.* Experimental Eye Research, 2020. **195**: p. 108031.

[20] Excellence, N.I.f.H. and Care, *Classification*. 2018: National Institute for Health and Care Excellence (UK).

[21] VanDenLangenberg, A.M. and M.P. Carson, *Drusen Bodies*, in *StatPearls*. 2020, StatPearls Publishing: Treasure Island (FL).

[22] Age-Related Eye Disease Study Research, G., *The Age-Related Eye Disease Study (AREDS): design implications. AREDS report no. 1.* Controlled clinical trials, 1999. **20**(6): p. 573-600.

[23] Fleckenstein, M., et al., *The Progression of Geographic Atrophy Secondary to Age-Related Macular Degeneration.* Ophthalmology, 2018. **125**(3): p. 369-390.

[24] Gehrs, K.M., et al., *Age-related macular degeneration--emerging pathogenetic and therapeutic concepts.* Ann Med, 2006. **38**(7): p. 450-471.

[25] Chew, E.Y., et al., *Ten-Year Follow-up of Age-Related Macular Degeneration in the Age-Related Eye Disease Study: AREDS Report No. 36.* JAMA Ophthalmology, 2014. **132**(3): p. 272-277.

[26] Soundara Pandi, S.P., et al., *Progress in developing rodent models of age-related macular degeneration (AMD)*. Exp Eye Res, 2020. **203**: p. 108404.

[27] Bryda, E.C., *The Mighty Mouse: The Impact of Rodents on Advances in Biomedical Research.* Missouri Medicine, 2013. **110**(3): p. 207-211.

[28] Fletcher, E.L., et al., *Studying age-related macular degeneration using animal models.* Optometry and vision science : official publication of the American Academy of Optometry, 2014. **91**(8): p. 878-886.

[29] Philips, T. and J.D. Rothstein, *Rodent Models of Amyotrophic Lateral Sclerosis.* Curr Protoc Pharmacol, 2015. **69**: p. 5 67 1-5 67 21.

[30] Hadziahmetovic, M., et al., *The oral iron chelator deferiprone protects against iron overload-induced retinal degeneration.* Invest Ophthalmol Vis Sci, 2011. **52**(2): p. 959-968.

[31] Espinosa-Heidmann, D.G., et al., *Cigarette Smoke–Related Oxidants and the Development of Sub-RPE Deposits in an Experimental Animal Model of Dry AMD.* Investigative Ophthalmology & Visual Science, 2006. **47**(2): p. 729-737.

[32] Kelley, N., et al., *The NLRP3 Inflammasome: An Overview of Mechanisms of Activation and Regulation.* International journal of molecular sciences, 2019. **20**(13): p. 3328.

[33] Tarallo, V., et al., *DICER1 Loss and Alu RNA Induce Age-Related Macular Degeneration via the NLRP3 Inflammasome and MyD88.* Cell, 2012. **149**(4): p. 847-859.

[34] Bedell, M.A., et al., *Mouse models of human disease. Part II: recent progress and future directions.* Genes Dev, 1997. **11**(1): p. 11-43.

[35] Chintalapudi, S.R., et al., *Systems genetics identifies a role for Cacna2d1 regulation in elevated intraocular pressure and glaucoma susceptibility.* Nat Commun, 2017. **8**(1): p. 1755.

[36] Stiemke, A.B., et al., *Systems Genetics of Optic Nerve Axon Necrosis During Glaucoma.* Front Genet, 2020. **11**: p. 31.

[37] Geisert, E.E. and R.W. Williams, *Using BXD mouse strains in vision research: A systems genetics approach.* Mol Vis, 2020. **26**: p. 173-187.

[38] Muraoka, Y., et al., *Real-Time Imaging of Rabbit Retina with Retinal Degeneration by Using Spectral-Domain Optical Coherence Tomography.* PLOS ONE, 2012. **7**(4): p. e36135.

[39] Qiu, G., et al., *A new model of experimental subretinal neovascularization in the rabbit.* Experimental Eye Research, 2006. **83**(1): p. 141-152.

[40] Moshiri, A., et al., *A nonhuman primate model of inherited retinal disease.* The Journal of Clinical Investigation, 2019. **129**(2): p. 863-874.

[41] Picaud, S., et al., *The primate model for understanding and restoring vision.* Proceedings of the National Academy of Sciences, 2019. **116**(52): p. 26280-26287.

[42] Group*, T.A.-R.E.D.S.R., *Lutein + Zeaxanthin and Omega-3 Fatty Acids for Age-Related Macular Degeneration: The Age-Related Eye Disease Study 2 (AREDS2) Randomized Clinical Trial.* JAMA, 2013. **309**(19): p. 2005-2015.

[43] Yiu, G., et al., *In Vivo Multimodal Imaging of Drusenoid Lesions in Rhesus Macaques.* Scientific Reports, 2017. **7**(1): p. 15013.

[44] Flaxel, C.J., et al., *Age-Related Macular Degeneration Preferred Practice Pattern®.* Ophthalmology, 2020. **127**(1): p. P1-P65.

[45] *Promising New Treatments for AMD.* American Academy of Ophthalmology, 2020.

[46] Markham, A., *Brolucizumab: First Approval.* Drugs, 2019. **79**(18): p. 1997-2000.

[47] Chew, E.Y., et al., *Summary Results and Recommendations From the Age-Related Eye Disease Study.* Archives of Ophthalmology, 2009. **127**(12): p. 1678-1679.

[48] Brown, D.M., et al., *Ranibizumab versus Verteporfin for Neovascular Age-Related Macular Degeneration.* New England Journal of Medicine, 2006. **355**(14): p. 1432-1444.

[49] Rosenfeld, P.J., et al., *Ranibizumab for Neovascular Age-Related Macular Degeneration.* New England Journal of Medicine, 2006. **355**(14): p. 1419-1431.

[50] *Comparison of Anti-VEGF Treatments for Wet AMD.* American Academy of Ophthalmology, 2020.

[51] Comparison of Age-related Macular Degeneration Treatments Trials Research, G., et al., *Ranibizumab and bevacizumab for treatment of neovascular age-related macular degeneration: two-year results.* Ophthalmology, 2012. **119**(7): p. 1388-1398.

[52] Monés, J., et al., *Risk of Inflammation, Retinal Vasculitis, and Retinal Occlusion-Related Events with Brolucizumab: Post Hoc Review of HAWK and HARRIER.* Ophthalmology, 2020.

[53] Scholl, H.P., et al., *Systemic complement activation in age-related macular degeneration.* PLoS One, 2008. **3**(7): p. e2593.

[54] Akyol, E. and A. Lotery, *Gene, Cell and Antibody-Based Therapies for the Treatment of Age-Related Macular Degeneration.* Biologics, 2020. **14**: p. 83-94.

[55] Lois, N., et al., *Endothelial progenitor cells in diabetic retinopathy.* Frontiers in endocrinology, 2014. **5**: p. 44-44.

[56] Satarian, L., et al., *Intravitreal Injection of Bone Marrow Mesenchymal Stem Cells in Patients with Advanced Retinitis Pigmentosa; a Safety Study.* J Ophthalmic Vis Res, 2017. **12**(1): p. 58-64.

[57] Nebbioso, M., et al., *Therapeutic Approaches with Intravitreal Injections in Geographic Atrophy Secondary to Age-Related Macular Degeneration: Current Drugs and Potential Molecules.* Int J Mol Sci, 2019. **20**(7).

[58] Holz, F.G., et al., *Efficacy and Safety of Lampalizumab for Geographic Atrophy Due to Age-Related Macular Degeneration: Chroma and Spectri Phase 3 Randomized Clinical Trials.* JAMA Ophthalmology, 2018. **136**(6): p. 666-677.

[59] Yehoshua, Z., et al., *Systemic complement inhibition with eculizumab for geographic atrophy in age-related macular degeneration: the COMPLETE study.* Ophthalmology, 2014. **121**(3): p. 693-701.

[60] Novartis, P., *A Multicenter, Randomized, Sham-control, Proof-of-concept Study of Intravitreal LFG316 in Patients With Geographic Atrophy Associated With Age-related Macular Degeneration*. 2020, clinicaltrials.gov.

[61] Ho, A.C., et al., *Experience With a Subretinal Cell-based Therapy in Patients With Geographic Atrophy Secondary to Age-related Macular Degeneration.* Am J Ophthalmol, 2017. **179**: p. 67-80.

[62] Fuhrmann, S., et al., *Distribution of CNTF receptor alpha protein in the central nervous system of the chick embryo.* J Comp Neurol, 2003. **461**(1): p. 111-122.

[63] Li, S., et al., *Ciliary neurotrophic factor (CNTF) protects retinal cone and rod photoreceptors by suppressing excessive formation of the visual pigments.* The Journal of biological chemistry, 2018. **293**(39): p. 15256-15268.

[64] Kauper, K., et al., *Two-year intraocular delivery of ciliary neurotrophic factor by encapsulated cell technology implants in patients with chronic retinal degenerative diseases.* Invest Ophthalmol Vis Sci, 2012. **53**(12): p. 7484-7491.

[65] Chew, E.Y., et al., *Effect of Ciliary Neurotrophic Factor on Retinal Neurodegeneration in Patients with Macular Telangiectasia Type 2: A Randomized Clinical Trial.* Ophthalmology, 2019. **126**(4): p. 540-549.

[66] Iveric bio, I., *A Phase 2/3 Randomized, Double-Masked, Controlled Trial to Assess the Safety and Efficacy of Intravitreous Administration of Zimura™ (Anti-C5 Aptamer) in Subjects With Geographic Atrophy Secondary to Dry Age-Related Macular Degeneration*. 2020, clinicaltrials.gov.

[67] Apellis Pharmaceuticals, I., *A Phase II, Multicenter, Randomized, Single-Masked, Sham-Controlled Study of Safety, Tolerability and Evidence of Activity of Intravitreal APL-2 Therapy in Patients With Geographic Atrophy (GA)*. 2020, clinicaltrials.gov.

[68] Kassa, E., et al., *Complement inhibition as a therapeutic strategy in retinal disorders.* Expert Opin Biol Ther, 2019. **19**(4): p. 335-342.

[69] Alcon, R., *A Randomized, Multi-Center, Single Masked, Sham Controlled, Proof-of-Concept Study of Intravitreal CLG561 as a Monotherapy and in Combination With LFG316 in Subjects With Geographic Atrophy*. 2019, clinicaltrials.gov.

[70] Weiss, J.N. and S. Levy, *Stem Cell Ophthalmology Treatment Study (SCOTS): Bone Marrow-Derived Stem Cells in the Treatment of Age-Related Macular Degeneration.* Medicines (Basel, Switzerland), 2020. 7(4): p. 16.

[71] Hemera, B., *A Phase 1, Open-Label, Multi-Center, Dose-Escalating, Safety and Tolerability Study of a Single Intravitreal Injection of AAVCAGsCD59 in Patients With Advanced Non-Exudative (Dry) Age-Related Macular Degeneration With Geographic Atrophy*. 2019, clinicaltrials.gov.

[72] *History of Changes for Study: NCT03846193.*

[73] Campochiaro, P.A., et al., *The Port Delivery System with Ranibizumab for Neovascular Age-Related Macular Degeneration: Results from the Randomized Phase 2 Ladder Clinical Trial.* Ophthalmology, 2019. **126**(8): p. 1141-1154.

[74] Innovent Biologics Co, L., *A Dose Escalation Phase I Clinical Study to Evaluate the Tolerability and Safety of IBI302 in Patients With Wet Age-related Macular Degeneration (AMD)*. 2020, clinicaltrials.gov.

[75] Kunimoto, D., et al., *Efficacy and Safety of Abicipar in Neovascular Age-Related Macular Degeneration: 52-Week Results of Phase 3 Randomized Controlled Study.* Ophthalmology, 2020. **127**(10): p. 1331-1344.

[76] da Cruz, L., et al., *Phase 1 clinical study of an embryonic stem cell-derived retinal pigment epithelium patch in age-related macular degeneration.* Nat Biotechnol, 2018. **36**(4): p. 328-337.

[77] Salero, E., et al., *Adult human RPE can be activated into a multipotent stem cell that produces mesenchymal derivatives.* Cell Stem Cell, 2012. **10**(1): p. 88-95.

[78] Kendall, R.L. and K.A. Thomas, *Inhibition of vascular endothelial cell growth factor activity by an endogenously encoded soluble receptor.* Proc Natl Acad Sci U S A, 1993. **90**(22): p. 10705-10709.

[79] Regenxbio, I., *A Phase I/IIa, Open-label, Multiple-cohort, Dose-escalation Study to Evaluate the Safety and Tolerability of Gene Therapy With RGX-314 in Subjects With Neovascular AMD (nAMD)*. 2020, clinicaltrials.gov.

[80] GenVec, *An Open-label, Phase I, Single Administration, Dose-Escalation Study of AdGVPEDF.11D in Neovascular Age-related Macular Degeneration (AMD)*. 2011, clinicaltrials.gov.

[81] Campochiaro, P.A., et al., *Lentiviral Vector Gene Transfer of Endostatin/Angiostatin for Macular Degeneration (GEM) Study.* Hum Gene Ther, 2017. **28**(1): p. 99-111.

[82] Nadeau, J.H. and J. Auwerx, *The virtuous cycle of human genetics and mouse models in drug discovery.* Nat Rev Drug Discov, 2019. **18**(4): p. 255-272.

Section 5

Preclinal Model of Brucellar Spondylodiscitis

Chapter 11

Preclinical Models of Brucellar Spondylodiscitis

Xiaoyu Cai, Tao Xu, Maierdan Maimaiti and Liang Gao

Abstract

Brucellar spondylodiscitis, the most prevalent and significant osteoarticular presentation of human Brucellosis, is difficult to diagnose and usually yields irreversible neurologic deficits and spinal deformities. Relevant aspects of *Brucella* pathogenesis have been intensively investigated in preclinical models. Mice, rats, rabbits, and sheep are representing available models to induce Brucellosis. Evaluation of Brucellar spondylodiscitis may be performed using a large variety of methods, including plain radiography, computed tomography, magnetic resonance imaging, histological analysis, blood test, and bacteria culture. This chapter focuses on these preclinical models of Brucellar spondylodiscitis. The requirements for preclinical models of Brucellar spondylodiscitis, pearls and pitfalls of the preclinical model establishment, and comprehensive analyses of Brucellar spondylodiscitis in animals are also depicted.

Keywords: Animal models, Preclinical models, Brucellar spondylodiscitis, Brucellosis

1. Introduction

Brucellosis, an infectious disease caused by the *Brucella* bacteria in both humans and animals, leads to a significant impact on the public health and the animal industry [1]. Since 1950, comprehensive measures against Brucellosis were undertaken in China and a great number of achievements had been made in its prevention and control [2]. It, however, remains a serious public health issue, and much remains to be accomplished to reach the goal of controlling human and animal Brucellosis in China. As the most common and significant osteoarticular presentation of human Brucellosis, Brucellar spondylodiscitis has a variable course with a long latency between the onset of symptoms and the radiologic changes' appearance with and unspecific clinical symptoms, hindering an early intervention to prevent irreversible neurologic deficits and spinal deformities (**Figure 1**) [4, 5]. It is an endemic disease in areas of sheep farming, which is also widespread among farmers, animal breeders, veterinarians, and veterinary technicians as an occupational disease [6, 7]. Due to the late-onset radiological findings, slow growth rate in blood cultures, and complexity of the serodiagnosis, timely and accurate diagnosis of Brucellar spondylodiscitis is still a challenge for clinicians [8, 9].

Preclinical models exhibiting symptoms comparable to those in humans are essential for the translation of preclinical findings into clinical practice [10–13]. Relevant aspects of the Brucella pathogenesis have been intensively investigated in both *in vitro* and preclinical *in vivo* models. Several preclinical models are available to mimic Brucellar spondylodiscitis and provide beneficial platforms allowing the

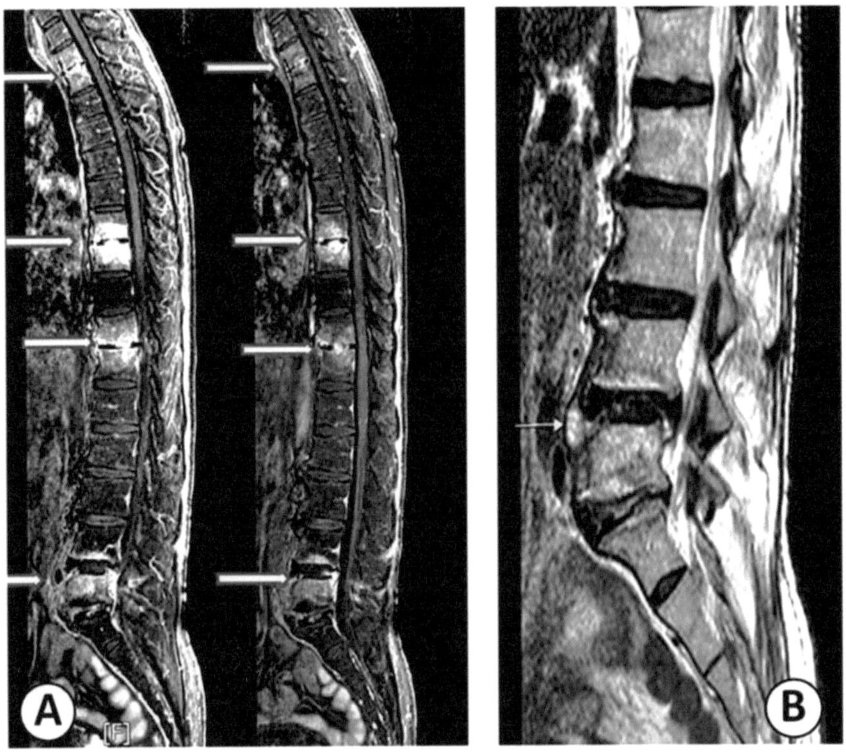

Figure 1.
A typical case of noncontiguous multiple-level Brucellar spondylodiscitis with an epidural abscess in a 57-year-old man with a 6-month history of low back pain, restricted range of motion, fever, chills, and night sweating. (A) the midsagittal magnetic resonance imaging revealed increased signal intensity (arrows) involving the T2-T3, T8–9, T11–12, and L4–5 disks and vertebral bodies. (B) Pathologic signal changes were identified, compatible with a 14 × 8-mm paraspinal abscess (L5), with low signal intensity on T1-weighted images, high signal intensity on T2-weighted images, and post-contrast peripheral enhancement (arrow) [3].

management and exploration of translational investigations of medical device and novel therapeutics [14–16].

This chapter focuses on these preclinical models of Brucellar spondylodiscitis. The requirements for preclinical models of Brucellar spondylodiscitis, pearls and pitfalls of the preclinical model establishment, and comprehensive analyses of Brucellar spondylodiscitis in animal models are also deliberated.

2. Requirements for preclinical models of Brucellar spondylodiscitis

Investigators have previously established Brucellosis models in many diverse animals [15], however the animal candidates for stimulating *in vivo* Brucellar spondylodiscitis should be suitable for both the implantation of the *Brucella* bacteria and the convenience for the anatomical morphology research (**Table 1**). Common requirements for preclinical models of Brucellar spondylodiscitis are diverse, including but not limited to:

1. The geometrical size and anatomical structure of the animal spine should be comparable to the human spine.

2. The biomechanical properties of the animal spine should be close to the human spine.

Species	Characteristics of spine	References
Mouse	Significantly smaller size than the human spine Different mechanical loading from the human spine Advantages of easy surgical manipulations	[17, 18]
Rat	Normalized disc height in rats higher than that in humans Vertebral dimensions varying more in rats than in humans Vertebrae slenderer in rats than in humans	[18, 19]
Rabbit	Seven lumbar vertebral segments in rabbit and the lowest segment connected to the sacrum (similar to humans) Biomechanical behavior of the lumbar spine comparable with the human lumbar spine	[18, 20, 21]
Sheep	Spine size larger than humans (particularly in vertebral body height and pedicle height) Similar increasing trend of spinal canal width and depth to humans	[22]

Table 1.
Comparison of the spine structure of animal models of brucellosis.

3. The model needs reflect the clinical nature of the Brucellar spondylodiscitis.

4. The radiographic characteristics of Brucellar spondylodiscitis in specific animals should be analogous to the human setting.

5. The generated preclinical data can be translated into the clinical situation and further benefit the clinical treatments.

3. Preclinical models of Brucellar spondylodiscitis

Mice, rats, rabbits, and sheep represent the available candidates to induce Brucellosis [23–26]. However, the preclinical model of Brucellar spondylodiscitis with a possible high translational efficiency has only been established in rabbits so far [14].

3.1 Mice

Mice are the most extensively used to investigate chronic infections of *Brucella* [15]. Enright and colleagues constructed the Brucellosis model with the mouse by intravenous injection of 5×10^4 colony forming units (CFU) of either *Brucella* attenuated strain 19 or *Brucella abortus* strain 2308 to confirm *Brucella abortus* produces a chronic granulomatous response in mice, and extend earlier studies in demonstrating that prominent acute and subacute inflammatory responses also occur [27]. Steven *et al.* made the mouse model with the method of intraperitoneal injections of 10^5 CFU of *Brucella* strain 2308 or 10^7 CFU of either strain 19 or RB51 [28]. Tobias' Brucellosis mouse model was built by intraperitoneally infected with 10^6 CFU of *Brucella abortus* strain 2308 [29]. The spleen is the most heavily colonized organ with voluminous histiocytic infiltrates and multifocal microgranulomas [27–29]. Besides the spleen, the liver is also a common site for colonization and replication of *Brucella* in the mice [27, 30, 31]. Mice infected with virulent strains of *Brucella* have mild to moderate hepatitis characterized by neutrophilic infiltrate at early stages of the infection, followed by histiocytic infiltrate with epithelioid cells and microgranulomas at its chronic stages [27, 29]. It is noteworthy that *Brucella* infection in mice results in lesions that mimic those described in chronic infections in humans, and patients with chronic Brucellosis may develop splenomegaly and hepatomegaly [32]. In addition, multifocal granulomas with epithelioid macrophages are also detected in the liver or spleen parenchyma of patients who were infected with *Brucella* [33, 34]. Chronic infection of the *Brucella* in humans may also yield osteoarticular alterations, including osteoarthritis and spondylodiscitis [35]. Rajashekara *et al.* reported that mice may develop bacterial colonization in periarticular tissues during the chronic stages of *Brucella melitensis* infection [36]. In mice surviving over 45 days after intraperitoneal infection of *Brucella melitensis*, the bioluminescent *Brucella melitensis* were detected in the vertebral joints of their tails, suggesting that the mice might be a useful model for the study of human osteoarticular diseases, including the Brucellar spondylodiscitis [16]. Comparisons of disease manifestations (e.g. timing of the disease onset, structural alterations of the spines, and definite localization of the bacterial foci) between animal and human Brucellar spondylodiscitis would be beneficial for evaluating its potential translational values and further recognizing specific histological, radiographic, and clinical signs, allowing for an early detection and intervention of human Brucellar spondylodiscitis.

The mouse model has been utilized for the evaluation of the efficiency of different pharmacotherapies for human Brucellosis [37–39]. Several lines of evidence suggest that mice treated with ciprofloxacin, by subcutaneous (40 mg/kg), digestive (200 mg/kg), or intraperitoneal (20 mg/kg) route, are not able to control the infection of *Brucella* melitensis. In contrast, mice treated with doxycycline (40 mg/kg) at 24 hours after infection efficiently clear the infection [38, 39]. Shasha *et al.* showed that mice administered intraperitoneally with doxycycline (40 mg/kg/day) or rifampin (25 mg/kg/day) had high levels of antibiotics in the blood following 1-hour postinjection (doxycycline: 5.4 μg/ml and rifampin: 18 μg/ml, respectively) and were able to clear the infection. The treatment regimen of the usage of doxycycline and rifampin is consistent with the therapeutic protocols of human Brucellosis.

3.2 Rats

The rats, more resistant to *Brucella* infection than the mice [15], can develop the persistent bacteremia, and do not have a spontaneous cure over the 1-month infection [23]. Therefore, rats can serve as a model candidate to evaluate the increased susceptibility to *Brucella* infection, which mimics the chronic symptoms in patients. Yumuk *et al*. analyzed the rat model by intraperitoneal injection of 2×10^5 to 4×10^5 CFU of *Brucella melitensis* strain 16 M [23]. Moreover, the rat model has also been used to analyze the efficacy of various antibiotics to treat Brucellosis [40–42] and to evaluate the pathological properties and clinical characters of *Brucella* infection during the pregnancy [43]. Also, the similar morphology of the spine at the axial plane between rats and humans supports their application as an applicable candidate for the spine research [19, 44]. Since patients with Brucellar spondylodiscitis are commonly detected at the late phase of the disease, rats, as the potential model of chronic Brucellar spondylodiscitis, may be beneficial to assist to exam specific remedies against those chronic manifestations within a clinically relevant setting.

The usefulness of pharmacotherapy has been investigated in the treatment for Brucellosis in the rat model. Geyik *et al*. reported that rats were administered orally with rifampicin (50 mg/kg/day) and doxycycline (40 mg/kg/day), or spiramycin (50 mg/kg/day), or a combination of spiramycin and rifampicin at the same dose for 21 days [40]. All the rats were cured with the treatment results that the effectivities of spiramycin and rifampicin plus spiramycin were similar to rifampicin plus doxycycline. This result is helpful for the effective alternative in the treatment of human Brucellosis. Furthermore, Sezak and colleagues proposed that moxifloxacin might be an alternative choice in the treatment of Brucellosis [42]. Doxycycline (10 mg/kg/day) plus rifampicin (6 mg/kg/day) were administered intragastrically in Yumuk's study [41]. In the experiment group, all the rats received a liquid diet containing ethanol. The cure rate was 64.71% in ethanol-fed and 100% in ethanol free group. The results suggest that ethanol ingestion diminishes the efficacy of doxycycline plus rifampicin combination therapy of rat Brucellosis model, which holds implications for the treatment programme for human Brucellosis.

3.3 Rabbits

Compared with other animals, rabbits are medium-sized animals which frequently used in spine research with various advantages [45]. The rabbit spine maintains considerable morphological and structural similarities to the human spine, and its body size allows for an adequate exposure during the surgical interventions [46, 47]. Furthermore, rabbits yield higher possibilities than rodents to successfully translate preclinical discoveries into humans [48, 49]. Similarly, compared with larger animals, radiographic analyses are largely convenient in rabbits particularly for *in vivo* explorations [50].

Age is a critical issue to be considered when establishing a rabbit model of local restricted Brucellar spondylodiscitis. The significant variance of the innate immune response between young and adult rabbits against infections of foreign microbes should be recognized [14]. Virus related studies highlighted the significantly superior innate immune system in young rabbits (<4 weeks) over adult rabbits, which contributed to their distinct susceptibility to virus infections [51–53]. These data may partially explain the fact that adult rabbits are only partially susceptible to *Brucella* infection [15], and about 20% of infected animals developed a very short and sporadic bacteremia [25]. In contrast, our previous experiment within young rabbits showed that 83.4% (10 out of 12) rabbits were successfully infected by the intraosseous injection of 3×10^7 CFU of *Brucella melitensis* strain M5–90 [14]. Moreover, to mimic a local restricted inflammation without systemic dissemination of the microbes, studies via a local injection intervention with a reduced dose within young rabbits can avoid the unanticipated animal death due to the local or systematic administration with a relatively larger dosage within adult rabbits. Therefore, even with a relatively smaller size of the spine than adult rabbits, young rabbits may be more suitable to establish such a local restricted model of Brucellar spondylodiscitis.

Of note, despite the animal model for Brucellar spondylodiscitis has been established in rabbits, no studies about its treatments are available for the rabbit Brucellosis.

3.4 Sheep

Although *Brucella* ovis is one of the few classical *Brucella* species that do not have zoonotic potential, this organism is considered a major cause of reproductive failure in sheep [54]. The attenuated vaccine strain *Brucella melitensis* Rev.1, against *Brucella* infection of sheep and goats, are still the most efficient ones available among living vaccines [55]. When the bacteria are administered by the classic subcutaneous method ($10^9 - 2 \times 10^9$ CFU) in the sheep, a long-lasting serologic response is subsequently yielded. Primary manifestations of *Brucella* ovis infection in sheep are lesions of the epididymis and testis in males (e.g., epididymitis and orchitis), placentitis and abortion in ewes, and occasionally perinatal death in lambs [56], as well as arthritis [57]. The sheep spine is relatively larger than humans, particularly in vertebral body width, which would be advantageous for the easier surgical operation [22]. However, sheep are expensive to house and the operation requires special settings, which also hinder the widely accessibility of this model [58].

Oxytetracycline combined with streptomycin were evaluated for eliminating *Brucella melitensis* from naturally infected sheep. The following treatment regiments were equally effective in eliminating *Brucella* in the sheep: oxytetracycline (20 mg/kg/day) intravenously daily for 6 weeks combined with streptomycin (20 mg/kg/day) intramuscularly for 3 weeks; long-acting oxytetracycline 20 mg/kg intramuscularly every 3 days for 6 weeks plus streptomycin 20 mg/kg intramuscularly every 3 days for 3 weeks; long-acting oxytetracycline mg/kg intramuscularly every 3 days for 6 weeks combined with streptomycin 20 mg/kg intramuscularly every 3 days for 3 weeks [59]. The data indicated the most effective and practical regimen for eliminating *Brucella* in the sheep.

4. Pearls and pitfalls of the preclinical model establishment

The key to establish the preclinical model is to implant the *Brucella* into the superior zone of the anterior column of lumbar vertebral body (**Figure 2**). In rabbits, to boost a localized inoculation into the vertebral body and minimize the vascular dissemination, the *Brucella* bacteria should be meticulously implanted within the superior zone of the anterior column of the L6 vertebral body of rabbits,

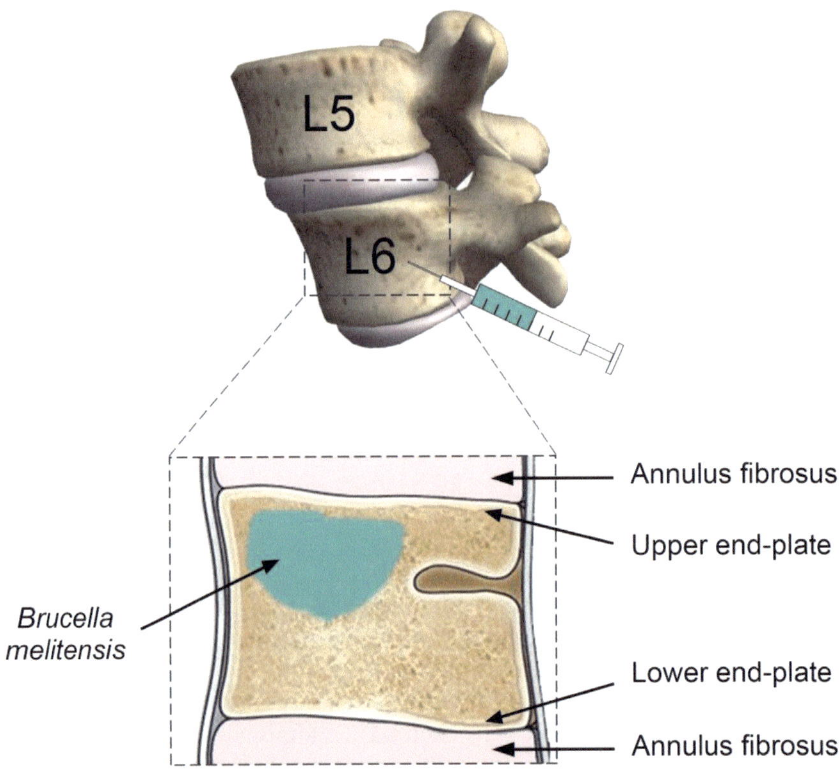

Figure 2.
Schematic of the experimental challenge injection with Brucella melitensis *into the 6th lumbar vertebrae (L6) of rabbits [14].*

where the direct vertebral body feeding capillaries scantily supplied [14]. During the procedure, the insertion site, direction, and drill depth of the Kirschner wire should be properly monitored. The open surgery is recommended to expose the target vertebrae for the intraosseous injection rather than the radiograph-guided percutaneous injection to ensure an accurate localization of the bacterial inoculation. Also, to avoid iatrogenic nerve injuries intraoperatively, the different patterns of the level of the nerve root origin and adjacent vertebra in animals from humans need to be recognized.

5. Comprehensive analyses of Brucellar spondylodiscitis in preclinical models

Several techniques can be applied for the evaluation of Brucellar spondylodiscitis in animals. To observe the targeted vertebral body and intervertebral disc

Classification	MRI characteristics
Discitis	Regional inflammation involving intervertebral disc Disc space narrowing Low signal on T1-weighted image mixing high signal on T2-weighted image
Spondylitis	Regional inflammation involving adjacent vertebrae Vertebrae diffuse marrow edema Homogeneous or uneven low signal on T1-weighted image of vertebrae
Paraspinal/ psoas abscess	Regional inflammation involving paraspinal or psoas Paravertebral abscess Psoas abscess
Appendicitis	Regional inflammation involving appendicitis Low signal on T1-weighted image High signal on T2-weighted image
Compound	Endemic inflammation involving two or more parts of vertebral and paravertebral structures T1-weighted image reveals incomplete heterogeneous hypointensity T2-weighted image reveals hyperintensity

Table 2.
Magnetic resonance imaging (MRI) classification of Brucellar spondylodiscitis adapted from [14].

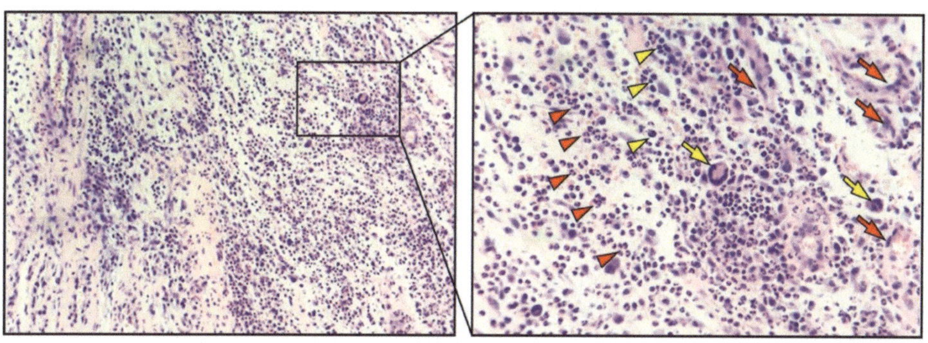

Figure 3.
Histological descriptions of the paravertebral soft tissue of Brucellar spondylodiscitis model in rabbits [14]. Hematoxylin and eosin staining features predominant lymphocyte and monocytes infiltration with sparsely distributed epithelioid cells and multinucleated giant cells. Yellow arrows indicate multinucleated giant cells and red arrows specify epithelioid cells. Yellow arrowheads define lymphocytes and red arrowheads display monocytes (magnification: (left) × 40; (right) × 100).

postoperatively, *in vivo* plain radiography, computed tomography, and magnetic resonance imaging (MRI) analyses should be performed under a general anesthesia. Specifically, the MRI findings were classified into five types, such as discitis type, spondylitis type, paraspinal/psoas abscess type, appendicitis type, and compound type, with a previously reported classification system (**Table 2**) [14]. Histological analysis for samples biopsied from the affected intervertebral disc, upper and lower end-plates, paravertebral soft tissue, psoas, and granulation tissue is highly recommended for identify the pathological pattern of the infection [60]. The pathological characteristics of Brucellar spondylodiscitis in rabbits are the massive inflammatory cell infiltration without evident bony erosions within the biopsied paravertebral structures, including lymphocytes, monocytes, and multinucleated giant cells (**Figure 3**) [61]. Blood test and bacteria culture can be done to further investigate the pathophysiological status of Brucellar spondylodiscitis.

6. Preclinical evaluation of therapeutic interventions and vaccines

Pharmacotherapy is the main therapeutic intervention for the treatment of human Brucellosis, including Brucellar spondylodiscitis. Ciprofloxacin, doxycycline, rifampin has been utilized for the evaluation of the efficiency of different pharmacotherapies for human Brucellosis [37–39]. Different combination of rifampicin, doxycycline, and spiramycin or moxifloxacin were analyzed in rat Brucellosis model for the potential therapeutic options [40, 42]. Oxytetracycline combined with streptomycin were evaluated in the sheep for the test of practical and cost-effective treatment regimen for Brucellosis [59]. Additionally, as a new antibiotic carrier, the microspheres have been used to test for a treatment effect of *Brucella* infection [62]. Microspheres based on poly (lactide-co-glycolide) wherein gentamicin entrapped have been tested to target gentamicin to the cells of the monocyte–macrophage system to reduce drug toxicity and control its release over several days [63]. However, Prior and colleagues reported that mice infected with virulent strains of *Brucella* and treated with three intraperitoneal doses of 100 μg gentamicin microspheres were not able to reduce bacterial load in the spleen after 1 and 3 weeks posttreatment [37].

Surgery should be performed to treat Brucellar spondylodiscitis if the pharmacotherapy is poorly done. The indications for surgery included the following: persistent pain due to spinal instability, severe or progressive neurologic dysfunction due to nerve root compression by inflammatory granuloma or epidural abscesses, and no response to antibiotic therapy [9, 64]. The preclinical model is critical for the research of the improvement of surgery protocols. However, the rabbit model was originally developed for the study of Brucellar spondylodiscitis. Future studies are needed to further refine the surgical procedures.

By far, the quality of live vaccines that are commercially used for preventing animal Brucellosis is evaluated in mouse models. Live *Brucella abortus* (strain S19), which is the most widely used vaccine in cattle, has been tested in mice. The mice were previously treated with 10^5 CFU of Brucella reference strain S19 vaccine [15]. All mice were injected intraperitoneally with 10^5 CFU of *Brucella* 30 days after the vaccination. The commercial vaccine is considered efficient when mice have a significantly lower bacterial load than the unvaccinated control group and when the vaccinated group has similar immunogenicity value to the mice group vaccinated with S19 reference strain [15]. Recently, a new candidate vector vaccine against human Brucellosis based on recombinant influenza viral vectors subtypes H5N1 expressing *Brucella* outer membrane protein (Omp) 16, L7/L12, Omp19 or copper/zinc superoxide dismutase proteins has been developed [65]. The effectiveness of the new anti-Brucellosis vector vaccine was determined by studying its protective effect after conjunctival, intranasal and sublingual administration in doses 10^5 50% egg infective dose (EID_{50}), 10^6 EID_{50} and 10^7 EID_{50} during prime and boost vaccinations of animals, followed by challenge with virulent strains of *Brucella* infection. Double intranasal immunization of guinea pigs at a dose of 10^6 EID_{50}, which provided 80% protection of guinea pigs from *Brucella* infection [65]. The proposed vaccine has achieved the best level of protection, which in turn provides a basis for its further promotion.

7. Challenges and outlooks

During the past decades, significant progresses to diagnose and treat the Brucellar spondylodiscitis have been achieved [66–69]. However, many obstacles still exist to be overcome in order to employ and utilize new strategies to refine early detection, diagnosis, therapy [70, 71]. Regarding the basic research, no appropriate vaccines exist due to an incomplete understanding of the mechanisms of human Brucellosis, including Brucellar spondylodiscitis. Clinically, the early and differential diagnosis of the Brucellar spondylodiscitis is challenging, especially in the early phases of the disease. Also, pharmacotherapy is the main clinical therapeutic modality for Brucellar spondylodiscitis and should be individually tailored; however, medication selection, administration, dosage, and duration are still largely debatable.

The ideal preclinical models should reflect the precise clinical characteristics of the human Brucellar spondylodiscitis and serve as a platform to explore the potential vaccines, examine novel diagnostic methods, and preselect innovative therapeutics [72–74]. More investigations in the future are still required to determine the optimal clinically relevant large preclinical model, to identify the efficacy-associated factors (e.g. age, joint size, gender, and dosage), to compare possible dissimilarities between models with local contained lesions or system atic spreading.

8. Conclusions

The pathogenesis, diagnosis, and treatment approach of Brucellar spondylodiscitis has recently become a clinical and research focus. Brucellar spondylodiscitis with highly variable clinical manifestations are practically challenging to be mimicked with laboratory preclinical models. More human-relevant preclinical models should be established to provide better insights into the sophisticated mechanism of human Brucellosis and early interventions of Brucellar spondylodiscitis.

Author details

Xiaoyu Cai[1,2,3], Tao Xu[1], Maierdan Maimaiti[1] and Liang Gao[2,3]*

1 Department of Spine Surgery, First Affiliated Hospital of Xinjiang Medical University, Urumqi, China

2 Sino Euro Orthopaedics Network (SEON), Berlin, Germany

3 Center for Clinical Medicine, Hua Tuo Institute of Medical Innovation (HTIMI), Wuhan, China

*Address all correspondence to: lianggao@web.de

References

[1] Nicoletti P. Brucellosis: past, present and future. Prilozi. 2010;31(1):21-32.

[2] Yang H, Zhang S, Wang T, Zhao C, Zhang X, Hu J, et al. Epidemiological Characteristics and Spatiotemporal Trend Analysis of Human Brucellosis in China, 1950-2018. Int J Environ Res Public Health. 2020;17(7).

[3] Tekin R, Cevik R, Nas K. Noncontiguous multiple-level brucellar spondylodiscitis with an epidural abscess. Rev Soc Bras Med Trop. 2015;48(5):638.

[4] Turgut M, Turgut AT, Koşar U. Spinal brucellosis: Turkish experience based on 452 cases published during the last century. Acta Neurochir (Wien). 2006;148(10):1033-1044; discussion 44.

[5] Bozgeyik Z, Ozdemir H, Demirdag K, Ozden M, Sonmezgoz F, Ozgocmen S. Clinical and MRI findings of brucellar spondylodiscitis. Eur J Radiol. 2008;67(1):153-158.

[6] Zileli M, Ebeoglu A. Brucellar spondylodiscitis. ArgoSpine News & Journal. 2011;23(3):99-104.

[7] Kutlu M, Ergonul O, Sayın Kutlu S, Guven T, Ustun C, Alp S, et al. Risk factors for occupational brucellosis among veterinary personnel in Turkey. Preventive veterinary medicine. 2014;117.

[8] Araj GF. Update on laboratory diagnosis of human brucellosis. Int J Antimicrob Agents. 2010;36 Suppl 1:S12-S17.

[9] Abulizi Y, Cai X, Xu T, Xun C, Sheng W, Gao L, Maimaiti M. Diagnosis and Surgical Treatment of Human Brucellar Spondylodiscitis. J Vis Exp. 2021:e61840.

[10] Gao L, Guo R, Han Z, Liu J, Chen X. Clinical trial reporting. Lancet. 2020;396(10261):1488-1489.

[11] Guo R, Gao L, Xu B. Current Evidence of Adult Stem Cells to Enhance Anterior Cruciate Ligament Treatment: A Systematic Review of Animal Trials. Arthroscopy. 2018;34(1):331-40.e2.

[12] Cai X, Gao L, Cucchiarini M, Madry H. Association of Nicotine with Osteochondrogenesis and Osteoarthritis Development: The State of the Art of Preclinical Research. J Clin Med. 2019;8(10).

[13] Gao L, Goebel LKH, Orth P, Cucchiarini M, Madry H. Subchondral drilling for articular cartilage repair: a systematic review of translational research. Dis Model Mech. 2018;11(6).

[14] Cai X, Xu T, Xun C, Abulizi Y, Liu Q, Sheng W, et al. Establishment and Initial Testing of a Medium-Sized, Surgically Feasible Animal Model for Brucellar Spondylodiscitis: A Preliminary Study. Biomed Res Int. 2019;2019:7368627.

[15] Silva TMA, Costa EA, Paixão TA, Tsolis RM, Santos RL. Laboratory Animal Models for Brucellosis Research. Journal of Biomedicine and Biotechnology. 2011;2011:518323.

[16] Rajashekara G, Glover DA, Banai M, O'Callaghan D, Splitter GA. Attenuated bioluminescent Brucella melitensis mutants GR019 (virB4), GR024 (galE), and GR026 (BMEI1090-BMEI1091) confer protection in mice. Infect Immun. 2006;74(5):2925-2936.

[17] Daly C, Ghosh P, Jenkin G, Oehme D, Goldschlager T. A Review of Animal Models of Intervertebral Disc Degeneration: Pathophysiology, Regeneration, and Translation to the Clinic. BioMed Research International. 2016;2016:5952165.

[18] O'Connell GD, Vresilovic Ej Fau - Elliott DM, Elliott DM. Comparison of

animals used in disc research to human lumbar disc geometry. (1528-1159 (Electronic)).

[19] Jaumard NV, Leung J Fau - Gokhale AJ, Gokhale Aj Fau - Guarino BB, Guarino Bb Fau - Welch WC, Welch Wc Fau - Winkelstein BA, Winkelstein BA. Relevant Anatomic and Morphological Measurements of the Rat Spine: Considerations for Rodent Models of Human Spine Trauma. (1528-1159 (Electronic)).

[20] Wu J, Xue J, Huang R, Zheng C, Cui Y, Rao S. A rabbit model of lumbar distraction spinal cord injury. (1878-1632 (Electronic)).

[21] Kroeber MW, Unglaub F Fau - Wang H, Wang H Fau - Schmid C, Schmid C Fau - Thomsen M, Thomsen M Fau - Nerlich A, Nerlich A Fau - Richter W, et al. New in vivo animal model to create intervertebral disc degeneration and to investigate the effects of therapeutic strategies to stimulate disc regeneration. (1528-1159 (Electronic)).

[22] Wilke HJ, Kettler A Fau - Wenger KH, Wenger Kh Fau - Claes LE, Claes LE. Anatomy of the sheep spine and its comparison to the human spine. (0003-276X (Print)).

[23] Yumuk Z, Küçükbasmaci Ö, Büyükbaba Boral Ö, Küçüker Anğ M, Dundar V. The effects of streptozotocin-induced diabetes on brucellosis of rats. FEMS Immunology & Medical Microbiology. 2003;39(3):275-278.

[24] If T, Na R. Comparative study of the susceptibility and infectious sensitivity of laboratory animals and sheep to different species of the causative agent of brucellosis. Zhurnal mikrobiologii epidemiologii i immunobiologii. 1971;48:97-101.

[25] Thorpe BD, Sidwell RW, Lundgren DL. Experimental studies with four species of Brucella in selected wildlife, laboratory, and domestic animals. Am J Trop Med Hyg. 1967;16(5):665-674.

[26] Huddleson IF, Hallman ET. The Pathogenicity of the Species of the Genus Brucella for Monkeys. The Journal of Infectious Diseases. 1929;45(4):293-303.

[27] Enright FM, Araya Ln Fau - Elzer PH, Elzer Ph Fau - Rowe GE, Rowe Ge Fau - Winter AJ, Winter AJ. Comparative histopathology in BALB/c mice infected with virulent and attenuated strains of *Brucella abortus*. (0165-2427 (Print)).

[28] Stevens MG, Olsen SC, Pugh GW, Jr., Palmer MV. Immune and pathologic responses in mice infected with Brucella abortus 19, RB51, or 2308. Infection and immunity. 1994;62(8):3206-3212.

[29] Tobias L, Cordes Do Fau - Schurig GG, Schurig GG. Placental pathology of the pregnant mouse inoculated with *Brucella abortus* strain 2308. (0300-9858 (Print)).

[30] Izadjoo MJ, Mense Mg Fau - Bhattacharjee AK, Bhattacharjee Ak Fau - Hadfield TL, Hadfield Tl Fau - Crawford RM, Crawford Rm Fau - Hoover DL, Hoover DL. A study on the use of male animal models for developing a live vaccine for brucellosis. (1865-1674 (Print)).

[31] Kahl-McDonagh MM, Arenas-Gamboa Am Fau - Ficht TA, Ficht TA. Aerosol infection of BALB/c mice with Brucella melitensis and *Brucella abortus* and protective efficacy against aerosol challenge. (0019-9567 (Print)).

[32] Young JD. Brucellosis with hepatomegaly and splenomegaly.

[33] Colmenero Jde D, Queipo-Ortuño Mi Fau - Maria Reguera J, Maria Reguera J Fau - Angel Suarez-Muñoz M, Angel

Suarez-Muñoz M Fau - Martín-Carballino S, Martín-Carballino S Fau - Morata P, Morata P. Chronic hepatosplenic abscesses in Brucellosis. Clinico-therapeutic features and molecular diagnostic approach. (0732-8893 (Print)).

[34] Akritidis N, Tzivras M, Delladetsima I, Stefanaki S, Moutsopoulos HM, Pappas G. The Liver in Brucellosis. Clinical Gastroenterology and Hepatology. 2007;5(9):1109-1112.

[35] Franco MP, Mulder M Fau - Gilman RH, Gilman Rh Fau - Smits HL, Smits HL. Human brucellosis. (1473-3099 (Print)).

[36] Rajashekara G, Glover Da Fau - Krepps M, Krepps M Fau - Splitter GA, Splitter GA. Temporal analysis of pathogenic events in virulent and avirulent Brucella melitensis infections. (1462-5814 (Print)).

[37] Prior S, Gander B, Irache JM, Gamazo C. Gentamicin-loaded microspheres for treatment of experimental Brucella abortus infection in mice. J Antimicrob Chemother. 2005;55(6):1032-1036.

[38] Shasha B, Lang R, Rubinstein E. Therapy of experimental murine brucellosis with streptomycin, co-trimoxazole, ciprofloxacin, ofloxacin, pefloxacin, doxycycline, and rifampin. Antimicrob Agents Chemother. 1992;36(5):973-976.

[39] Arda B, Tunçel M, Yaimazhan T, Gökengin D, Gürel O. Efficacy of oral levofloxacin and dirithromycin alone and in combination with rifampicin in the treatment of experimental murine Brucella abortus infection. Int J Antimicrob Agents. 2004;23(2):204-207.

[40] Geyik MF, Dikici B Fau - Kokoglu OF, Kokoglu Of Fau - Bosnak M, Bosnak M Fau - Celen MK, Celen Mk Fau - Hosoglu S, Hosoglu S Fau - Ayaz C, et al. Therapeutic effect of spiramycin in brucellosis. (1328-8067 (Print)).

[41] Yumuk Z, Dundar V. The effect of long-term ethanol feeding on efficacy of doxycycline plus rifampicin in the treatment of experimental brucellosis caused by Brucella melitensis in rats. (1120-009X (Print)).

[42] Sezak N, Kuruuzum Z Fau - Cakir N, Cakir N Fau - Yuce A, Yuce A. Comparison of rifampicin and moxifloxacin efficacy in an experimental model of animal brucellosis. (1973-9478 (Electronic)).

[43] Siddiqur RM, Kirl BB. Clinical and pathological findings in experimental brucellosis in pregnant rats. (1972-2680 (Electronic)).

[44] Oláh T, Michaelis JC, Cai X, Cucchiarini M, Madry H. Comparative anatomy and morphology of the knee in translational models for articular cartilage disorders. Part II: Small animals. Ann Anat. 2021;234:151630.

[45] Subbian S, Bandyopadhyay N, Tsenova L, O'Brien P, Khetani V, Kushner NL, et al. Early innate immunity determines outcome of Mycobacterium tuberculosis pulmonary infection in rabbits. Cell Commun Signal. 2013;11:60.

[46] Wu J, Xue J, Huang R, Zheng C, Cui Y, Rao S. A rabbit model of lumbar distraction spinal cord injury. Spine J. 2016;16(5):643-658.

[47] Grilló MJ, Blasco JM, Gorvel JP, Moriyón I, Moreno E. What have we learned from brucellosis in the mouse model? Vet Res. 2012;43(1):29.

[48] Denayer T, Stöhr T, Van Roy M. Animal models in translational medicine: Validation and prediction. New Horizons in Translational Medicine. 2014;2(1):5-11.

[49] Mak IW, Evaniew N, Ghert M. Lost in translation: animal models and clinical trials in cancer treatment. (1943-8141 (Print)).

[50] Sobajima S, Kompel Jf Fau - Kim JS, Kim Js Fau - Wallach CJ, Wallach Cj Fau - Robertson DD, Robertson Dd Fau - Vogt MT, Vogt Mt Fau - Kang JD, et al. A slowly progressive and reproducible animal model of intervertebral disc degeneration characterized by MRI, X-ray, and histology. (1528-1159 (Electronic)).

[51] Marques RM, Teixeira L Fau - Aguas AP, Aguas Ap Fau - Ribeiro JC, Ribeiro Jc Fau - Costa-e-Silva A, Costa-e-Silva A Fau - Ferreira PG, Ferreira PG. Immunosuppression abrogates resistance of young rabbits to Rabbit Haemorrhagic Disease (RHD). (1297-9716 (Electronic)).

[52] Neave MJ, Hall RA-O, Huang N, McColl KA, Kerr P, Hoehn M, et al. Robust Innate Immunity of Young Rabbits Mediates Resistance to Rabbit Hemorrhagic Disease Caused by Lagovirus Europaeus GI.1 But Not GI.2. LID - 10.3390/v10090512 [doi] LID - 512. (1999-4915 (Electronic)).

[53] Trzeciak-Ryczek A, Tokarz-Deptuła B, Deptuła W. Expression of IL-1β, IL-2, IL-10, TNF-β and GM-CSF in peripheral blood leukocytes of rabbits experimentally infected with rabbit haemorrhagic disease virus. (1873-2542 (Electronic)).

[54] Blasco JM. Brucella ovis. Animal brucellosis. 1990;8:9-12.

[55] Blasco JM, Molina-Flores B. Control and eradication of Brucella melitensis infection in sheep and goats. Vet Clin North Am Food Anim Pract. 2011;27(1):95-104.

[56] Garin-Bastuji B, Blasco JM, Marín C, Albert D. The diagnosis of brucellosis in sheep and goats, old and new tools. Small Ruminant Research. 2006;62(1):63-70.

[57] Alhamada AG, Habib I, Barnes A, Robertson I. Risk Factors Associated with Brucella Seropositivity in Sheep and Goats in Duhok Province, Iraq. Veterinary sciences. 2017;4(4):65.

[58] Oláh T, Cai X, Michaelis JC, Madry H. Comparative anatomy and morphology of the knee in translational models for articular cartilage disorders. Part I: Large animals. Ann Anat. 2021;235:151680.

[59] Radwan AI, Bekairi SI, Mukayel AA. Treatment of Brucella melitensis infection in sheep and goats with oxytetracycline combined with streptomycin. Rev Sci Tech. 1992;11(3):845-857.

[60] Wang F, Ni B, Zhu Z, Liu F, Zhu YZ, Liu J. Intra-discal vancomycin-loaded PLGA microsphere injection for MRSA discitis: an experimental study. Arch Orthop Trauma Surg. 2011;131(1):111-119.

[61] Hull NC, Schumaker BA. Comparisons of brucellosis between human and veterinary medicine. Infect Ecol Epidemiol. 2018;8(1):1500846.

[62] Prior S, Gander B, Lecároz C, Irache JM, Gamazo C. Gentamicin-loaded microspheres for reducing the intracellular Brucella abortus load in infected monocytes. J Antimicrob Chemother. 2004;53(6):981-988.

[63] Prior S, Gander B, Blarer N, Merkle HP, Subirá ML, Irache JM, et al. In vitro phagocytosis and monocyte-macrophage activation with poly(lactide) and poly(lactide-co-glycolide) microspheres. Eur J Pharm Sci. 2002;15(2):197-207.

[64] Katonis P, Tzermiadianos M, Gikas A, Papagelopoulos P, Hadjipavlou A. Surgical treatment of

spinal brucellosis. Clin Orthop Relat Res. 2006;444:66-72.

[65] Bugybayeva D, Kydyrbayev Z, Zinina N, Assanzhanova N, Yespembetov B, Kozhamkulov Y, et al. A new candidate vaccine for human brucellosis based on influenza viral vectors: a preliminary investigation for the development of an immunization schedule in a guinea pig model. Infect Dis Poverty. 2021;10(1):13.

[66] Hammami F, Koubaa M, Feki W, Chakroun A, Rekik K, Smaoui F, et al. Tuberculous and Brucellar Spondylodiscitis: Comparative Analysis of Clinical, Laboratory, and Radiological Features. Asian Spine J. 2020.

[67] Unuvar GK, Kilic AU, Doganay M. Current therapeutic strategy in osteoarticular brucellosis. North Clin Istanb. 2019;6(4):415-420.

[68] Liang C, Wei W, Liang X, De E, Zheng B. Spinal brucellosis in Hulunbuir, China, 2011-2016. Infect Drug Resist. 2019;12:1565-1571.

[69] Zhang Y, Zhang Q, Zeng Z. Histopathological findings of nucleus pulposus in lumbar brucellar spondylodiscitis. Rev Soc Bras Med Trop. 2019;52:e20180108.

[70] Lee H, Hur J, Lee J, Lee S. Brucellar Spondylitis. Journal of Korean Neurosurgical Society. 2008;44:277-279.

[71] Zileli M, Ebeoglu A. Brucellar spondylodiscitis. ArgoSpine News & Journal. 2011;23.

[72] Zhang N, Fang M, Chen H, Gou F, Ding M. Evaluation of spinal cord injury animal models. Neural Regen Res. 2014;9(22):2008-2012.

[73] Sheng SR, Wang XY, Xu HZ, Zhu GQ, Zhou YF. Anatomy of large animal spines and its comparison to the human spine: a systematic review. Eur Spine J. 2010;19(1):46-56.

[74] Zhang Y. Animal models of inflammatory spinal and sacroiliac joint diseases. Rheum Dis Clin North Am. 2003;29(3):631-645.